THE
HORMONE
DIET

THE HORMONE DIET

A 3-Step Program to Help You Lose Weight, Gain Strength, and Live Younger Longer

NATASHA TURNER, ND

RODALE.

This is a reprint of a book first published in 2009 by Random House Canada,
a division of Random House of Canada Limited.

Trade hardcover published in May 2010.
Trade paperback published in April 2011.

Rodale books may be purchased for business or promotional use or for special sales.
For information, please write to:
Special Markets Department, Rodale Inc., 733 Third Avenue, New York, NY 10017

Printed in the United States of America
Rodale Inc. makes every effort to use acid-free ⊗, recycled paper ⊗.

Book design by Terri Nimmo

Photos © Sam Gibbs

Library of Congress Cataloging-in-Publication Data

Turner, Natasha (Natasha S.)
The hormone diet : a 3-step program to help you lose weight, gain strength, and live
younger longer / Natasha Turner.
     p.   cm.
Originally published : Canada : Random House, 2009.
Includes bibliographical references and index.
ISBN-13 978–1-60529–402–5 hardcover
ISBN-13 978–1–60961–141–5 paperback
    1. Reducing diets—Popular works.   2. Hormone therapy—Popular works.   3. Diet
therapy—Popular works. I. Title.
RM222.2T84 2009
615.5'35—dc22   2010012657

Distributed to the trade by Macmillan

2   4   6   8   10   9   7   5   3   paperback

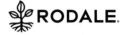

We inspire and enable people to improve their lives and the world around them.
www.rodalebooks.com

For my husband,
"Hey Tim," thank you for believing in me.
I am so blessed to share my life with you.

For Mom,
Thank you for your continued reminders to keep things simple,
be positive, make time for others, live life to the fullest, and
to never take it or your loved ones for granted.
Your courage, strength, wisdom, and humor
inspire me—always. I love you.

CONTENTS

INTRODUCTION

If you are looking for a big opportunity, seek out a big problem.

H. JACKSON BROWN JR.

My Story of Hormonal Havoc

Just a few months had passed since I had graduated from college in 1993. I was 22. I arrived home one day from my summer job in tears and feeling overwhelmed. I felt weak and feverish. I couldn't think—my head was buzzing with confusion. I couldn't understand people when they spoke to me. I couldn't seem to process information fast enough to make sense of anything. My best friend, Lise, who was living with me at the time, was talking to me about some mundane household incident and all I could do was stare blankly back at her. She said, "Don't worry, I can tell you're just not getting it. It's okay." I started to cry again. I thought I was going crazy and was certain I had a serious neurological disease.

Later that day, I wound up in the emergency room, where the doctors found I indeed had a fever, along with severe anemia. They told me to take some iron and to go home and rest, which was about all I was capable of doing. I would wake up feeling okay, but within minutes the confusion and fogginess in my head would return. I couldn't even watch TV.

When I thought about it as best I could, I realized something had been off for months before my breaking point. I had needed so much sleep—over 16 hours a day—and was too tired to go to the gym, even though I was an exercise fanatic. I was gaining weight—25 pounds, a lot for my small frame—and I felt fat and unattractive. My periods were irregular and I was losing fistfuls of hair. I had chalked it all up to the stress of finishing school and ending a relationship with my boyfriend at the time.

Thank heavens the emergency room doctor who treated me decided to investigate more thoroughly into why I was so anemic and tested my blood to rule out hypothyroidism. Days later, I received a call letting me know my TSH was over 25; a normal level is considered to be less than 4.7, and an optimal level is less than 2. (TSH is a hormone that increases when the thyroid is not functioning well.) I was severely hypothyroid, with extremely low iron levels. Confusion was overcoming me because my brain function was slowing down along with the rest of me. I started taking thyroid medication immediately. Within a week I felt like a completely different person, and I continue to take thyroid medication today.

Looking back, I know I had the telltale symptoms of hypothyroidism as early as age 13. I remember waking up with my pillow *covered* in my hair and being taken to dermatologists for hair loss, but nothing those doctors proposed ever helped. I remember feeling tired all the time and having horrible menstrual issues, including pain, cramping, and irregular cycles. I always had belly fat and would *never* wear a two-piece bathing suit. I hated my body.

Now I know my disease was missed because I seemed to be slim. Because my weight appeared "normal," my doctors did not think of looking for hypothyroidism, a condition commonly found in noticeably overweight people.

Fast forward to 2000. After finishing 4 years of training, I began my practice as a naturopathic doctor. Between patients, I was skipping out to buy cookies or muffins because I craved them so badly. I never used to like these foods, though I sure had to have them now. But within about 20 minutes of the last sugary bite, I would be falling asleep in a "carb coma." Still, I couldn't stop my seemingly insatiable snack habit. At the same time, my periods were becoming more irregular, my breasts were shrinking, my waist was getting wider, and I was losing hair—again.

On a professional hunch, I underwent a thorough investigation involving blood work and ultrasounds. My suspicions were confirmed—I had polycystic ovarian syndrome (PCOS). PCOS is a condition characterized by irregular periods, hair loss, acne, and weight gain; it's also linked to an increased risk of breast cancer, infertility, and diabetes. So I now had not one, but two metabolic diseases. My family doctor, Dr. Tammy Hermant, suggested the diabetes medication metformin, along with the birth control pill, in an attempt to regulate my periods.

Since PCOS is associated with insulin resistance, the underlying cause of type 2 diabetes, insulin sensitizing medications such as metformin are regularly prescribed to treat it. And I was definitely insulin resistant. Besides the high insulin levels detected by my blood work, my cravings, constant hunger, fatigue after eating, and fat gain around my abdomen were obvious signs. But I was truly not interested in taking the metformin. I also had high levels of testosterone and dehydroepiandrosterone (DHEA), which explained my hair loss, dwindling breasts, and bulking waistline. I was also not interested in taking the birth control pill. Given my training, I wanted to figure out how to manage my health—threatened as it was—in a more safe and natural way.

The Genesis of the Hormone Diet Approach

I had already begun to research hormones and hormonally related conditions. I was fascinated by their interconnectedness and the number of bodily functions they influenced. The standard treatment for a seemingly uncomplicated hormonal issue such as hypothyroidism—simply replacing thyroid hormone—was by no means the complete solution. In fact, it was frighteningly inadequate in many cases.

Today, when I see cases of hypothyroidism in my clinical practice at Clear Medicine, I rarely rush to treat the thyroid deficiency right away. (I make exceptions, of course, when a patient's TSH reading is sky-high or the patient already is taking a strong dose of thyroid medication and is still experiencing symptoms.) Instead I start by working to detoxify the patient's liver and digestive system; to balance his or her stress hormone levels with good sleep and stress management; to use foods that level out blood sugar and insulin; to replenish the nutrients needed to make thyroid hormone; and to treat PMS or any other signs of sex hormone imbalance. If the patient is still experiencing unresolved symptoms, *only then* do I address the thyroid.

I believe this approach provides a lasting health fix because each one of these factors influences the thyroid. Jumping right into treating the thyroid would be like building a house on sand. The foundation would constantly be shifting and would require constant repair. Helping a person achieve overall hormonal balance makes specific treatment for the thyroid unnecessary in some cases. While in other cases, body imbalances commonly associated with hypothyroidism, such as low stomach acid (which can reduce nutrient absorption), iron deficiency, high cholesterol, and adrenal (stress) gland fatigue, must be addressed as well.

My multifaceted approach to thyroid treatment has helped me garner a listing as a "Top Thyroid Doctor" on www.thyroid-info.com. But my approach to hormonal balance goes far beyond treating thyroid patients.

Through my years of clinical practice, I have gained a much clearer view of the *real* big picture. Exploring the interrelationship between our hormones and so many functions in the body, I began to realize that a step-by-step approach needed to be followed *in order* to restore total balance and long-term health. I knew that veering from this course would make lasting results next to impossible. I also knew my approach would not necessarily be the quickest, but it would be the most effective.

And so *The Hormone Diet* was born. I have been working on the ideas and treatments described in this book since 2000. In the field of hormones, new information is discovered weekly. I am sure by the time this book hits the press, I will already have more to add.

The Hormone Diet Is for Men and Women of All Ages

The mere mention of "hormones" can conjure images of menopausal women or nefarious food additives. Indeed, many patients come to me seeking to address these specific concerns. But this book is definitely not only for those with hormonal issues. It is not even strictly directed at people seeking to lose weight. I have used the approach outlined in these pages to successfully treat thousands of patients with a broad spectrum of health goals. Some needed to gain much-needed muscle. Others wanted healthier looking skin. Still others wanted to get rid of headaches, improve their sleep, ease their digestion, increase their energy, improve their fertility, or sharpen their memory.

So many of us believe we can get healthy by losing weight. The truth is *we must be healthy to lose weight*. When you complete the steps outlined in Part Two of this book, you will optimize your hormonal balance, lose unwanted fat, and restore your health in the process. Unlike so many other "diet" books lining the shelves these days, *The Hormone Diet* offers a complete wellness plan that addresses *every* cause of obesity. It promotes healthy bodily function from head to toe, inside and out.

Truly Solving Obesity Means Understanding Why We're Fat

Oversecretion of insulin is considered by many experts to be the primary cause of obesity today. Because our body secretes insulin in response to carbohydrates, many experts suggest that simply removing carbohydrates from our diet is the solution. Some researchers go further, suggesting that we should not exercise because it only serves to stimulate our appetite.

I couldn't disagree more strongly. The recommendation to not exercise literally puts lives in danger. Also, if we know that limiting simple carbohydrates reduces insulin and that exercise improves insulin sensitivity, which also reduces insulin—then why not recommend both?

Dieting alone—restricting calories and carbohydrates—does nothing to build metabolically active muscle, a necessary health reserve for our later years. Combine diet and exercise, however, and you will lose the fat and save your muscle. *The number on the scale is by no means your most significant indicator of health.* It does *nothing* to identify how much muscle you have or *where* you carry your fat—both more important factors for wellness than how much you weigh. Instead, the complete Best Body Assessment I have outlined in Chapter 6 will give you clear and easy-to-follow methods for measuring *all* the factors that determine your health and wellness.

The type of exercise we choose is also critical. I would argue that 30 years of regular jogging won't help you attain an optimal body composition, and by increasing physical stress on the body, could potentially accelerate the natural loss of metabolically active muscle we all experience as we age. Doing cardiovascular exercise alone might be just as bad as not exercising at all—we need to add strength training into the mix as well. Strength training and dieting together is *the* answer for achieving a lean, toned body, balancing our hormones and addressing many of the major causes of obesity. I believe you need cardio only once a week! Add in the benefits of sleep, stress management, health-promoting supplements, and an anti-inflammatory detox, and you've got the winning combination I outline later for you in my three-step, 6-week health fix.

As you read on, you'll learn that excess insulin is just *one* of the culprits behind obesity, albeit a big one. Several more of the most common fat-packing imbalances cannot be solved by dieting alone. *These imbalances can prevent successful fat loss even when great diet and exercise plans are in place.* They include:

1. Inflammation
2. Insulin resistance
3. Low serotonin, which leads to cravings, depression, or anxiety
4. Chronic stress
5. Estrogen dominance (a state arising from relative excess of estrogen to progesterone, which is known to cause weight gain and to increase the risk of PMS and breast cancer)
6. Menopause
7. Andropause
8. Hypothyroidism

As a society, we are trained to consult our doctors about the long-term outcome of these imbalances, such as high blood pressure, obesity, diabetes, cancer, arthritis, and heart disease. We are, however, much less likely to consult our doctors for the "less" serious conditions of fatigue, memory loss, low libido, poor concentration, or difficulty managing weight—the first true indicators of potential major health issues that affect a majority of the population today. My hope is that this book will encourage you to *think* and *act* differently about your health.

A Proven Method for Lasting Fat Loss

The guidelines in this book are really quite simple. You'll learn how to sleep soundly, detoxify your body, subdue stress, eat well, take the right supplements, exercise, and enjoy fulfilling sex. As a bonus, I'll teach you about the benefits of safe, natural skin care. Believe me, none of this is rocket science—but they are practices few of us are coordinating well in our busy, stress-filled lives.

The innovative aspect is the *way* I suggest you undertake these steps, the *science* in which they are rooted, and the *effects* they will have on your body. The intricacies and subtleties behind this wellness plan are *vast*. My approach doesn't involve rushing toward an instant cure; it involves gentle preparation, a step-by-step approach, and clever refinements. It makes *The Hormone Diet* perfectly suited to you and to everyone you know, regardless of specific health goals.

If you've tried every diet and they've all failed you, *it's not your fault*. This plan is different and will help you to realize why your past efforts were doomed to fail *unless* they took into account the complex chemicals that are really running the show—your hormones!

More Than Just Another Diet Book

Although this book is written with a slant toward losing fat, it's really about restoring your total health. If you take me up on *The Hormone Diet* challenge, you'll embark on a program that's far more than just an eating plan. It's a total wellness program that differs from other diets. It offers the potential for *lifelong results* because it fixes every reason why we are fat. Before giving a moment's thought to your exercise routine, you will spend the first 4 weeks concentrating on *preparing* your body for lasting weight loss. Only after you have set the foundation for hormonal balance will you begin concentrating on what you do in the gym, which will then restore your metabolism. The preparatory steps are key to addressing *all* potential causes of excess weight and obesity, not just the ones trumpeted by the diet and exercise industries.

How to Use This Book

Read Part One to understand your muscle, your fat, and your metabolism, all of which speak directly to your hormones. Complete your Hormonal Health Profile to discover whether one or more hormonal imbalances have been compromising your health or weight loss efforts.

Use Part Two, the three-step fix, to restore your hormonal balance and total wellness.

Helping You Take Control of Your Health

I am thrilled to have the opportunity to share *The Hormone Diet* with you which, amazingly, became a #1 national bestseller 1 week after its release in Canada. I believe it provides answers to the questions many people are searching for—including why they feel the way they feel and, most importantly, why they can't lose weight.

I wrote this book and founded Clear Medicine because my goal is to bring preventive medicine to anyone who has a desire to achieve better health. When I first began to practice naturopathic medicine years ago, I always had to explain to people exactly what I did for a living. Occasionally, I still do, but today I find people are more aware, as they are looking for answers to support and maintain their wellness.

Someone once told me that the best motivation for living healthily is to develop a chronic disease. Believe me, I've been there, I've witnessed family members in the same position, and I *don't* want this to be your motivation for change. Instead, I wish to inspire you to take *complete responsibility* for your health and to think of managing your wellness with the same eye to the future as you apply to managing your finances. Without your health, all the money in the world means nothing.

Strive for strength and harmony. They are magnificent attributes that will help you in all aspects of your life.

Wishing you perfect balance,

Natasha Turner, BSc, ND
Toronto, December 2009

PART ONE

YOUR HORMONES, YOUR BODY

Life is not a path of coincidence, happenstance, and luck,
but rather an unexplainable, meticulously charted course for one to
touch the lives of others and make a difference in the world.

BARBARA DILLINHAM

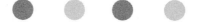

CHAPTER 1

THE NEW FORMULA FOR FAT LOSS

Here's what you can expect to learn in this chapter:
- How to set the stage for successful fat loss
- The facts about hormones
- Why dieting can cause hormonal havoc
- How hormones boost metabolic rate and fat burning
- How inflammation causes obesity and hormonal imbalance
- How to control appetite with the help of hormones
- How hormones affect sexual appetite
- The road to safe weight loss

For decades, an endless stream of well-marketed diets and new-fangled exercise programs have been promising an easy path to a leaner, trimmer you. Every year, it seems, we are enticed to drop all "bad carbs" or to purchase the latest piece of home gym equipment and good health and happiness will surely be ours. But the rules of fat loss have changed from what we once thought them to be. No longer can we rely on diet alone to shed unwanted weight. Nor can we simply exercise the pounds away. Certainly, poor eating habits and lack of physical activity are two of the biggies when it comes to explaining escalating obesity rates. But they are by no means the only culprits.

Today's headlines read like a laundry list of previously overlooked factors that can impede successful weight loss—from lack of sleep and excess stress to the chemicals in our soaps. With so many lifestyle influences to consider, all the calorie-cutting and exercise in the world, in isolation, will not provide the golden key to achieving the lasting change we desire.

Until now, the prevailing approach to conquering obesity has been like putting a broken arm in a sling without first resetting the bone. Yes, weight loss happens when we burn more calories—via exercise and basic life functions such as breathing and digesting—than we take in. But there's another absolutely critical, routinely ignored variable that must be integrated into this equation: *our hormones*. These wondrous, unseen chemicals are produced by our bodies to manage everything from breathing to digestion to sexual responses and more. At the same time, our hormones are influenced by a myriad of factors, including exercise, diet, sleep, stress, and even the seemingly innocuous, everyday chemicals in cosmetics.

What Are Hormones?

What are you thinking right now? Do you feel happy or anxious? What did you eat for your last meal? Is it noisy where you are? How deeply or quickly are you breathing? Did you exercise today? How many cups of coffee have you had? Do you like the person beside you at the moment? Have you enjoyed sex lately?

The answer to every one of these questions has an impact on your hormones. As your five senses delicately interact with and respond to your environment, your nervous system is continuously communicating with your endocrine system—a series of glands and tissues constantly at work manufacturing, delivering, and processing a wide assortment of hormones to maintain body balance. Even the emotions you experience have the potential to influence your hormones—and vice versa.

Hormones are essentially tiny chemical messengers that spark communication processes throughout your body. They play an enormous role in influencing almost every aspect of your well-being, including your thoughts and feelings. Whether you feel the need to sleep, warm up, cool down, eat jelly beans, grab a coffee, or have a quickie, your desires and actions can be traced back to your hormonal activity.

Hormones also directly affect your appearance. Besides body composition, the look and feel of your skin and hair are influenced by hormones. If you want to look fresher, stimulate your metabolism, lose fat, feel calmer, sleep better, get stronger, feel sexier, and focus better, gaining control over your hormonal balance is truly the key.

Since hormones control our appetites and stimulate metabolism, achieving and maintaining hormonal balance plays an *essential* role in achieving lasting fat loss. Yes, diet and exercise are important, but so are sleeping well, reducing toxin exposure, maintaining healthy liver function, optimizing digestion, limiting stress, and conquering inflammation. All of these factors can influence our hormonal activity—and weight-loss success—in truly dramatic ways.

Our hormones dictate where we store fat and how we will lose it. Research from the *Journal of the American Medical Association* (April 2007) suggests our hormones also determine our success with different diets. Dr. David Ludwig, director of the obesity program at Children's Hospital Boston, found that people who rapidly secreted large amounts of the hormone insulin in response to consumption of sugar or carbohydrates tended to achieve better weight-loss results on a low-glycemic diet that restricted starches and sugars than they did on a low-fat diet. He also discovered that they carried more weight around the waist (the so-called apple shape) compared with those who secreted less insulin and tended to store their excess fat around their hips (the pear shape).

THE ENDOCRINE SYSTEM

While the nervous system coordinates rapid responses to outside stimuli, the endocrine system controls slower, longer-lasting responses to
your environment. The link between these two systems is the hypothalamus, a small, almond-sized gland located in the brain.

Functioning as an endocrine gland, the hypothalamus
secretes hormones that stimulate the pituitary gland to release
other hormones into the bloodstream. The pituitary is often
referred to as the "master gland," since its hormones act on the
thyroid, ovaries, testes, and adrenal glands to regulate growth,
reproduction, nutrient absorption, and metabolism.

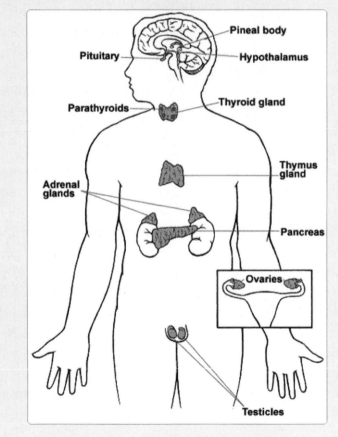

Each of these glands responds to instructions from the pituitary and secretes hormones specific to its unique function in the body. The ovaries and testes, for instance, secrete the sex hormones estrogen, progesterone, and testosterone. The adrenal glands release the stress hormone cortisol and antistress hormone DHEA. The thyroid releases thyroid hormones to manage your metabolic rate.

Many more hormones are produced without the direction of the pituitary gland by other tissues and glands of the endocrine system, including the pancreas, thymus gland, digestive tract, fat cells, adrenal glands, pineal gland, and the brain. Moreover, hormonal messages from other sources are relayed *back to* the hypothalamus to alter our behavior or actions. The hormone leptin is a good example of this type of hormonal control. This substance travels from fat cells through the bloodstream to the hypothalamus to regulate appetite.

Most bodily tissues are targets for one or more hormones released from the pituitary gland. According to Mary Dallman, a professor of physiology at the University of California who studies the effects of stress on appetite and obesity, two predominant endocrine hormones, cortisol and insulin, heavily influence caloric intake by acting on the brain. The stress hormone cortisol, in particular, activates a strong response in the brain to match our perceived stress with a desire to eat comfort foods—the tasty treats we associate with pleasant experiences, often from childhood. Unfortunately, consuming comfort foods, which are typically high in carbohydrates and fat, can cause a resulting spike in our insulin level, leading to the accumulation of belly fat.

Working together, the endocrine, nervous, and digestive systems can either help or hamper your weight-loss and wellness goals. Once you understand these complex systems and get them communicating optimally with one another, you will be well on your way to hormonal bliss and lifelong health.

The pear-shaped subjects fared equally well on both types of eating programs, but they tended to *gain back over half the weight* they lost on the low-fat diet after the study was completed. The apple-shaped people who followed the low-fat regimen also regained their weight, but kept it off after the low-glycemic diet.

Knowing your current hormonal state can help you select the eating plan that will work best for you. In Part Two, I'll tell you about a simple blood test that can provide you with not only a sense of your hormonal profile but also a strong indication of your potential for fat loss and aging well.

Hormonal Imbalance As a Cause of Obesity

The human body is a truly phenomenal machine that naturally strives to remain in a balanced state. When we're cold, we shiver. When we're thirsty or hungry, the brain gives us the appropriate signals to drink or grab a bite to eat. When our hormones and bodily responses are thrown out of balance, stress is the result. The body then miraculously offers a wide range of alerts, which can be as subtle as an increase in thirst or as severe as diabetes.

Consider these alarming statistics:

- An estimated 65 million Americans have metabolic syndrome, a set of underlying risk factors for type 2 diabetes and heart disease.
  - By the age of 30, 1 in 4 people has an associated risk factor, such as abdominal fat or insulin resistance.
  - By the age of 60, 3 out of 4 people have one or more of the associated factors.
- One in 13 people suffers from hypothyroidism. Some sources say up to 30 percent of the population has a thyroid disorder and an estimated 13 million cases may remain undiagnosed each year.

- Forty-three percent of women ages 18 to 59 report experiencing sexual dysfunctions at some point in their life.
- About 75 percent of women experience premenstrual syndrome (PMS).
- Seventy-five percent of menopausal women in North America experience life-disrupting symptoms.
- Andropause, also known as male menopause, affects 30 to 40 percent of aging men.
- An estimated 30 percent of men and 40 percent of women suffer from insomnia, a statistic that increases with age.
- Seventy-four percent of adults are chronically sleep deprived.
- The World Health Organization reports that by 2020 depression will become the number two cause of disability and premature death for men and women of all ages.
- An estimated 80 to 90 percent of all disease is caused by stress.

What's the unifying factor among all these conditions? Every one of them is spurred by an underlying hormonal imbalance. Sadly, the signs and symptoms of hormonal imbalances are so widespread that they barely register as blips on our radar screens. Many of us have hormone-related health conditions that interfere with our quality of life, and we're not even aware of them. In fact, we're so imbalanced, I fear most of us don't even know what "normal" feels like anymore!

At the same time, we are in the midst of an obesity epidemic. More than 61 percent of Americans are overweight (BMI greater than 25), a number that continues to escalate each year. According to National Center for Health 2005/2006 statistics, more than 34 percent of Americans are obese (BMI greater than 30) compared to 32.7 percent who are overweight. Just under 6 percent are extremely obese. Data from the National Institutes of Health (NIH) show obesity and related conditions alone account for more than $100 billion in health-care expenses annually in the United States.

Setting the Stage for Fat-Loss Success

What does hormonal havoc mean to you? Some women might immediately think of hot flashes or the emotional meltdown they experienced before their last period. Men might think back to what it was like being 17, when they could think of nothing but sex, sex, and more sex. Both these situations involve hormones that are out of whack, as do hypothyroidism, infertility, diabetes, stress, insomnia, depression, anxiety, obesity, irregular periods, low libido, memory loss, and a lengthy list of other conditions brought on by hormonal mix-ups.

But maybe you just feel tired all the time. Or you notice fat hanging around that seems impossible to lose. Perhaps your cravings for sweets, carbs, or salt will not let up, your skin is not as bright as it once was, or the texture of your hair has changed. These much subtler signs can also signal a state of hormonal upheaval.

When you complete your Hormonal Health Profile in the next chapter, you will see there are many symptoms of hormonal imbalance. No matter how an imbalance manifests on the outside, the internal reality remains the same—*any and all hormonal imbalance leads to difficulty losing weight, increased risk of obesity and unhealthy aging.* Long-term weight loss and wellness are *next to impossible* until you bring your hormones back into balance.

The New Equation for Fat Loss:

$$\text{Hormonal Balance} + \left(\text{Calories Taken In} - \text{Calories Burned} \right) = \text{Lasting Fat Loss}$$

Boost Metabolism with Help from Your Hormones

One of the primary factors determining body weight is metabolism, the internal furnace that regulates fat burning. Everyone's metabolism is different, which is why some people appear to be able to eat just about anything and remain lean while others seem to pack on pounds easily. But being overweight doesn't necessarily mean you have a slow metabolism, and there are five major factors that affect our metabolic rate.

1. THE THYROID: YOUR INTERNAL THERMOSTAT

The thyroid controls the metabolic rate of every single cell in the body and also maintains body temperature. Without enough thyroid hormone, all our bodily functions slow down. We feel tired and lethargic, gain weight, experience constipation, feel cold, and are prone to depression.

2. THE RUSH OF ADRENALINE

A quick release of adrenaline is the body's first response to stress. This hormone provides a short-term metabolic boost because it draws on the body's fat stores to provide that burst of energy we feel in a "fight-or-flight" situation.

3. MARVELOUS MUSCLE

Muscle tissue is metabolically active at rest, as well as during use. So the more muscle you have, the more calories you'll burn, even while sleeping or watching TV. This metabolic factor is the easiest to control with the right wellness plan. Unfortunately, loss of muscle is a normal part of aging. My three-step plan in Part Two of this book shows you how to slow this process and maximize muscle growth, even as you age.

4. THE THERMIC EFFECT OF EATING

Thermic pertains to heat. Thermic or "thermogenic" foods literally heat you up and raise your metabolism. The thermic effect happens as your body burns calories, simply by digesting and absorbing the food. Yes, even the very act of eating stimulates your metabolism, especially when you consume protein, which has the highest thermic effect of any food group. There's another metabolic benefit of protein: Eating it also helps to support metabolically active muscle growth, especially if you are practicing strength training. And strength training helps to increase the thermic effect! A study published in the *Medicine and Science in Sports and Exercise Journal* found the thermic effect of the same meal was 50 percent greater in men who engaged in regular weight training versus those who were sedentary. This certainly helps to illustrate why strength training is so important for optimal calorie burning.

5. YOUR LOVELY LIVER

While your muscle is your primary fat-burning tissue, your liver is your master fat-burning organ. Knowing this, it makes good sense to adopt detoxification and other habits that promote healthy liver function.

All these metabolism factors involve, or are influenced by, your hormones. In each case, an appropriate hormonal balance is the key to ensuring optimal metabolic function.

How Hormones Power Up Your Fat-Burning Pathways

Have you ever thought about all the wonderful things your peroxisome proliferator-activated receptors (PPARs)* do for you? I know—it's a mouthful! You very likely have never even heard of them, but everyone has PPARs, the key regulators of fat burning,

---

* There are different types of PPARs—gamma, delta, alpha—located in different tissues, such as those in the liver (alpha) or the muscle (gamma). Their functions, however, are similar in that they regulate the storage and burning of fat. For the purposes of this book, I have chosen not to differentiate between the types. This subject matter is complicated enough!

blood sugar levels, and the balance of energy within your cells. Naturally present in the liver, fat cells, heart muscles, and skeletal muscles, PPARs are also known to improve cellular response to insulin, a critical factor in successful fat loss. Because the muscles and liver contain fat-burning PPARs, plenty of muscle tissue and optimal liver function are essential to your fat-loss success as well.

After you eat, PPARs react to the presence of fat and sugar in your bloodstream by sending messages to your cells to crank up your fat-burning metabolism. PPARs are also fired up when you exercise. If you are currently overweight and low on lean muscle mass, your PPARs are likely not functioning at their best.

Many factors can interfere with PPARs, but the two biggest influences are *inflammation* and *hormonal imbalance*. Dysfunctional PPARs are also considered key culprits in the development of insulin resistance and obesity. Several pharmaceutical companies are currently investigating drugs that work directly on these receptors to aid fat loss and prevent diabetes.

Since hormones influence PPARs, hormones are directly linked to fat burning and weight loss, right down to the cellular level. For you to lose fat, your hormones have to help open up the PPARs' fat-burning pathways in your liver and muscles. The catch is that this process will not happen successfully until the fires of inflammation are extinguished. Researchers are aggressively searching for ways to tackle inflammation as an underlying cause of disease and obesity. Findings at the Joslin Diabetes Center in Boston, for example, have already led to a clinical trial of an anti-inflammatory agent for treating type 2 diabetes. Six years ago, Dr. Steven Shoelson, a professor at Harvard Medical School, reported that very high doses of aspirin, a known anti-inflammatory, proved effective in improving insulin-glucose tolerance, boosting insulin sensitivity, and lowering blood lipid levels.

All of this is precisely why an anti-inflammatory detox is the essential first step of the Hormone Diet. This may sound like a complicated biology lesson, but my point is simply to let you know that this plan is specifically designed to get your fat-burning PPARs revving!

A FAT-PACKING HORMONAL IMBALANCE

CONDITION 1
The Internal Fire of Inflammation

This concept [inflammation as a cause of disease] is so intriguing because it suggests a new and possibly much simpler way of warding off disease. Instead of different treatments for, say, heart disease, Alzheimer's, and colon cancer, there might be a single, inflammation-reducing remedy that would prevent all three . . . it appears that many of the attributes of a Western lifestyle— such as a diet high in sugars and saturated fats, accompanied by little or no exercise—also make it easier for the body to become inflamed.

Christine Gorman, Alice Park, and Kristina Dell, "The Fires Within" [cover story], *Time* (February 23, 2004)

The last time you suffered through a sinus infection, sprained an ankle, or felt the irritating itch of a mosquito bite, you experienced the effects of inflammation. Infections or injuries trigger a chain of events called the inflammatory cascade. The normal, familiar signs of inflammation, such as redness, pain, swelling, and fever, are the first signals that our immune system is being called into combat mode. Behind the scenes, the body strives to maintain a critical balance between the signals that sustain this protective response and the signals that announce the battle has been won. Eventually, the inflammatory response eases as the body's powerful natural anti-inflammatory compounds move in to initiate the healing phase.

Within a well-balanced immune system, inflammation ebbs and flows as needed. Clearly, a certain degree of inflammation is a basic mechanism of a healthy immune system, just as the proper balance of cholesterol is vital to our cellular health. But, in the same way that surplus cholesterol can block an artery, excessive or persistent inflammation leads to tissue destruction and disease.

Chronic activation of the inflammatory response takes a heavy toll on the body and has recently been recognized as the root cause of most diseases associated with aging. Besides a typical inflammatory illness such as arthritis, the list of conditions spurred by inflammation includes cancer, heart disease, obesity, osteoporosis, Alzheimer's disease, autoimmune disease, diabetes, stroke, and even the wrinkling of our skin.

Inflammation and Obesity
Reducing inflammation is an absolutely vital step in allowing the body to lose unwanted fat. Remember the PPARs, the masters of the fat-burning pathways in our liver and muscle cells? They influence the tight interaction between our insulin sensitivity, inflammation, and weight. A PPAR imbalance contributes to inflammation, obesity, and insulin resistance. Because of this interaction, anti-inflammatory supplements and insulin-sensitizing lifestyle habits, which help to optimize the fat-burning capabilities of our PPARs, can be highly beneficial in the fight against obesity.

Causes of Chronic Inflammation

Widespread inflammation triggers a cascade of problems that seriously weaken the very foundations of our health and well-being. The following are some of the main causes of chronic inflammation.

- **Poor digestive health:** A whopping 60 percent of the immune system is clustered around the digestive tract. Compromises to digestion, including food allergies, bacterial imbalance, deficiency of enzymes or acids, yeast overgrowth, parasites, and stress, negatively affect not only the process of digestion but also our entire immune system. I begin the treatment of every patient by focusing on digestion simply for these reasons. Painful conditions such as gas, bloating, heartburn, reflux, constipation, diarrhea, irritable bowel syndrome, Crohn's disease, and ulcerative colitis are all related to inflammation in the digestive system.
- **An immune system gone awry:** Many experts now view inflammation as a symptom of an immune system in constant overdrive. When the body is stuck in this state, even ordinarily mild stressors such as viral infections, emotional stress, or exposure to household chemicals can cause the immune system to wildly overreact. Allergies, autoimmune disease, and tissue destruction can result when our immune system is working too hard to protect us.
- **Poor nutritional habits:** I discuss this topic in more detail in Chapter 10, Nasty Nutrition, but Dr. Paresh Dandona, a professor of medicine at the State University of New York at Buffalo who specializes in the topic of metabolism and inflammatory stress, found that overconsumption of any macronutrient—protein, carbohydrate, or fat—can contribute to inflammation. He and his team of researchers also identi-

fied immediate effects of specific foods on inflammation. Orange juice, for instance, was shown to have anti-inflammatory properties. Red wine was found to be neutral, whereas cream promoted inflammation. The team also discovered that overweight test subjects experienced significant changes in free radical stress indicators and inflammation just *1 week* after starting a more nutritious diet. Considering the long-term health benefits of reducing inflammation, this rapid change is extremely encouraging. You can also expect these benefits within the first 2 weeks of your three-step action plan.

- **Lack of exercise:** Since exercise increases the body's natural production of anti-inflammatory compounds, a lack of exercise can leave us prone to inflammation.
- **Abdominal obesity and insulin resistance:** Preexisting inflammation can also cause both of these conditions. That's right, not only does preexisting inflammation cause both of these conditions, but abdominal obesity and insulin resistance actually cause inflammation! A vicious circle indeed!
- **Estrogen decline:** Menopause appears to be linked to an increase in inflammation, especially due to waning estrogen. Progesterone is also important for keeping the immune system in check.
- **Environmental toxicity, liver toxicity, and fatty liver:** Compromised liver function not only interferes with the body's ability to burn fat, but it also hinders the elimination of toxins.
- **Depression and stress:** Depression in obese men is significantly associated with increased levels of C-reactive protein (CRP), an inflammatory marker in the blood, as shown by a 2003 German study published in the journal *Brain, Behavior, and Immunity.* This research supports the strong link between our emotions, our hormones, and inflammation. In another

study conducted in 2004 and published in *Archives of Internal Medicine,* a similar link was found between depression and higher levels of inflammation (as denoted by CRP) in both men and women. The link, however, was stronger in men than in women. In fact, the men with the most recent bouts of depression showed the highest CRP values.

Are You a Hotbed of Inflammation?
Inflammation is a health concern for everyone, but particularly for those who suffer from digestive disorders, allergies, auto-immune disease, arthritis, heart disease, asthma, eczema, acne, obesity, abdominal fat, headaches, joint stiffness, depression, and sinus disorders. The results of your Hormonal Health Profile may help you to assess the presence of inflammation in your body and as a factor interfering with your fat loss. In Appendix A, I also outline all the procedures involved in testing for inflammation, though two blood tests for highly sensitive C-reactive protein and homocysteine are the simplest and best diagnostic tools currently available to assess inflammation.

Your Body Shape and Hormonal Balance

As human beings, we are all unique and each one of us stores fat differently. Are you plagued by love handles, belly fat, or bra fat? Do excess pounds tend to cling to your hips and thighs? The very shape of your body can reveal a lot about what's going on inside of you because hormones also control where your fat accumulates. In Chapter 5 you will learn about healthy body composition and how different hormones contribute to the accumulation of fat in all our favorite places. My most important message to you on this subject is that you can *change your body shape* by bringing your hormones into proper balance.

Hormonal Balance and Appetite Control

As the medical community frantically searches for solutions to the growing obesity epidemic, exciting research in the area of appetite control is building every day. Mounting evidence shows that besides their ability to boost metabolism, many hormones and neurotransmitters (chemical messengers that work within the brain) are involved in appetite control by acting on the hypothalamus gland, the part of the brain that governs feelings of hunger and fullness. By collecting and processing information from the digestive system, the internal biological clock, fat cells, stress-controlling mechanisms, and other sources within the body, the hypothalamus acts as the master switch that tells us to eat more or to put the fork down.

By following my three steps, you can gain control of your hormones, which in turn tames your appetite. Besides what and when you eat, typically overlooked factors such as the amount of sleep you get, your thoughts, and your emotions can influence the hormones that flip the appetite switch one way or the other. Once you understand this guiding principle, you can use it to your advantage for successful weight loss and optimal health.

Hormones and Your Sexual Appetite

Research reveals that 43 percent of women and about 30 percent of men experience a form of sexual dysfunction at some time in their lives. A lack of desire, erectile dysfunction, and inability to orgasm are just a few of the complaints that cause people to lose that loving feeling. These findings are certainly not surprising, though. Many of us are overweight, overtired, stressed-out, and burned-out. No wonder we do not feel up for sex!

Besides all the wonderful weight-loss benefits I've been telling you about, balancing your hormones can also help boost your sex drive and enhance your sexual enjoyment while you trim your waistline. Believe it or not, some of the hormones that control fat storage and the ability to lose weight are the very same ones that influence sexual desire and performance.

Good sex is good for you and for weight loss, too. One of the goals of the *Hormone Diet* is to help you achieve and maintain hormonal balance with the help of more pleasurable sex, more often. This just might be my favorite piece of advice to share.

Dieters Beware: Counting Calories Causes Hormonal Chaos

After everything I've told you so far, you can see why typical weight-loss diets simply do not work. Just look at what happens to your body—and your hormones—when you excessively restrict calories or skip meals.

- You feel hungrier because your body responds to restricted caloric intake by releasing hormones that stimulate appetite.
- Your level of thyroid hormone drops, causing a slowdown in your metabolism.
- Your level of stress hormone increases in response to the physical stress of skipping meals or insufficient carbohydrate intake.
- Reproductive function slows because your sex hormones change due to insufficient caloric intake.
- Growth functions such as cell regeneration and tissue repair are inhibited.

When your hormones are thrown into a state of chaos, your tendency to overeat kicks in. Then, when your caloric intake starts to yo-yo, your metabolism suffers through a dangerous series of highs and lows. The end results of all this havoc include weight gain (exactly what you did *not* want); cravings and mood imbalances; a damaged metabolism; and the loss of precious, metabolically active muscle tissue.

Most important, extreme caloric restriction is not an effective long-term fat-loss solution because it's just not sustainable. The short-term victories achieved with this type of eating are *always* followed with rebound weight gain because, whether we like it or not, hormones will kick in to return the body to status quo. Furthermore, the increase in stress hormones caused by excessive caloric restriction is highly destructive and will actually cause you to want to eat and eat—and eat some more.

Dieting Alone Is Not an Effective Weight-Loss Solution

Stroll through your local bookstore and you'll find volume after volume promising *the* diet plan that will help you melt away unwanted pounds. In truth, medical research reveals that just about every one of today's popular diets offers the same potential outcome as the next. *Sticking* to the diet is actually what yields optimal results. A 2005 study reported in the *Journal of the American Medical Association* found sticking to a diet was a far greater determinant of successful weight loss than the type of diet the person stuck to. When researchers compared popular programs such as Weight Watchers, Atkins, the Zone Diet, and the Ornish Diet, weight loss and changes in cardiovascular disease risk factors were similar among all the diets after a 1-year period.

But most of us can't stick to a diet. In 2007, Traci Mann, an associate professor of psychology at UCLA, led a team of researchers in a comprehensive and rigorous analysis of diet programs using 31 long-term studies. Their results, presented in the *Journal of the American Psychological Association,* weren't encouraging. Mann's team found that most people regained the 5 to 10 pounds they lost, and more. Only a *small minority* of participants experienced sustained weight loss.

The conclusion is clear: *For most people, diets do not lead to sustained weight loss and health benefits.* The UCLA study tells us that most people would be *better off not dieting,* since the practice itself is a predictor of future weight gain! Repeatedly losing and gaining weight is also linked to cardiovascular disease, stroke, diabetes, and altered immune function.

> *We are recommending that Medicare should not fund weight-loss programs as a treatment for obesity. The benefits of dieting are too small and the potential harm is too large for dieting to be recommended as a safe, effective treatment for obesity.*
>
> TRACI MANN,
> associate professor of psychology, *UCLA*

Should we in the health-care profession start recommending against dieting because of its potential health risks? Possibly. Certainly good eating habits are important for weight loss, but exercise is important, too. In fact, people who exercise and basically watch what they eat (rather than follow strict diets) have the greatest weight-loss success. The same UCLA study found exercise to be the key factor leading to sustained weight loss. Dr. Edward Weiss, of Saint Louis University's Doisy College of Health Sciences, goes a step further, suggesting that exercise should be chosen *over* dieting for weight loss if we must choose one or the other.

What's more, Weiss studied two groups of overweight but otherwise healthy adults ages 50 to 60 who followed either a reduced-calorie diet or an exercise program that involved 60 minutes of walking, six times a week. Although both groups lost 9 to 10 percent of their body weight, *those who dieted lost muscle.* Those who exercised did not lose any muscle. Since muscle is so crucial to our metabolic rate, weight gain naturally tends to follow a loss of muscle mass. The loss of muscle mass that naturally occurs with aging is one of the reasons why our metabolic rate decreases as we advance in years.

If we want to optimize weight loss and avoid premature aging, we clearly need to stay away from practices that compromise muscle tissue.

Eating for Hormonal Health

If losing weight is tough, maintaining our goal weight is far tougher. Your odds of losing the pounds and maintaining your optimal weight, however, can be dramatically improved by combining the hormonal benefits of sleep, stress management, detoxification, and exercise with healthy eating. But what is the right diet solution for hormonal balance and good health? I believe the answer lies somewhere between the food selections of a Mediterranean diet and the principles of glycemically balanced eating, or the "Glyci-Med" approach, as I have termed it—the foundation of the *Hormone Diet* nutrition plan.

A Groundbreaking Dietary Approach

Although the Mediterranean diet isn't new, talk of its protective role against many conditions and metabolic syndrome is. Studies conducted over the past 10 years show that the foods of the Mediterranean diet offer protection from a multitude of metabolic disorders including obesity and high blood pressure, as well as heart disease and various types of cancer. It's commonly characterized by daily olive oil consumption and a ratio of monounsaturated to saturated fats that's much higher than in other places in the world. In addition, the Mediterranean diet features the following:

- Daily consumption of unrefined cereals and products (whole grain bread, pasta, rice, etc.)
- Vegetables (2 or 3 servings per day), fruits (4 to 6 servings per day), and fat-free or low-fat dairy products (1 or 2 servings per day). Although intake of milk is limited, cheese and yogurt consumption is relatively high. Feta cheese, for example, is regularly added to stews and salads.

- Moderate consumption of wine (1 or 2 glasses per day), mainly during mealtimes
- Weekly consumption of potatoes (4 or 5 servings per week), fish (4 or 5 servings per week), and olives and nuts (more than 4 servings per week)
- Consumed more rarely are poultry and eggs (1 to 3 servings per week)
- Sweets (1 to 3 servings per week)
- Red meat and meat products are consumed only a few times each month.

Less familiar than the Mediterranean diet are the principles of glycemically balanced eating. The term "glycemic" refers to the presence of sugar in the blood. Glycemically balanced eating means following a diet that focuses on leveling out blood sugar, which in turn prevents the release of excess insulin. Maintaining consistent blood sugar and insulin is one of the most important steps to balancing all hormones in the body and ensuring that your metabolism stays in high gear. Glycemically balanced eating helps you achieve these goals because it means (1) eating frequently and at the right times; (2) eating enough; and (3) consuming protein, fat, fiber, and carbohydrates together at every meal.

You'll find more details in Part Two, but the Mediterranean diet becomes glycemically balanced (to form the Glyci-Med approach) by choosing the right foods at the right times and by tweaking the Mediterranean food selections ever so slightly in this way:

- More vegetables (6 to 10 servings) are consumed than fruits (3 servings) each day.
- Eggs and poultry are eaten more often (3 to 5 servings per week).
- Whey protein and other portable protein sources are recommended, such as a protein bar (1 serving a day).

- Nuts are consumed more often (daily).
- Whole grains are consumed in limited amounts (1 to 3 servings a day, depending on your gender and activity level).
- Potatoes are consumed less frequently (a maximum of once a week).
- Sweets are enjoyed only once a week (rather than 1 to 3 times a week).

Together with exercise, the Glyci-Med dietary approach will help to keep your body at its healthy set point—a body weight that remains consistent, usually within a 5-pound range. Your metabolism will naturally work to preserve your set point with the help of your hormones by either turning up your calorie-burning engines or slowing them down, as needed.

Three Simple Steps to Total Wellness and Fat Loss

STEP 1: RENEW AND REVITALIZE. First, you will revitalize your body and mind as you recuperate from the harmful effects of sleep deprivation and stress. You will cool the fire of chronic inflammation, one of the primary causes of aging, disease, and obesity. Finally, you will maximize the function of your liver—an essential first step for safe, lasting fat loss. By the end of Step 1, you'll have quieted three factors that cause obesity and interfere with weight loss: sleep deprivation, chronic stress, and toxicity—and will have lost 5 to 12 pounds.

STEP 2: REPLENISH YOUR BODY AND BALANCE YOUR HORMONES. Next, you will begin to restore hormonal balance by choosing the right foods at the right times and in the right amounts. You will enhance your efforts by taking the five key supplements we all need in order to maintain health and prevent nutrient deficiencies that can interfere with your metabolism and cause hormonal chaos.

Step 2 also offers targeted fixes for specific hormonal imbalances, *if you need them.* Using the results of your Hormonal Health Profile, the Hormone Diet approach will show you how to take the necessary steps to treat your specific signs of imbalance *in precise order to ensure lasting weight loss, hormonal balance, and health.*

For instance, you will first add extra insulin-sensitizing supplements, if they are needed, to get you back in balance. At the same time, I'll suggest remedies for signs of anxiety, depression, or other brain chemistry imbalances. Your mood and emotional state are directly linked to your total wellness and sleep quality, as well as your cravings and your ability to stick to healthy food choices. By this stage, you'll have successfully tackled two more causes of obesity—insulin resistance and serotonin deficiency. Sound exciting?

Eating regularly and sleeping well help in the war on stress, but if your body is showing signs that it needs extra support to cope, adapt, and refill your energy reserves, subduing excess stress hormones is the next path to follow. Your stress hormones also influence your sex hormones, so the key to restoring your libido and sex hormone balance is tackling excess stress. More specifically, the anti-aging, antistress hormone DHEA increases estrogen and muscle-building testosterone, whereas the long-term stress hormone cortisol can depress progesterone and testosterone. Interestingly enough, an imbalance of estrogen, progesterone, or testosterone interferes with fat loss and muscle building, *even* with the perfect diet and exercise plan. And excess cortisol, insulin, or both can cause abdominal fat, even when you are otherwise thin!

Once your sex hormones are back in balance, you'll feel them work their metabolic magic because each of these hormones influences the master of metabolism, thyroid hormone. By addressing these hormones, you will have removed the last of the possible fat-packing factors—low thyroid, menopause, andropause, and estrogen dominance.

STEP 3: RESTORE STRENGTH, VIGOR, AND RADIANCE. The final step is to address the hormones that maximize strength and renewal—growth hormone, melatonin, and acetylcholine—with hormone-enhancing exercise (and supplements, if you find they are required). These are the hormones that fine-tune your body composition by building muscle, shrinking fat cells, and slowing the effects of aging. This step will revive your metabolism and keep it revving.

This systematic approach is my secret to restoring total hormonal balance. Where other diets may stall, are not sustainable, or simply fail, this key aspect of the Hormone Diet plan will restore your metabolism and keep your fat-loss hormones primed—for life!

If you've never been able to lose those last 5 to 25 pounds, now you will. If you've never dieted but want to feel toned and strong, this is your solution. If you already have good health but want to feel even better, this is the fix for you. If you're on your way to obesity, diabetes, heart disease, or rapid aging, this is the plan that will finally help you restore hormonal balance and turn your health around.

Most of my patients, and readers who have shared their success stories, lose 5 to 9 pounds in their very first week. Although these results provide a wonderful source of motivation, it is the improvement in their overall well-being that inspires them to keep going. Now you, too, can experience what it feels like to be in *perfect balance.*

CHAPTER 2

ARE YOU IN BALANCE?
THE HORMONAL HEALTH PROFILE

If you can uncover the subtle signs and symptoms of imbalance, you can take the right steps to fix it and increase your chances of losing fat and keeping it off. To help you do this, I have created the Hormonal Health Profile.

This easy-to-follow checklist is designed to help you identify hormonal imbalances in the quickest way possible. If you have struggled with weight loss in the past, my bet is that your profile results will be extremely valuable in helping you to figure out why.

With your answers in hand, you will be able to fine-tune your plan by adding specific foods and supplements to address your unique hormone-balancing needs. In some cases, this tool may also encourage you to search out a health-care provider, should you wish to have additional medical treatment to get control of your hormones.

The Hormonal Health Profile
How to Complete It

In the following pages, you'll find a series of checklists of symptoms and conditions arranged into groups. Each numbered group pertains to a specific hormonal imbalance or condition that can, in one way or another, impede your weight loss and increase the negative effects of aging.

As you go through the lists, check off all of the symptoms and signs you are currently experiencing within each group. Add up your total for each group and record it in the box provided at the bottom of the list, or keep track on a separate sheet of paper.

Since more than one hormone can cause similar symptoms, you will find a lot of repetition among the different groups. Just keep going and do your best to be consistent with your answers throughout the entire profile. You want to create the most complete picture of your current state of hormonal wellness.

Next, transfer your scores from each group of questions in the profile to the matching numbered space within the Treatment Pyramid on page 53.

YOUR HORMONAL HEALTH PROFILE

Check off all that apply to you and total your scores in each group.

INFLAMMATION	
Sagging, thinning skin or wrinkling	
Spider veins or varicose veins	
Cellulite	
Eczema, skin rashes, hives, or acne	
Menopause (women); andropause (men)	
Heart disease	
Prostate enlargement or prostatitis	
High cholesterol or blood pressure	
Loss of muscle tone in arms and legs; difficulty building or maintaining muscle	
Aches and pains	
Arthritis, bursitis, tendonitis, or joint stiffness	
Water retention in hands or feet	
Gout	
Alzheimer's disease	
Parkinson's disease	
Depression	
Night eating syndrome (waking at night to binge eat)	

INFLAMMATION (continued)	
Fibromyalgia	
Increased pain or poor pain tolerance	
Headaches or migraines	
High alcohol consumption	
Bronchitis, allergies (food or environmental), hives, or asthma have worsened or developed	
Autoimmune disease	
Fat gain around "love handles" or abdomen	
Loss of bone density or osteoporosis	
Generalized overweight/weight gain/obesity	
Fatty liver (diagnosed by your doctor)	
Diabetes (type 2)	
Sleep disruptions or deprivation	
Irritable bowel or inflammatory bowel disease	
Frequent gas and bloating	
Constipation, diarrhea, or nausea	
TOTAL (Warning score: > 11)	

HORMONAL IMBALANCE 1: EXCESS INSULIN	
Age spots and wrinkling	
Sagging skin	
Cellulite	
Skin tags	
Acanthosis nigricans (a skin condition characterized by light brown to black patches or markings on the neck or underarm)	
Abnormal hair growth on face or chin (women)	
Vision changes or cataracts	
Infertility or irregular menses	
Shrinking or sagging breasts	
Menopause (women); andropause or erectile dysfunction (men)	

HORMONAL IMBALANCE 1: EXCESS INSULIN (continued)	
Heart disease	
High cholesterol, high triglycerides, or high blood pressure	
Burning feet at night (especially while in bed)	
Water retention in the face/puffiness	
Gout	
Poor memory, concentration, or Alzheimer's disease	
Fat gain around "love handles" and/or abdomen	
Fat over triceps	
Generalized overweight/weight gain/obesity	
Hypoglycemia; cravings for sweets, carbohydrates or constant hunger or increased appetite	
Fatigue after eating (especially carbohydrates)	
Fatty liver (diagnosed by your doctor)	
Diabetes (type 2)	
Sleep disruption or deprivation	
TOTAL (Warning score: > 9)	

HORMONAL IMBALANCE 2: LOW DOPAMINE	
Fatigue, especially in the morning	
Poor tolerance for exercise	
Restless leg syndrome	
Poor memory	
Parkinson's disease	
Depression	
Loss of libido	
Feeling a strong need for stimulation or excitement (foods, gambling, partying, sex, etc.)	
Addictive eating or binge eating	
Cravings for sweets, carbohydrates, junk food, or fast food	
TOTAL (Warning score: > 4)	

HORMONAL IMBALANCE 3: LOW SEROTONIN	
PMS characterized by hypoglycemia, sugar cravings, sweet cravings, and/or depression	
Feeling wired at night	
Lack of sweating	
Poor memory	
Loss of libido	
Depression, anxiety, irritability, or seasonal affective disorder	
Loss of motivation or competitive edge	
Low self-esteem	
Inability to make decisions	
Obsessive-compulsive disorder	
Bulimia or binge eating	
Fibromyalgia	
Increased pain or poor pain tolerance	
Headaches or migraines	
Cravings for sweets or carbohydrates	
Constant hunger or increased appetite	
Inability to sleep in, no matter how late going to bed	
Less than 7.5 hours of sleep per night	
Irritable bowel	
Constipation	
Nausea	
Use of corticosteroids	
TOTAL (Warning score: > 7)	

HORMONAL IMBALANCE 4: LOW GABA	
PMS characterized by breast tenderness, water retention, bloating, anxiety, sleep disruptions, or headaches	
Feeling wired at night	
Aches and pains or increased muscle tension	
Irritability, tension, or anxiety	
Difficulty falling asleep or staying asleep	
Less than 7.5 hours of sleep per night	
Irritable bowel	
Frequent gas and bloating	
TOTAL (Warning score: > 3)	

HORMONAL IMBALANCE 5: EXCESS CORTISOL	
Wrinkling, thinning skin or skin that has lost its fullness	
Hair loss	
Infertility or absent menses (unrelated to menopause)	
Feeling wired at night	
Heart palpitations	
Loss of muscle tone in arms and legs	
Cold hands or feet	
Water retention in face/puffiness	
Poor memory or concentration	
Loss of libido	
Depression, anxiety, irritability, or seasonal affective disorder	
High alcohol consumption	
Frequent colds and flus	
Hives, bronchitis, allergies (food or environmental), asthma, or autoimmune disease	
Fat gain around "love handles" or abdomen	
A "buffalo hump" of fat on back of neck/upper back	
Difficulty building or maintaining muscle	
Loss of bone density or osteoporosis	
Cravings for sweets or carbs, hypoglycemia, or constant hunger	
Difficulty falling asleep	
Difficulty staying asleep (especially waking between 2 and 4 a.m.)	
Less than 7.5 hours of sleep per night	
Irritable bowel or frequent gas and bloating	
Use of corticosteroids	
TOTAL (Warning score: > 8)	

HORMONAL IMBALANCE 6: LOW DHEA	
Dry skin	
Heart disease	
Erectile dysfunction	
Andropause	
Feeling wired at night	
Poor tolerance for exercise	
Loss of muscle tone in arms and legs	
Poor memory or concentration	
Irritability or easily agitated	
Loss of libido	
Depression	
Loss of motivation or competitive edge	
Autoimmune disease	
Fat gain around "love handles"	
Fat gain over triceps	
Fat gain around abdomen	
Difficulty building or maintaining muscle	
TOTAL (Warning score: > 6)	

HORMONAL IMBALANCE 7: EXCESS ESTROGEN	
Spider or varicose veins	
Cellulite	
Heavy menstrual bleeding	
PMS characterized by breast tenderness, water retention, bloating, swelling, and/or weight gain	
Fibrocystic breast disease	
Prostate enlargement	
Erectile dysfunction	
Breast growth (men)	
Loss of morning erection	
Irritability, mood swings, or anxiety	
Headaches or migraines (especially in women before their menses)	
High alcohol consumption (> 4 drinks per week for women and > 7 drinks per week for men)	
Autoimmune disease or allergies	
Fat gain around "love handles" or abdomen (men)	
Fat gain at hips (women)	
Current use of hormone replacement therapy or birth control pills	
TOTAL (Warning score: > 6)	

HORMONAL IMBALANCE 8: LOW ESTROGEN	
Dry or sagging skin	
Thinning skin or skin has lost its fullness	
Hair loss	
Dry eyes or cataracts (women)	
PMS characterized by depression, hypoglycemia, sugar cravings, and/or sweet cravings	
Infertility or absent menses (not related to menopause)	
Painful intercourse and/or vaginal dryness	
Shrinking or sagging breasts	
Urinary incontinence (stress or otherwise)	
Menopause	
Fatigue	
Hot flashes	
Poor memory or concentration	
Irritability	
Loss of libido	
Depression or mood swings	
Headaches or migraines	
Fat gain around "love handles" or abdomen (menopausal women)	
Loss of bone density or osteoporosis	
Difficulty falling or staying asleep	
TOTAL (Warning score: > 8)	

HORMONAL IMBALANCE 9: LOW PROGESTERONE	
Dry skin or skin that has lost its fullness	
Spider or varicose veins	
Hair loss	
Short menstrual cycle (< 28 days) or excessively long bleeding times (< 6 days)	
PMS characterized by breast tenderness, anxiety, sleep disruptions, headaches, menstrual spotting, water retention, bloating, and/or weight gain	

HORMONAL IMBALANCE 9: LOW PROGESTERONE (continued)	
Infertility or absent menses (not related to menopause)	
Fibrocystic breast disease	
Menopause (women); andropause (men)	
Prostate enlargement	
Hot flashes	
Lack of sweating	
Feeling cold and/or cold hands or feet	
Heart palpitations	
Water retention	
Irritability and/or anxiety	
Loss of libido	
Headaches or migraines	
Autoimmune disease, hives, asthma, or allergies	
Loss of bone density or osteoporosis	
Difficulty falling or staying asleep	
TOTAL (Warning score: > 6)	

HORMONAL IMBALANCE 10: EXCESS PROGESTERONE	
Acne	
PMS characterized by depression	
Infertility	
Water retention	
Depression	
Frequent colds and flus	
Weight gain or difficulty losing weight	
Current use of hormone replacement therapy or birth control pills	
TOTAL (Warning score: > 4)	

HORMONAL IMBALANCE 11: LOW TESTOSTERONE	
Dry skin	
Thinning skin or skin has lost its fullness	
Painful intercourse	
Heart disease (men)	
Erectile dysfunction	
Andropause (men)	
Loss of morning erection	
Fatigue	
Poor tolerance for exercise	
Loss of muscle tone in arms and legs	
Poor memory or concentration	
Loss of libido	
Depression or anxiety	
Loss of motivation or competitive edge	
Headaches or migraines (men)	
Fat gain around "love handles" or abdomen (men and women)	
Difficulty building or maintaining muscle	
Loss of bone density or osteoporosis (men and women)	
Sleep apnea (men)	
Use of corticosteroids	
TOTAL (Warning score: > 7)	

HORMONAL IMBALANCE 12: EXCESS TESTOSTERONE	
Acne	
Acanthosis nigricans (women)	
Hair loss (scalp)	
Abnormal hair growth on face (women)	
Infertility	
Shrinking or sagging breasts	
Prostate enlargement	

HORMONAL IMBALANCE 12: EXCESS TESTOSTERONE (continued)	
Irritability, aggression, or easily agitated	
Fat gain around abdomen (women)	
Cravings for sweets or carbohydrates (women)	
Constant hunger or increased appetite (women)	
Fatty liver (women)	
TOTAL (Warning score: > 4)	

HORMONAL IMBALANCE 13: LOW THYROID	
Dry skin and/or hair	
Acne	
Hair loss	
Brittle hair and/or nails	
PMS, infertility, long menstrual cycle (> 30 days), or irregular periods	
Abnormal lactation	
Fatigue	
Lack of sweating, feeling cold, or cold hands and feet	
High cholesterol	
Poor tolerance for exercise	
Heart palpitations	
Outer edge of eyebrows thinning	
Aches and pains	
Water retention/puffiness in hands or feet	
Poor memory	
Loss of libido	
Depression	
Loss of motivation or competitive edge	
Iron deficiency anemia	
Hives	
Generalized overweight/weight gain/obesity	
Constipation	

HORMONAL IMBALANCE 13: LOW THYROID (continued)	
Use of corticosteroids	
Current use of synthetic hormone replacement therapy or birth control pills	
TOTAL (Warning score: > 8)	

HORMONAL IMBALANCE 14: LOW ACETYLCHOLINE	
Poor tolerance for exercise	
Loss of muscle tone in arms and legs or poor muscle function/strength	
Poor memory or concentration, decrease in memory or recall	
Alzheimer's disease	
Difficulty building or maintaining muscle	
Difficulty falling asleep or staying asleep, disrupted sleep patterns	
Irritable bowel	
Constipation	
TOTAL (Warning score: > 3)	

HORMONAL IMBALANCE 15: LOW MELATONIN	
Andropause (men); menopause (women)	
Night eating syndrome (waking at night to binge eat)	
High alcohol consumption	
Cravings for sweets or carbohydrates; increased appetite	
Difficulty falling asleep	
Failing to sleep in total darkness	
Difficulty staying asleep (especially waking between 2 and 4 a.m.)	
Sleep apnea	
Less than 7.5 hours of sleep per night	
Use of corticosteroids	
TOTAL (Warning score: > 3)	

HORMONAL IMBALANCE 16: LOW GROWTH HORMONE	
Dry skin	
Thinning skin or skin has lost its fullness	
Sagging skin	
Menopause (women); andropause (men)	
Lack of exercise	
Loss of muscle tone in arms or legs	
High alcohol consumption	
Fat gain around "love handles" or abdomen	
Difficulty building or maintaining muscle	
Loss of bone density or osteoporosis	
Generalized overweight/weight gain/obesity	
Failing to sleep in total darkness	
Difficulty staying asleep (especially waking between 2 and 4 a.m.)	
Sleep apnea	
Use of corticosteroids	
TOTAL (Warning score: > 5)	

After you have completed your profile, go ahead and transfer your scores from each group to the appropriate space in the Treatment Pyramid on the opposite page.

Interpreting Your Scores

For each group of profile questions, I have listed a score in parentheses next to the box for your total—the *warning score*. If your score is *the same or higher than* the warning score, you likely have an imbalance. For each of your high scores, refer to the noted sections of the book to learn about the specific imbalance and its impact on your health.

You also have to transfer your scores to the second Treatment Pyramid on page 281 in Chapter 13. It's here that the *treatment solutions* to your imbalances are provided, should you choose to use them as part of your three steps. This pyramid shows how to "tweak" your action plan in order to meet your individual needs, especially if you discover that you have more than one imbalance. The precise order of treatment presented in the pyramid is definitely my *secret to restoring hormonal balance,* as each level builds upon the next.

What Do Your Results Mean?

Even though I have listed a warning score for each group, ultimately it's up to you to decide on a course of action or whether a particular imbalance warrants further investigation. True diagnosis is not something you can do at home. A high score in *any one of the groups* suggests to me, however, that you would benefit from completing *all three steps* of the Hormone Diet. And I am confident you will yield even greater results by *choosing specific treatments* to address your imbalances once you reach Step 2.

As I mentioned, if your profile results reveal that you *do* have hormonal imbalances, you may want to focus on specific sections of the following two chapters. If you wish, you can read both chapters from start to finish. Or, you can focus strictly on the imbalances that apply to you, then get right to the "skinny" on your fat in Chapter 5.

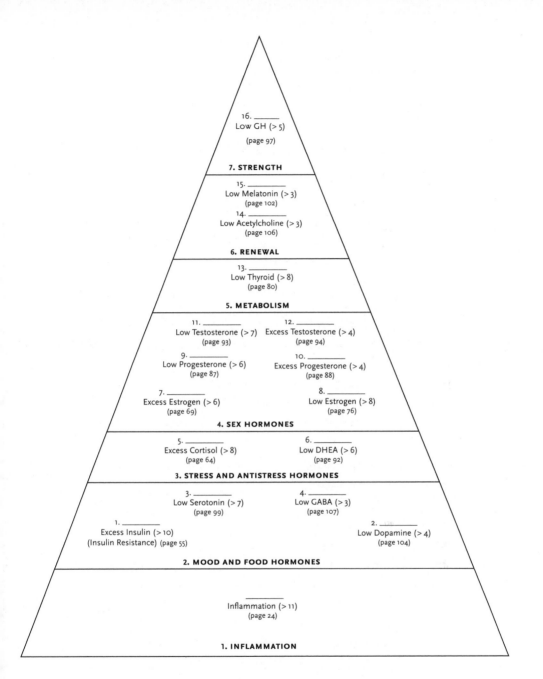

16. _____
Low GH (> 5)
(page 97)

7. STRENGTH

15. _____
Low Melatonin (> 3)
(page 102)

14. _____
Low Acetylcholine (> 3)
(page 106)

6. RENEWAL

13. _____
Low Thyroid (> 8)
(page 80)

5. METABOLISM

11. _____   12. _____
Low Testosterone (> 7)   Excess Testosterone (> 4)
(page 93)   (page 94)

9. _____   10. _____
Low Progesterone (> 6)   Excess Progesterone (> 4)
(page 87)   (page 88)

7. _____   8. _____
Excess Estrogen (> 6)   Low Estrogen (> 8)
(page 69)   (page 76)

4. SEX HORMONES

5. _____   6. _____
Excess Cortisol (> 8)   Low DHEA (> 6)
(page 64)   (page 92)

3. STRESS AND ANTISTRESS HORMONES

3. _____   4. _____
Low Serotonin (> 7)   Low GABA (> 3)
(page 99)   (page 107)

1. _____   2. _____
Excess Insulin (> 10)   Low Dopamine (> 4)
(Insulin Resistance) (page 55)   (page 104)

2. MOOD AND FOOD HORMONES

_____
Inflammation (> 11)
(page 24)

1. INFLAMMATION

THE TREATMENT PYRAMID

CHAPTER 3

YOUR FAT-LOSS FOES:
THE HORMONES THAT PACK ON POUNDS

Losing weight is a cascade of many steps, beginning with the production of certain hormones and continuing with their action in the brain. Some people are resistant to these hormones, just as other people are insulin-resistant. These people never receive the message from the brain that tells them they're full.

ELVIRA DE MEJIA, assistant professor of food science and human nutrition, University of Illinois

Here's what you will learn about in this chapter:
- The four hormones that are our fat-loss foes because they interfere with fat burning, boost appetite, and cause weight gain
- Three fat-packing hormonal imbalances: insulin resistance, chronic stress, and estrogen dominance

Although I could easily dedicate a full chapter to each individual hormone, I have chosen instead to divide them into two basic groups: those that are our fat-loss foes and those that are our fat-loss friends.

This chapter focuses on four fat-packing hormones: insulin, cortisol, estrogen, and ghrelin. When not in proper balance, these substances can absolutely sabotage your fat-loss success.

Besides revealing how individual hormones can either help

or hinder your fat loss, I also wish to explain that no hormone works in isolation. All of these fascinating substances interact with and influence each other, which is why a spike in one hormone typically causes a drop in another. This complex interplay is part of the body's incredible mechanism for coping with an imbalanced state. Too much or too little of any one hormone can interfere with your metabolism, accelerate aging, and compromise your overall wellness.

For your quick reference, I have clearly marked my discussions of each hormone in this chapter and Chapter 4 with the numbers matching the relevant group of questions in the Hormonal Health Profile in Chapter 2 (i.e., as Hormonal Imbalance 1, Hormonal Imbalance 2, etc.). You may choose to concentrate only on the sections that pertain to your specific imbalance(s). Or you can certainly read everything covered in these two chapters and return, if necessary, for a review each time you complete the profile. Choose the option that works best for you—there is a lot of information here to take in!

Hormonal Imbalance 1—Excess Insulin
The Ins and Outs of Insulin

Insulin is an essential substance whose main function is to process sugar in your bloodstream and carry it into your cells to be used. The carbohydrates you eat are broken down into sugar (glucose) through the process of digestion, which begins in your mouth and ends in your small intestine. Once sugar enters your bloodstream from your digestive tract, it triggers your pancreas to release the hormone insulin. Insulin is released in proportion to the amount of sugar in the bloodstream (i.e., more sugar = more insulin).

Once insulin is released, the sugar in your bloodstream can be directed in three ways.

1. **Immediate use as a fuel source.** It is burned off right away, particularly by your brain and kidneys.
2. **Stored as glycogen in the liver or muscles for later use as an energy source.** Just as a glass can hold only so much water, the body's capacity to store glycogen is limited. For this reason, only a finite amount of the carbohydrates we consume can be used in this way. Because most of us consume plenty of carbs daily, our glycogen stores tend to fill up quickly (though exercise is one of the best ways to free up more storage space because it causes the body to draw on glycogen for energy).
3. **Stored as fat.** If all your glycogen storage sites are full and the excess sugar isn't used right away, the body will convert the leftovers to fat, a much longer-term fuel source that's far more difficult to burn off. Now you can see why limiting your intake of high-sugar, high-carb foods is beneficial. In doing so, you'll limit the amount of insulin released and, ultimately, the amount of sugar your body will store as fat.

Insulin and Abdominal Fat

Although insulin plays an essential role in healthy body function, an excess of this hormone will certainly make you gain weight. Not only does too much insulin encourage your body to store unused glucose as fat, but it also *blocks* the use of stored fat as an energy source. For these reasons, an abnormally high insulin level makes losing fat, especially around the abdomen, next to impossible.

Insulin and Appetite

To make matters worse, too much insulin can cause you to consume more calories. According to Dr. Robert Lustig, a pediatric endocrinologist at the University of California San Francisco Children's Hospital whose work was published in the August 2006 edition of the journal *Nature Clinical Practice Endocrinology & Metabolism,* insulin stimulates appetite by working on the brain in two ways. First, it blocks signals to the brain by interfering with the appetite-suppressing hormone leptin, causing us to eat more and become less active. Second, it causes a spike in dopamine, the hormone that signals the brain to seek rewards. Dopamine spurs a desire to eat in order to achieve a pleasurable rush—the same rush we may get from addictive behaviors. No wonder putting down the fork is so tough. We are addicted to food!

Balanced Insulin Does Your Body Good

Maintaining the correct amount of insulin offers tremendous benefits. Insulin is one of the body's main anabolic hormones, meaning it initiates the metabolic pathways that rebuild body proteins while preventing protein breakdown. It also promotes the use of sugar as an energy source. In this manner, the right amount of insulin encourages the growth of your muscles and the refilling of your glycogen stores. We can use these effects to our advantage, especially immediately after exercise—one of the few times when eating carbs and having an insulin spike is beneficial. Right after a workout, it promotes the entry of glucose and amino acids into muscle tissue to support repair and growth.

Insulin may also help prevent further breakdown of muscle tissue after a workout through its enhancing action on testosterone. The male sex hormone testosterone is vital to the growth and maintenance of muscle tissue. In the right amount, insulin prevents the body from breaking down proteins, such as those found in muscle tissue, for energy during times of stress. Without it, your cells would not have access to amino acids, glucose, and fatty acids to survive, let alone to grow, heal, and repair. This is precisely why those living with type 1 diabetes must take insulin by injection when the pancreas fails to manufacture it naturally. The problem of excess fat storage arises only when our insulin level is too high.

Causes of Insulin Overload

There are several reasons for excess insulin, but these are the main culprits:

- Consuming too many nutrient-poor carbohydrates—the type found in processed foods, sugary drinks, and sodas; foods containing high-fructose corn syrup; packaged low-fat foods; and artificial sweeteners
- Insufficient protein intake
- Inadequate fat intake
- Deficient fiber consumption
- Chronic stress
- Lack of exercise
- Overexercising or other activities that compromise muscle tissue
- Steroid-based medications
- Poor liver function and toxin exposure
- Aging

Besides turning you into a walking fat-storage facility, excess insulin will also make you feel just plain *bad*. Heart palpitations, sweating, poor concentration, weakness, anxiety, fogginess, fatigue, irritability, or impaired thinking are common side effects. These symptoms are particularly prevalent in the "crash" you tend to experience following a high-carbohydrate meal or the consumption of a lot of alcohol, both of which cause irregular peaks and valleys in your insulin level.

To make matters worse, our bodies typically respond to these unpleasant feelings by making us think we're hungry, which in turn causes us to reach for more high-sugar foods and drinks. And then we end up in a vicious cycle of hormonal imbalance, not to mention weight gain.

But wait, there's more. Since insulin also influences sodium uptake in the kidneys, an excess of this hormone can cause you to retain water, experience swelling, and look like that famous little dough boy. He's cute, but definitely not anyone's top choice as a physique role model.

Excess insulin can affect men and women in different ways. For men, a high insulin level typically sparks heightened activity of an aromatase enzyme in your fat cells, which causes more of your masculinizing hormone, testosterone, to be converted into the feminizing hormone estrogen. If this trend continues long-term, you'll see increased fat deposits in "female" areas, such as your abdomen and even your chest (as breasts), not to mention a negative impact on your sex drive and erectile function.

Women are just as vulnerable. The same aromatase enzyme boosts conversion of estrogen to testosterone. As a result, high insulin can lead to such lovely effects as increased fat storage in the abdomen, shrinking and sagging breasts, abnormal hair growth, acne, and even male-pattern hair loss. Not good.

A FAT-PACKING HORMONAL IMBALANCE

HORMONAL IMBALANCE 1: EXCESS INSULIN
(Insulin Resistance and Metabolic Syndrome)
When excess insulin is present over a long period, our cells start to grow accustomed to having so much of it around all the time. As a result, our cellular response to insulin becomes blunted and our

pancreas is called upon to step up its insulin production in an attempt to maintain a normal blood sugar level. This *decrease* in insulin sensitivity is called insulin resistance.

Imagine insulin as a truck carrying sugars into our cells. The truck enters the cells using a special garage-door opener. If the opener stops working, the truck is stuck in the driveway. Soon after, another truck will pull up behind the first one and they'll both become trapped. Eventually a whole fleet of trucks will be backed up, causing a major traffic jam throughout the body—or chronically high insulin. All of this happens because the garage-door opener (aka the insulin receptor) is no longer responding to the presence of the truck (aka insulin).

Insulin resistance primarily develops in the skeletal muscle cells, but it can also occur in fat cells, the liver, and other tissues. Once our cells become resistant to insulin, losing weight becomes harder than ever. Moreover, physiological changes start to occur in the body, signaling a condition called metabolic syndrome, the clinical manifestation of insulin resistance.

THE INCIDENCE OF METABOLIC SYNDROME

At the 2007 Postgraduate Nutrition Symposium at Harvard University, researchers revealed findings suggesting that inflammation and insulin resistance are *the* major contributors to rising rates of type 2 diabetes and the overall fattening of North America. The diagram on the opposite page, adapted from the Centers for Disease Control and Prevention (CDC), illustrates the current epidemic of insulin resistance and diabetes across the nation.

Medical experts estimate that 40 percent of the US population will be obese by the year 2009. Forty percent! Wow! Simply eating too much (i.e., "super-sizing") or routinely making bad

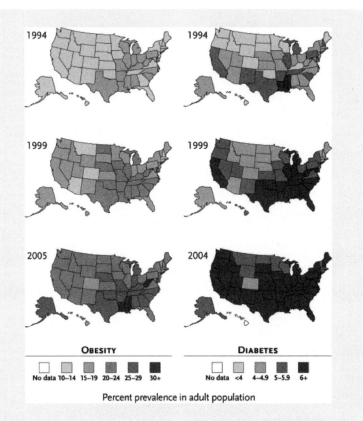

1994   1994

1999   1999

2005   2004

OBESITY   DIABETES

No data 10–14 15–19 20–24 25–29 30+   No data <4 4–4.9 5–5.9 6+

Percent prevalence in adult population

THE PROGRESSION OF INSULIN RESISTANCE AND DIABETES IN THE UNITED STATES FROM 1994 TO 2004

Source: http://focus.hms.harvard.edu/2007/040607/metabolism.shtml

food choices leads to the consumption of hundreds of excess calories daily. The Centers for Disease Control and Prevention reported that in 2007 23.6 million children and adults in the United States—7.8 percent of the population—had diabetes. Each year, 1.6 million new cases of diabetes are diagnosed in people ages 20 years and older, with the vast majority between 40 and 59 years of age. In addition, an estimated 65 percent of the American population has one or more components of meta-bolic syndrome (listed below), which is a known precursor to diabetes. Even teens are at risk. A study reported in the April 2005 edition of *Circulation*, an American Heart Association journal, described obesity and insulin resistance as a menacing tag team that dramatically accelerates cardiovascular risk in teenagers.

Insulin resistance is now an epidemic of *massive* proportion, one that is overloading our medical-care systems. We must change our perspective from disease treatment to prevention, the exact objective you can expect to achieve with the help of the *Hormone Diet* three-step system.

ASSESSING YOUR INSULIN SENSITIVITY AND RISK OF METABOLIC SYNDROME

Before you can address a potential problem, you need to gain a better understanding of your current health picture. Your answers to the Hormonal Health Profile may have provided you with a good indication of your insulin sensitivity. In addition, as part of the preparation stage of your three steps (see Chapter 6), I recommend a blood test to assess your insulin sensitivity.

If, in the meantime, you're wondering whether you are insulin resistant or insulin sensitive, take a good look at your waist and pinch your love handles. If you carry excess fat in this area, you may be insulin resistant. If you're naturally lean, your insulin sensitivity is likely in good shape.

A full workup to establish a treatment plan and definite diagnosis for metabolic syndrome includes blood tests, blood pressure readings, and, in some cases, additional exams such as an abdominal ultrasound to assess the liver. Should you wish to talk to your health-care provider about this type of investigation, I have outlined all the tests involved in a complete investigation of insulin resistance. (See Appendix A, "Understanding Blood Tests.")

According to the current medical definition, metabolic syndrome is diagnosed when *three or more* of the following risk factors are identified after a clinical evaluation has been completed:

- Low levels of "good" cholesterol (HDL)
- High levels of "bad" cholesterol (LDL)
- Elevated triglycerides (unsaturated fats)
- Increased waist-to-hip ratio, since fat accumulates around the abdomen and "love handle" areas rather than the hips
- High blood pressure (i.e., above 130/85, according to the National Cholesterol Education Program)
- Elevated blood sugar levels (i.e., greater than 110 mg/dL)

WHAT DOES A DIAGNOSIS OF METABOLIC SYNDROME MEAN FOR YOUR HEALTH?

Metabolic syndrome is associated with increased risk of type 2 diabetes, obesity, high blood pressure, stroke, and coronary heart disease. New research has also uncovered a link between elevated insulin levels and certain types of malignancies, including breast cancer. Furthermore, insulin resistance is associated with higher risk of four of the top five leading causes of death in the United States (as reported by the American Heart Association 2003 Heart and Stroke Statistical Update), including cancer, heart disease, diabetes, and Alzheimer's disease.

On the upside, even severe instances of metabolic syndrome can be improved with better lifestyle habits. Going back to the analogy of a fleet of insulin trucks backed up in the bloodstream, the problem can be alleviated in two ways. First, we can restore the function of the garage door with lubricant so it responds more easily to the opener. Exercise and insulin-sensitizing supplements are highly effective for this purpose. Second, we can lessen the traffic load in the first place by reducing the number of insulin trucks in the fleet. In other words, better nutritional habits lead to an overall reduction in the release of insulin. The three-step plan will give you the tools you need to implement both these solutions, as it has for so many of my patients already. Depending on the results of your Hormonal Health Profile, you may also choose to add supplements, described in Chapter 13, to your program.

Hormonal Imbalance 5—Excess Cortisol
Another Culprit of Unsightly Ab Fat

Our bodies provide us with uniquely designed mechanisms to cope with immediate and chronic stress. Our nervous system drives our immediate stress response, while our chronic stress response is handled by our endocrine system.

Right Here, Right Now: Immediate Stress Response and the Nervous System

Two guys are hiking along a trail in the woods when a huge grizzly bear suddenly appears on the path in front of them. One of the men drops to the ground and starts ripping off his boots and frantically putting on his running shoes. The other man sees what his friend is up to and exclaims, "What are you doing? You can't out-

run that bear!" To which the first man replies, "I know. But I can outrun you."

Fortunately, our bodies are physiologically well-adapted to handle a situation as stressful as crossing paths with a grizzly bear. Our hearts race, breathing becomes rapid and shallow, blood pressure rises, our pupils dilate, digestion slows, and our hands become cold or clammy as bloodflow is directed to our limb muscles in preparation for a speedy getaway. Blood sugars also increase, while a hefty shot of adrenaline sparks the release of stored fats to quickly provide our bodies with the burst of energy we need for a successful escape.

Normally these changes are temporary and are only necessary for those few moments when we're face-to-face with extreme stress. These responses tend naturally to be followed by a period of relaxation, especially after physical exertion (like running away from a bear). Physical exertion also helps to burn up all the sugar and fat our bodies release to help us escape the stress. If there's no physical exertion to burn up that excess fuel, the extra sugars and fats can pose a problem, especially around our waistlines.

Constant stimulation of your nervous system, either through your thoughts or information taken in via your five senses, is one of *the* major causes of hormonal imbalance and weight gain. Your brain responds to stress by encouraging a high intake of fatty and sugary foods—the so-called comfort foods that cause stubborn weight gain. So taking active steps to beat stress and calm your nervous system is *essential* for fat loss.

Here for the Long Haul: Cortisol, Our Long-Term Stress Response

The good thing about short-term stress, such as finding a bear in your path, is that it comes, you deal with it, and it goes. It's the unrelenting stress that comes with worries about finances, a divorce, a job you despise, chronic illness, or generally feeling overwhelmed with your life that can cause lasting damage.

Persistent or chronic stress involves a different physiological process in your body. Under situations of chronic stress—whether the stress is physical, emotional, mental, or environmental, *real or imagined*—your body releases high amounts of the hormone cortisol. For instance, cold, hunger, low blood pressure, pain, broken bones, injuries, inflammation, our sleep-wake cycle, intense exercise, and emotional upsets all cause the brain to activate our stress pathway and increase cortisol production by the adrenal glands (two glands that sit on top of your kidneys and also produce adrenaline).

If you have a mood disorder such as anxiety, depression, post-traumatic stress disorder, or exhaustion, or if you have a digestive issue such as irritable bowel syndrome, you can bet your stress response pathway is in overdrive, cranking up your cortisol. If you routinely have anxiety-provoking or upsetting thoughts racing through your mind, your stress systems will constantly be working overtime.

Mental and emotional stress may be *most* injurious because they're usually not followed by a relaxation response the way most physical stress is. As long as the perceived stressful event remains constantly in your mind, your body cannot fully achieve a relaxed, healthy, balanced state. When prolonged, this state of imbalance leads to permanent physiological changes.

But cortisol, just like insulin, isn't all bad. We need it to survive and to adapt to stressful situations. It also maintains our blood pressure and body temperature, controls inflammation, and allows other hormones (such as adrenaline) to take effect quickly as they provide us with energy by breaking down fat.

A FAT-PACKING HORMONAL IMBALANCE

HORMONAL IMBALANCE 5: EXCESS CORTISOL

(Chronic Stress or Anxiety)

HOW DOES STRESS MAKE YOU FAT?

Unlike adrenaline, which draws on your fat stores for energy during stressful situations, cortisol consumes your muscle tissue for fuel. Prolonged stress can lead to muscle wasting and high blood sugar simply because your body is struggling to adapt. When these conditions take over, stress becomes extremely destructive to your metabolism, body composition, and wellness.

Another stress hormone called NPY (neuropeptide Y) also plays an important role in controlling your eating habits by working in your brain. Once released, NPY *decreases* your metabolic rate, causes more belly fat storage, and also fuels your appetite for sugary foods and carbohydrates—a triple-whammy for your waistline.

So many side effects of stress conspire to make you fat! Together, high cortisol and elevated NPY impact your metabolism, appetite, and body composition in the following nasty ways:

- Cortisol depresses your metabolic rate by interfering with thyroid hormone
- Cortisol and NPY fuel your desire for fatty foods and carbohydrates
- Both boost abdominal fat storage
- Cortisol depletes your happy hormone, serotonin, causing depression and more carbohydrate cravings
- Cortisol can cause blood sugar imbalance, resulting in hypoglycemia and symptoms of shakiness, irritability, fatigue, and headaches between meals
- Cortisol causes you to eat more than you need to by stimulating appetite-boosting NPY and blocking appetite-suppressing leptin

- Cortisol saps testosterone, which can result in languishing libido and a host of serious health risks
- Cortisol eats away at muscle and slows repair of metabolically active muscle cells
- Excess cortisol leads to sleep disruption, a known cause of weight gain
- Cortisol blunts the growth hormone that helps build metabolically active muscle, aids tissue rejuvenation, and slows the effects of aging
- Cortisol and NPY both decrease cellular sensitivity to insulin, resulting in elevated insulin levels, insulin resistance, and accumulation of abdominal fat

Through a complicated network of hormonal interactions, prolonged stress results in a raging appetite, metabolic decline, loads of belly fat, and a loss of hard-won, metabolically active muscle tissue. In other words, stress makes us soft, flabby, and much older than we truly are!

HOW DO YOU KNOW WHETHER YOUR STRESS IS OUT OF CONTROL?

Since symptoms of stress vary widely, pinpointing whether or not it's the main culprit behind specific health problems can be difficult. The Hormonal Health Profile may certainly help you to assess whether excess cortisol is having negative effects on your health and hormones. And I have outlined specific tests to assess your stress in Appendix A, should you wish to investigate your situation further with the help of your doctor. At this time, there is no lab test for measuring NPY. If you are under severe emotional stress, however, your NPY is likely on the high side. You can assess your cortisol using a salivary cortisol profile test that collects saliva at four different points during the day. When properly balanced, your cortisol should be highest at around 6 a.m. and lowest at night.

I typically see three common patterns of cortisol imbalance in my patients. In some cases, cortisol is elevated at all points of collection. In others, the normal cortisol pattern is reversed so that it's highest in the evening and lowest in the morning. The latter condition is characterized by extreme difficulty getting up in the morning, fatigue during the day, and difficulty falling asleep at bedtime. Low cortisol at all points of collection suggests total adrenal gland burnout.

You must control your cortisol if you want to achieve lasting health and a strong, lean body, which is why thinking positively and managing *all types* of stress are included as the first of the three steps. In fact, all of the steps of the Hormone Diet aim to control cortisol.

Hormonal Imbalance 7—Excess Estrogen
Too Much or Too Little Can Make You Fat

In women, estrogen is produced primarily by the ovaries in response to follicle-stimulating hormone (FSH), manufactured by the pituitary before menopause and by the adrenal glands and fat cells afterwards. Estrogen is the dominant hormone for the first 2 weeks or so after menstruation, when it stimulates the buildup of tissue and blood in the uterus, and the ovarian follicles simultaneously begin their development of the egg. The level of hormone peaks and then tapers off just as the follicle matures before ovulation.

Although estrogen is typically considered a female hormone, a certain amount of it is natural and important for men as well. Excess body fat in men, however, spurs an unhealthy rise in estrogen levels because fat cells are involved in converting testosterone to estrogen. Alcohol consumption and a high-fat diet have also been shown to increase estrogen levels in both men and women. Then there's the natural aging process in men, which tends to bring about a drop in testosterone production and a parallel increase in estrogen. I often say women and men seem to switch hormonal roles with age; men experience an increase in estrogen, whereas women lose it!

The Three Types of Estrogen

Though estrogen is often referred to as a single substance, it's actually made up of three hormones: estradiol, estrone, and estriol. In most cases, the term "estrogen" is used to refer to estradiol (as is the case in this book, unless I note otherwise).

1. **Estradiol** is the strongest and most prevalent estrogen hormone and plays a surprising number of critical roles in the body. This important substance is the primary hormone of the menstrual cycle and dictates the thickness of the uterine wall. Besides controlling vaginal moisture and lubrication, it enhances libido and sexual enjoyment and prevents urinary tract infections and urinary incontinence. It stimulates the cells that build bone and also aids the bone-edifying processes of calcium, magnesium, and zinc absorption. Estradiol supports cardiovascular health by dilating the blood vessels, increasing "good" HDL cholesterol, and lowering "bad" LDL cholesterol. It influences insulin response and aids blood sugar balance. Estradiol also has positive effects on the brain and nervous system, including improving memory, aiding sleep, and protecting nerve cells. This multitasking substance keeps our eyes moist and is also the secret to glowing skin, as it prevents wrinkling by maintaining skin tone, texture, and thickness. It is a potent antioxidant, especially for skin and brain cells.

2. **Estrone** is the second most potent estrogen and is often labeled the "bad" estrogen. It has earned this reputation because an excess is harmful to breast and uterine cells and is also thought to lead to cancer. Before menopause, the ovaries, liver, and fat cells produce estrone. After the onset of menopause, this hor-

mone is naturally produced in the fat cells. Women with excess body fat are, therefore, more likely to be estrone dominant. Regardless of age, estrone dominance is further intensified by high alcohol consumption (i.e., more than four drinks a week for women; more than seven for men), which is also known to boost cancer risk. Furthermore, abnormally high estrone blocks the beneficial effects of estradiol in the body, especially in the brain, and increases the risk of blood clots, toxic fat gain, gallstones, and stress on the liver.

3. **Estriol** is the weakest of the estrogens and is produced when estradiol and estrone convert to estriol. This hormone is often referred to as the "good" estrogen because it appears to block the harmful effects of estrone on breast cells. New research has also found that estriol may have positive effects on autoimmune functions. Although not as strong as estradiol, estriol still offers significant benefits when used as a supplement during menopause. It is very useful on its own for relieving vaginal dryness and for the treatment and prevention of urinary tract infections. Or, when mixed with estradiol in the form of Bi-est (80 percent estriol, 20 percent estradiol), it aids other symptoms of menopause such as hot flashes and insomnia. Unlike estradiol, estriol does not have the documented benefits on heart health, bones, or the brain, so mixing the two types of estrogen can be beneficial.

HOT HORMONE FACT

Estriol, naturally produced only during pregnancy, is thought to play a crucial role in preventing the mother's body from attacking the fetus as foreign tissue. In a similar manner, estriol may help patients suffering with multiple sclerosis (MS) by preventing an overactive immune system from destroying myelin. A 2002 study by UCLA neuroscientists showed that oral supplementation of estriol decreased the size and number of MS-related brain lesions and increased protective immune responses in patients with relapsing-remitting MS.

A FAT-PACKING HORMONAL IMBALANCE

HORMONAL IMBALANCE 7: EXCESS ESTROGEN
(Estrogen Dominance)

Estrogen balance is essential for achieving and maintaining fat loss. In men and premenopausal women, too much estrogen, a condition called estrogen dominance, causes toxic fat gain, water retention, bloating, and a host of other health and wellness issues. Whereas premenopausal women with too much estrogen tend to have the pear-shaped body type with more weight at the hips, both men and menopausal women with this condition exhibit an apple shape with more fat accumulation in the abdominal area. Researchers have now identified excess estrogen to be *as great a risk factor for obesity*—in both sexes—as poor eating habits and lack of exercise.

Estrogen dominance, a term coined by Dr. John R. Lee, a family physician and author of many books on natural progesterone therapy for menopausal women, can occur in two ways. It may arise when an imbalance of "good" estrogen relative to the "bad" is present, or when the total amount of estrogen is excessive in relation to its natural hormonal opponent, progesterone, which balances estrogen's effects.

Estrogen dominance can also be an issue for men, as testosterone and progesterone naturally decline with age or stress, and estrogen conversely rises. Statistics show that shockingly high numbers of men who live to the age of 65 and older will develop prostate cancer, likely due to estrogen exposure.

CAUSES OF ESTROGEN DOMINANCE

There are only two ways to accumulate excess estrogen in the body: We either produce too much of it on our own or acquire it from our environment or diet. We are constantly exposed to estrogenlike compounds in foods that contain toxic pesticides, herbicides, and growth hormones. Many of these toxins are known to cause weight gain, which serves to fuel the production of more estrogen from our own fat cells. More weight gain then leads to insulin resistance, which, you guessed it, increases the risk of estrogen dominance.

Pharmaceutical hormones such as those used in hormone replacement therapy (HRT) or the birth control pill also increase estrogen, whether we take them actively or absorb them when they make their way into our drinking water. Dr. Richard Stahlhut, a preventive medicine resident at the University of Rochester, writes, "Low-dose exposures to phthalates and other common chemicals [with estrogenic activity] may be reducing testosterone levels or function in men, and thereby contributing to rising obesity rates and an epidemic of related disorders, such as type 2 diabetes."

We are living in a virtual sea of harmful estrogens, and researchers are only beginning to identify the effects of this exposure on health in humans and even other species.

Estrogen dominance has many disturbing causes.

1. **Xenoestrogens:** These harmful compounds mimic estrogen. They make their way into the body from hormones added to foods, especially dairy and beef. They can also be present in pesticides, herbicides, plastics, and even cosmetics.
2. **Stress:** As the body responds to high levels of stress, it "steals" progesterone to manufacture the stress hormone cortisol, often leaving a relative excess of estrogen.
3. **Impaired liver function:** Since the liver breaks down estrogen, alcohol consumption, drug use, a fatty liver, liver disease, and

any other factor that impairs healthy liver function can cause an estrogen buildup.

4. **Poor digestion:** Insufficient dietary fiber, bacterial imbalance in the gut, and other problems that compromise digestion interfere with the proper elimination of estrogen from the body via the digestive tract.

5. **Alcohol consumption:** Research shows that even one alcohol drink can spark an increase in estrogen production.

6. **A high-fat diet:** High intake of saturated or polyunsaturated fat spurs the body's own production of estrogen.

7. **Nutrient deficiencies:** The body requires sufficient intake of zinc, magnesium, vitamin B_6, and other essential nutrients not only to support the breakdown and elimination of estrogen, but also to aid the function of enzymes responsible for the conversion of testosterone to estrogen.

8. **Obesity:** In both men and women, obesity increases the production of bad estrogen, encourages the storage of estrogen in fat cells, and causes a decline in sex-hormone-binding globulin (SHBG). When SHBG drops, more estrogen is left free in the body to bind with tissues in the breasts, ovaries, and fat cells. Obesity also accelerates estrogen production in men because fat cells influence the conversion of testosterone and androsterone into estrogen, which in turn stimulates unfavorable growth of the prostate gland.

9. **Lack of exercise:** One more reason why exercise is so essential for reducing the risk of breast cancer and other malignancies.

10. **Sleep deprivation:** Maintaining habits that prevent sufficient, quality sleep causes a reduction in the hormone melatonin, which helps protect against estrogen dominance.

WHAT DOES ESTROGEN DOMINANCE LOOK LIKE?

If you are a premenopausal woman with estrogen dominance, you likely have PMS, too much body fat around the hips, and difficulty losing weight. Perhaps you have a history of gallstones, varicose veins, uterine fibroids, cervical dysplasia, endometriosis, or ovarian cysts. For all you men out there, low libido, poor motivation, depression, loss of muscle mass, and increased belly fat are big red flags. You may even notice breast development. These symptoms are very similar to those that result from low testosterone, since estrogen dominance is usually accompanied with a low testosterone level.

In both sexes, estrogen dominance is thought to be responsible for many types of cancers. This particular hormone imbalance is currently estimated to be one of the leading causes of breast, uterine, and prostate cancer.

HOW DO YOU KNOW IF YOU ARE ESTROGEN DOMINANT?

Besides checking yourself for the very telling signs and symptoms outlined above, you can further assess your risk of estrogen dominance with your doctor using the tests I have outlined in Appendix A. You can also investigate the Estronex test from Metametrix labs. This test measures the ratio of two critical estrogen metabolites from a single urine specimen. One metabolite, 2-hydroxyestrone (2-OHE1), tends to inhibit cancer growth. Another, 16-alpha-hydroxyestrone (16-A-OHE1), actually encourages tumor development and is associated with estrogen dominance.

Hormonal Imbalance 8—Low Estrogen
Low Estrogen = More Belly Fat for Women

Too little estrogen also has negative impacts on health and appearance. As estrogen levels drop off, especially during menopause, many women find themselves battling that oh-so-lovely shift in body fat from the hips to the waist. Since estrogen helps our cells respond better to insulin, a plunge in estrogen also tends to cause an unwelcome increase in insulin. To make matters worse, the onset of menopause also brings about a decline in the neurotransmitter serotonin. This drop tends to fuel carbohydrate cravings, propelling insulin production even further. Combined with the loss of the cardio-protective benefits of estrogen, these hormonal and body-shape changes definitely contribute to an increased risk of heart disease at menopause.

Estrogen deficiency can affect women at any age. Major causes include the following:

- Aging/menopause
- Premature ovarian failure
- Surgical menopause (removal of the ovaries)
- Smoking
- High levels of stress
- Low-fat diets
- Exceedingly low body fat

The Trouble with Ghrelin

When the digestive system is empty, the stomach and upper intestine produce the hormone ghrelin to stimulate appetite. When you feel hungry and your stomach starts to sound like a grizzly bear, ghrelin is being produced. This hormone does the

SYMPTOMS OF ESTROGEN IMBALANCE

TOO MUCH ESTROGEN (Estrogen Dominance) (Hormonal Imbalance 7)		TOO LITTLE ESTROGEN (Hormonal Imbalance 8)	
Women	Men (Almost always accompanied by testosterone deficiency)	Women	Men
Depression and poor concentration	Prostate enlargement	Vaginal dryness	Loss of bone density
Headaches or migraines	Increased risk of prostate cancer	Memory loss and brain fog	Fatigue
Tendency toward toxic fat gain	Increased toxic abdominal fat	Depression and/or anxiety	Memory not as sharp
Water retention, bloating, puffiness	Breast enlargement	Decreased tolerance for pain	
Weight gain, especially at the hips and thighs	Low sex drive	Increased risk of Alzheimer's disease	
Fibrocystic breasts	Depression	Hair loss	
Uterine fibroids	Erectile dysfunction	Low sex drive	
Low sex drive	Low motivation	Dry eyes	
PMS	Hair loss	Urinary urgency and infections	
Increased risk of breast and uterine cancer	Bloating or puffiness	Thinning and wrinkling of the skin	
Increased risk of autoimmune disease	Increased risk of heart disease and stroke	Increased weight gain at the waist	
Hypothyroidism	Loss of muscle mass	Loss of bone density	
Mood swings	Fatigue	Increased risk of heart disease, high cholesterol, and high blood pressure	
Cervical dysplasia (abnormal PAP tests)	Sleep disruption	Night sweats and hot flashes (which can occur with any change in estrogen level, not just deficiency)	
Heavy periods		Sleep disruption	
Breast swelling and enlargement		Decrease in breast size	
Endometriosis		Increased risk of cataracts	
Ovarian disease		Increased cravings for carbohydrates	
Spider veins and varicose veins			
Cellulite			
Increased risk of gallstones			

important job of letting us know when it is mealtime. But it can also create challenges for us when we attempt to lose weight because it makes us feel hungry when we try to reduce our caloric intake. Research at Oregon Health & Science University has shown that ghrelin activates specialized neurons in our hypothalamus involved in weight regulation and appetite control. Upon reaching the brain, ghrelin also appears to stimulate the release of growth hormone, which in turn promotes the discharge of peptides, especially the stress hormone neuropeptide Y (NPY), which stimulates our desire to eat.

One of the reasons gastric bypass surgery (commonly referred to as stomach stapling) works so well for weight loss is that patients who undergo this procedure lose half of the source tissue that produces ghrelin, and less ghrelin means a lot less of an urge to eat.

Wow, that was a lot of information to process! You have just finished one the most information-dense chapters of the book. Now you can sit back, relax, take a deep breath, and let it sink in before moving on to the next chapter: Your Fat-Burning Friends.

CHAPTER 4

YOUR FAT-BURNING FRIENDS: THE HORMONES THAT HELP YOU LOSE WEIGHT

Here's what you will learn about in this chapter:
- The hormones that control your appetite, boost your metabolism, and aid fat loss
- Three more fat-packing hormonal imbalances that interfere with successful weight loss: hypothyroidism, menopause, and depression

So far I have painted a somewhat negative picture of the influences hormones have on your successful weight-loss journey. But there are indeed hormones inside you that actually help curb your appetite and improve your fat-loss prospects.

Your fat-burning friends are hormones that:

I. DIRECTLY STIMULATE METABOLISM
- Thyroid hormones
- Adrenaline
- Glucagon
- Progesterone

2. STIMULATE FAT LOSS BY SUPPORTING THE GROWTH OF METABOLICALLY ACTIVE MUSCLE
- DHEA

- Testosterone
- Growth hormone

3. CONTROL YOUR APPETITE AND PERFORM OTHER FUNCTIONS
THAT FUEL FAT LOSS
- Serotonin
- Melatonin
- Dopamine
- Acetylcholine
- Gamma-aminobutyric acid (GABA)
- Leptin
- Vitamin D_3

So get comfortable. I've filled this chapter with a whole lot of information that can make an enormous difference to your weight-loss efforts and to your quality of life.

1. THE HORMONES THAT DIRECTLY STIMULATE YOUR METABOLISM

Hormonal Imbalance 13—Low Thyroid
Thyroid Hormones: Masters of Your Metabolic Rate
The thyroid is a gland in the front of your neck, just below the Adam's apple. This critical gland produces thyroid hormones that influence every cell, tissue, and organ in your body.

Thyroid hormones regulate our metabolism and organ function, and directly affect heart rate, cholesterol levels, body weight, energy, muscle contraction and relaxation, skin and hair texture, bowel function, fertility, menstrual regularity, memory, mood, and other bodily processes. Normal levels of thyroid hormone are essential to the development of a baby's brain. In fact, women with low levels of thyroid hormone during pregnancy have been shown to give birth to babies with lower IQs.

The Four Types of Thyroid Hormone

1. TSH (THYROID-STIMULATING HORMONE): This substance is produced by the pituitary gland under direction from the hypothalamus. A high TSH suggests that your thyroid gland is not responding properly to signals from your pituitary telling it to make more hormones.

2. FREE T4 (THYROXINE): T4 is the thyroid hormone produced directly by your thyroid gland under stimulation of TSH. It's the major form of thyroid hormone in your bloodstream.

3. FREE T3 (TRIIODOTHYRONINE): T4 is converted to T3 in the cells of the body. T3 is the thyroid hormone that directly influences the metabolism of every single cell, tissue, and organ in your body.

4. REVERSE T3 (rT3): Under periods of stress or with a deficiency of the trace mineral selenium, your body may produce increased levels of rT3. A high level of rT3 is usually a signal of an underactive thyroid.

The levels of T3 and T4 in your body act as negative feedback mechanisms to the pituitary to stop the production of thyroid hormone until it's needed again. So, low levels of T3 and T4 will stimulate increased TSH production. Here's an analogy to make this clearer: imagine the pituitary as the boss and the thyroid as the worker. If the worker starts to slack off, the boss's demands for more work get louder and louder. If the worker is productive, there's less instruction from above.

Thyroid Hormone Imbalance

Like so many other hormones, thyroid hormones must be present in the appropriate balance in order to ensure optimal health. Too much thyroid hormone leads to hyperthyroidism, a condition that throws the metabolism into chronic high gear. Those with hyperthyroidism feel hot and experience a rapid heart rate, weight loss (or weight gain, if they eat a lot more due to increased appetite), irritability, insomnia, shakiness, and digestive troubles. Sufferers can also feel hyper, although fatigue is very common as well. Over time, hyperthyroidism can be extremely detrimental to bone density and muscle mass.

Hypothyroidism is caused by a deficiency of thyroid hormone. This condition affects 1 in 13 people, making it much more common than hyperthyroidism. Without enough thyroid hormone, every system in the body slows down. Those who suffer from hypothyroidism feel tired and tend to sleep a lot. Their digestion slows and weight gain typically occurs. They can also experience extremely dry skin, hair loss, and slower mental processes.

A FAT-PACKING HORMONAL IMBALANCE

HORMONAL IMBALANCE 13: LOW THYROID HORMONE (Hypothyroidism)

An estimated 13 million Americans have underactive thyroid function, only half of whom have been properly diagnosed. Women are five times more likely than men to be diagnosed with hypothyroidism.

WHAT CAUSES HYPOTHYROIDISM?

Hypothyroidism is a complex disorder that can stem from a number of different causes. Factors include the following:

• The thyroid failing to produce enough thyroid hormone. This deficiency is possibly caused by an autoimmune response against the thyroid or other problems with the function of the thyroid gland itself.

- The pituitary gland or the hypothalamus failing to send a critical signal to the thyroid instructing it to produce thyroid hormone.
- Thyroxine (T4) produced by the thyroid may not convert properly to its active form, triiodothyronine (T3), which ultimately influences the metabolism of every cell.
- The adrenal hormones cortisol and DHEA influence thyroid function. A deficiency of DHEA and excessive amounts of the stress hormone cortisol may inhibit thyroid hormone function.
- Toxic levels of mercury, typically resulting from mercury fillings in the mouth or consuming large amounts of mercury-laden ocean fish, may inhibit thyroid gland function.
- High levels of estrogen or a converse deficiency of progesterone inhibits thyroid function. Many menopausal women using estrogen replacement therapy may develop the symptoms of an underactive thyroid. Menopausal women who are already taking medication for hypothyroidism may also need to increase their dosage if they choose to use hormone replacement therapy (HRT).
- The excessive consumption of soy-based foods and beverages may decrease the activity of thyroid hormone in the body.
- Some studies suggest that ingestion of excess fluoride from drinking water and toothpaste may inhibit thyroid gland function. Pesticides in water and occupational exposure to polybrominated biphenyls and carbon disulfide have also been associated with decreased thyroid function.
- Nutritional deficiencies may prevent the proper manufacture or function of thyroid hormone in the body. Iodine and L-tyrosine are necessary for the formation of thyroid hormone, while selenium is necessary for the normal function of thyroid hormone.

Many individuals with decreased thyroid hormone levels also have a zinc deficiency.

• Certain medications may induce hypothyroidism. Lithium carbonate, a medication used to treat manic depression, is one of the most common medications known to cause hypothyroidism. Others include amiodarone hydrochloride (Amiodarone, Cordarone, and Pacerone), interferon-alfa (Infergen, Rebetron, and Wellferon), nitroprusside, perchlorate, and sulfonylureas.

WHAT ARE THE SYMPTOMS OF HYPOTHYROIDISM?

The symptoms of underactive thyroid disease can vary, and not all individuals will present in the same way.

The Hormonal Health Profile may have helped you to determine whether you show signs of a sluggish thyroid; the following are additional symptoms to watch for:

• Frequently feeling cold or having an intolerance for cold temperatures
• Dry skin, brittle hair, and splitting nails
• Lack of or diminished ability to sweat during exercise
• Hair loss
• Irregular menses or heavy menstrual bleeding
• Poor memory
• Depression
• Decreased libido
• Constipation
• Unexplained fatigue or lethargy
• Unexplained weight gain or an inability to lose weight
• Many individuals with hypothyroidism have associated iron deficiency anemia and/or high cholesterol

HOW IS HYPOTHYROIDISM DIAGNOSED?

In Appendix A, I outline the tests you may want to request from your doctor to fully assess the condition of your thyroid. Thyroid disease is diagnosed with blood tests. Four tests—for TSH, free T3, free T4, and thyroid antibodies—should be completed to get the most accurate picture of your thyroid health.

Some important notes on testing: In my practice, I often find thyroid antibodies register as abnormal long before the other three parameters, so these should be assessed. Many health-care providers also share concerns about the currently accepted normal reference ranges for TSH. US health professionals have recently reduced the upper range to 3. However, many integrated health practitioners feel it should be less than 2.0, and I agree.

Ultimately, this discrepancy means that many people suffering with the symptoms of an underactive thyroid may go without proper treatment. If you suspect you have a thyroid condition, make sure your doctor assesses you and your full range of symptoms, *not just your blood work*. Even a modest increase in TSH has been proven to accelerate weight gain and to interfere with a healthy metabolic rate in both men and women.

WHY IS HYPOTHYROIDISM A SERIOUS CONDITION IF LEFT UNTREATED?

A thyroid condition must be treated correctly and quickly to stave off further serious complications. Left untreated, thyroid conditions may lead to an increased risk of cardiovascular disease, infertility, premature ovarian failure, breast cancer, osteoporosis, obesity, goiter, and diabetes.

Adrenaline and Noradrenaline:
Your "Fight-or-Flight" Hormones

When present in the right amounts, adrenaline is very useful in supporting fat loss. It causes the body to free up stored fats and sugars to provide us with the burst of energy we need to escape or face danger, while sparing metabolically active muscle protein. Believe it or not, having a cup of coffee before your workout may offer an extra fat-burning boost simply because caffeine sparks adrenaline production.

Along with adrenaline, noradrenaline (NA, or norepinephrine) is released by nerve cells and the adrenal glands. NA also stimulates energy-expending fight-or-flight responses. Although it's typically not produced in as high a quantity as adrenaline, noradrenaline has very similar effects on physiology, including increasing the heart rate, raising blood sugar, and increasing tension in the skeletal muscles. It also stimulates the brain and helps us to think quickly when we are in tricky situations.

Glucagon: Converting Carbs into Energy

Glucagon works directly opposite to insulin in that it raises our blood sugar. When we exercise, consume protein, or experience a dip in blood sugar, glucagon kicks in to aid fat loss by instructing the body to use stored fat and sugars for fuel. Glucagon release is inhibited, however, when high amounts of sugar and insulin are present in our bloodstream. Another reason to keep that insulin level in check!

Since protein consumption stimulates glucagon activity, eating substantial amounts of meat, dairy, soy, or fish seems like a great approach to weight loss, right? Not necessarily. Your body much prefers carbohydrates over protein for use as an energy source. In fact, we want the body to choose sugar over protein for fuel because the latter process can break down muscle. Excess glucagon can also destroy precious muscle tissue that we work so hard to build and maintain.

The key to maintaining a stable blood sugar level, while also preventing the breakdown of muscle tissue, is to balance protein consumption with low-glycemic carbohydrates, such as fruits, vegetables, and whole grain breads and cereals—carbohydrates that limit insulin secretion. This combination of foods will promote glucagon release while also providing your body with sufficient fuel. If you consume too many carbohydrates or fail to eat enough protein, you will not benefit from the fat-burning effects of glucagon.

Hormonal Imbalance 9—Low Progesterone
Progesterone: Why Too Much or Too Little Makes You Fat

Progesterone is produced by the ovaries before menopause and in small amounts after menopause by the adrenal glands. Opposite to estrogen, progesterone is naturally higher in the second half of the menstrual cycle, when it causes thickening of the uterine wall in preparation for implantation of a fertilized egg. If no implantation occurs, progesterone levels decline, triggering the beginning of the menstrual flow. If implantation does occur, progesterone levels increase steadily during pregnancy. Together with estriol, progesterone helps prevent the mother's immune system from attacking the fetus as foreign tissue. Men also produce progesterone from the testes and the adrenal glands, but in much lower amounts than women.

Progesterone has many beneficial effects. It's a natural diuretic, sleep aid, antianxiety compound, and stimulator of metabolism (because it supports thyroid hormone). It's also considered to be thermogenic because it raises body temperature, just like when we eat protein. Progesterone may help to build bone density, reduce blood pressure, lower LDL cholesterol, improve the appearance and texture of hair and skin, aid libido, and prevent PMS. When balanced properly with estrogen, it's protective against breast and prostate cancer. This multifunctional hormone also aids fertility and helps to balance the immune system, thereby reducing the risk of auto-immune disease.

Progesterone inhibits the enzyme that causes the conversion of testosterone to dihydrotestosterone (DHT), the type of testosterone that contributes to hair loss in both men and women and prostate enlargement in men. As with all hormones, however, more is not necessarily better!

Progesterone tends to decline in women beginning in their 30s and in men after 60. When progesterone is stolen or decreased, estrogen dominance can arise. This imbalance is very common in women in their 30s and 40s.

Progesterone deficiency may arise for many different reasons.

- **Stress:** More stress means lower progesterone, as the body steals progesterone to increase cortisol production.
- **Lack of ovulation:** May occur with conditions such as polycystic ovarian syndrome (PCOS).
- **Low levels of luteinizing hormone (LH):** Released by the brain, LH triggers the production of progesterone.
- **Hypothyroidism:** An underactive thyroid gland.
- **Excess prolactin:** The hormone prolactin stimulates breast development during pregnancy and milk production during nursing. Too much prolactin can suppress progesterone production and can cause infertility and menstrual disorders. Prolactin levels can also increase with hypothyroidism and pituitary disorders.

Hormonal Imbalance 10—Excess Progesterone
Progesterone: Why Too Much or Too Little Makes You Fat

As is the case with its estrogen counterpart, progesterone must be balanced in order to help us maintain a lean body. Progesterone excess is rare, though I often see it in individuals who use progesterone creams or pills. Too much progesterone is troublesome and can cause acne, bloating, water retention, depression, and weight gain.

TOO LITTLE PROGESTERONE (Hormonal Imbalance 9)		TOO MUCH PROGESTERONE (Hormonal Imbalance 10)	
Women	Men	Women	Men
Anxiety	Prostate enlargement	Depression	Low libido
Sleep disruption	Sleep disruption	Weight gain and increased fat storage	Weight gain and increased fat storage
PMS	Increased body fat	Water retention and bloating	Water retention and bloating
Hair loss	Hair loss	Poor blood sugar balance, cravings, and increased appetite	Poor blood sugar balance, cravings, and increased appetite
Sluggish metabolism, increased risk of hypothyroidism	Bone density loss/osteoporosis	Increased stress hormones and possibly excess testosterone	Increased stress hormones and possibly excess testosterone
Bone density loss/osteoporosis	Increased risk of prostate cancer	Constipation	Suppression of the immune system; more frequent colds and flus
Autoimmune disease		Low libido	Possible infertility (some suggestion that excess progesterone may interfere with sperm production)
Periods that come too soon or spotting between periods		Suppression of the immune system; more frequent colds and flus	
Infertility or lack of menstruation		Increased risk of breast and uterine cancer	
Headaches, especially before menses		Increased risk of diabetes	
Increased allergies		Infertility	
Night sweats			
Miscarriage			
Water retention			
Swollen, tender, cystic breasts			

A FAT-PACKING HORMONAL IMBALANCE

MENOPAUSE
(Low Estrogen, Progesterone, and/or Testosterone)

According to US census data, there are about 37.5 million women at or near menopause. Menopause, which can begin as early as 40 years of age, is not just about estrogen decline. Supplies of progesterone, testosterone, and DHEA also tend to dry up, right along with the skin, hair, eyes, and libido!

At first I wasn't going to include menopause as one of the conditions of hormonal imbalance and weight gain because it is, after all, a natural and inevitable part of aging. I changed my mind, however, because so many women come through the doors of my office intensely frustrated with the unwelcome changes in their body during this phase of life. One of the biggies, which I mentioned in the previous chapter, is that annoying thickening of the waistline that occurs when estrogen drops. Although some women pass through menopause with few, if any, side effects, others experience life-disrupting symptoms that last for months or even years.

The trying symptoms of menopause stem from an imbalance of estrogen, progesterone, and testosterone. The results of your Hormonal Health Profile will help you discover whether you have specific signs of an imbalance associated with each of these hormones. And, of course, I will provide you with plenty of suggestions to correct specific imbalances to ease your menopausal discomfort in Chapter 13.

The most common symptoms of menopause include:

- Hot flashes
- Difficulty sleeping
- Emotional changes, including depression, anxiety, and irritability
- Headaches
- Heart palpitations
- Poor memory and concentration
- Urinary urgency or incontinence

- Vaginal dryness
- Weight gain around the waist
- Changes in the appearance of your skin and hair

HOW DO YOU KNOW IF YOU'RE MENOPAUSAL?

Clinically, a diagnosis of menopause is made when the menses have been absent for 1 year. But if you've noticed a missed period and are experiencing the symptoms noted above, you may have reached perimenopause. Your doctor can order blood work to determine whether you're menopausal or not. Most doctors will measure levels of FSH, LH, estradiol, and progesterone, though more tests are outlined in Appendix A for your reference.

MORE THAN JUST DISCOMFORT: WHY YOU NEED TO MANAGE MENOPAUSE

After the onset of menopause, a woman's risk of Alzheimer's disease, osteoporosis, heart disease, and cancer significantly increases. But good lifestyle habits (my three steps!), supplements, and bioidentical hormone replacement (BHRT) can help mitigate these risks.

Bioidentical hormones are derived from natural sources outside the body, such as soy and other plants. They function just as effectively as our own hormones, without the potentially harmful side effects of animal hormones or the synthetic hormones used in traditional HRT (such as Premarin). BHRT works wonderfully to restore perfect hormonal balance in menopause. This type of therapy works even better when the foundation for hormonal balance is first set with the help of detoxification, exercise, and good nutrition.

If you wish to try BHRT, be sure to seek out a practitioner who specializes in this area. Regular testing of your hormone levels and proper follow-up are essential when using any type of hormone replacement therapy. Furthermore, high doses of hormones should not be the aim. Instead, the goal should be to replenish hormonal deficiencies and return levels to those we normally experience in middle age, not high school!

2. HORMONES THAT STIMULATE FAT LOSS BY SUPPORTING THE GROWTH OF METABOLICALLY ACTIVE MUSCLE

Hormonal Imbalance 6—Low DHEA
Everyone Digs DHEA: The Antistress, Antiaging Hormone

Produced by the adrenal glands, dehydroepiandrosterone (DHEA) is a precursor to the sex hormones estrogen and testosterone and is one of the most abundant hormones in your body. This hormone with the very long name has a big list of benefits to match. It's known to support healthy immunity (particularly for the prevention of autoimmune imbalances), aid tissue repair, improve sleep, and counteract the negative effects of cortisol. It influences our ability to lose fat and gain muscle. It boosts libido and helps us feel motivated, youthful, and energetic—just a few of the reasons why DHEA is often touted as the antiaging hormone. DHEA naturally declines with age, stress, and illness and is often taken in supplements.

If your DHEA levels are too low, you may experience the following:

- Increased body fat and weight gain
- A decrease in muscle mass
- Loss of a sense of well-being
- Bone density depletion
- Low libido
- Poor ability to handle stress

I support the use of DHEA supplements, but only in low doses and only when a true deficiency has been definitively diagnosed via blood or saliva testing. Taking too much DHEA can trigger an unwelcome increase in testosterone and estrogen, which leads to increased cancer risk, hair loss, anger, aggression, and acne in both men and women.

Women may also experience effects such as a deeper voice, hair loss, and abnormal growth of facial hair.

Hormonal Imbalance 11—Low Testosterone
Testosterone: The Master Muscle-Building Hormone

Testosterone is an androgen—a masculinizing hormone—produced by the ovaries in women, the testes in men, and the adrenal glands in both sexes. Testosterone enhances libido, bone density, muscle mass, strength, motivation, memory, fat burning, and skin tone. In men, it influences sperm production, causes growth of the prostate gland, and is especially important for maintaining motivation and mood.

As with so many other hormones, testosterone levels tend to taper off with aging, obesity, and stress. Exposure to pesticides and toxins also negatively impacts the production of testosterone in the testes. Today, men are experiencing testosterone decline much earlier in life, and overall levels appear to be dropping.

Dr. Antti Perheentupa, a specialist in reproductive medicine at the University of Turku in Finland, presented evidence of this decline at an Endocrine Society meeting in the summer of 2006, reporting that a man born in 1970 has about 20 percent *less* testosterone at age 35 than a man of his father's generation had at the same age. Quite an alarming finding, considering low testosterone has been linked to depression, obesity, osteoporosis, heart disease, *and even death.* Many researchers pin this decline on environmental factors. Dr. Mitchell Harman, an endocrinologist at the University of Arizona College of Medicine, blames the proliferation of endocrine-suppressing, estrogenlike compounds used in pesticides and

> **TEST YOUR TESTOSTERONE**
> Recent studies have found that a decrease in testosterone in men at any age increases the risk of osteoporosis, heart disease, and even death. For this reason alone, having your levels of free testosterone tested in the blood or saliva at least once a year is incredibly important.
>
> HOT HORMONE TIP

other farming chemicals for the downward trend in male testosterone levels. Phthalates, commonly found in cosmetics, soaps, and most plastics (including, ahem, sex toys), are another known cause of testosterone suppression.

Loss of testosterone can lead to andropause, often referred to as male menopause. This condition is estimated to affect about 30 percent of aging men, although actual numbers may be much higher because the widely varying symptoms make a diagnosis difficult. The chart of symptoms of testosterone imbalance (page 96) illustrates how testosterone decline tends to cause an increase in body fat and loss of muscle mass. I should add that these effects can arise *in both men and women, even with dieting and exercise,* when a marked deficiency of testosterone exists.

Hormonal Imbalance 12—Excess Testosterone
Too Much of a Good Thing?

While excess testosterone is not very common in men, it affects about 10 percent of women. A surplus of female testosterone is typically a result of increased production by the adrenal glands and is associated with polycystic ovarian syndrome (PCOS) and hirsutism (excess hair growth). Besides causing acne, facial hair growth, and even male pattern hair loss in women, too much testosterone increases insulin resistance and weight gain (causing the apple body type).

I've had great success returning testosterone to normal levels in patients with PCOS or fertility concerns by using the Hormone Diet approach. The key to lowering testosterone is stress management (i.e., balancing cortisol) and controlling insulin levels through glycemically balanced eating, exercise, and insulin-sensitizing supplements. All of these strategies are included in my three steps.

In some cases, my approach can even restore testosterone to normal levels in men *without* the use of testosterone supplementation. This was the case with 37-year-old Max.

Max had been using testosterone replacement therapy for over 3 years when he came to see me. After we spoke, I failed to find any of the readily recognizable causes of low testosterone. He wasn't overweight, had no history of trauma to the testicles, wasn't reporting feeling overly stressed, had no history of sleep apnea, and had only mildly elevated cholesterol. Of course, my first thought was, Why the low testosterone at his age?

I was especially concerned for him because low testosterone can cause an increase in the risk of heart disease. Even worse, his father had had bypass surgery in his mid-forties; so I investigated the risk factors for heart disease closely. Max's cholesterol was only mildly elevated, his blood pressure was normal, and he was not overweight. Then I tested his homocysteine—it was 20, which is over *three times* the accepted optimal value of 6.3!

I concluded that high homocysteine (a protein known to cause hardening of the arteries), along with his slightly elevated cholesterol, was probably causing obstruction of the bloodflow to the testicles, and the manifestation of this was decreased testosterone production. It was fortunate we found this when we did. In 10 to 20 years he would not only be suffering with low testosterone, but most likely a heart attack as well. And

> **SKIP THE STATINS AND SAVE YOUR TESTOSTERONE**
>
> Some cholesterol-lowering medications, especially statins such as Lipitor and Zocor, may decrease your production of testosterone and bring about the harmful effects of low testosterone. You may be better off selecting natural cholesterol-reducing alternatives to statins, such as policosanols, omega-3 fish oils, garlic, red yeast extract, or coenzyme Q10. These compounds improve cholesterol and cardiovascular health without the potential negative side effects.
>
> HOT HORMONE TIP

guess what? Today Max's testosterone levels are normal—without the use of hormone replacement—and he's the father of twins!

This is a clear illustration of the need for a new, more comprehensive approach to health and hormonal balance—beyond being thin.

SYMPTOMS OF TESTOSTERONE IMBALANCE

TOO LITTLE TESTOSTERONE (Hormonal Imbalance 11)		TOO MUCH TESTOSTERONE (Hormonal Imbalance 12)	
Women	Men	Women (PCOS or Hirsutism)	Men (Andropause)
Muscle loss	Increased abdominal fat, muscle loss	Increased abdominal fat, insulin resistance	Aggression
Decreased libido	Impotence, erectile dysfunction, decreased libido	Acne	Acne
Fatigue	Increased risk of heart disease, fatigue	Irregular periods	Increased hair loss
Bone density loss	Increased risk of death, bone density loss	Increased risk of breast cancer	Possible increased risk of prostate enlargement or cancer
Decreased vitality	Sleep disruption, decreased vitality	Hair loss (scalp)	Increased hemoglobin
Increased body fat	Prostate problems (men treated with natural testosterone have been shown to have improvements in prostate health)	Increased hair growth (face and body)	
Depression and low motivation	Depression	Irritability	
Hair loss	Hair loss	Anger	
Dry skin and poor elasticity	Dry skin and poor elasticity	Decrease in breast size; sagging breasts	
Possibly hypothyroidism	Possibly hypothyroidism		

Hormonal Imbalance 16—Low Growth Hormone
Growth Hormone: In Charge of Growth and Repair

Growth hormone affects just about every cell in the body. Not surprisingly, it also has a major effect on our feelings, actions, and appearance. Because this regenerative hormone tends to decline with age, growth hormone supplements are often promoted as a way to slow the effects of aging.

Growth hormone is released during deep sleep and while we exercise. It's essential for tissue repair, muscle building, bone density, and healthy body composition. When we sleep in total darkness, melatonin is released, triggering a very slight but critical cool-down in the body. As body temperature drops, growth hormone is released and works its regenerative magic. If we sleep with lights on or eat too close to bedtime, the natural cool-down process will not take place, putting us at risk of low levels of both melatonin and growth hormone. At the same time, we lose the important effects of sleep on fat loss.

Once released into the bloodstream, growth hormone has a very short life—only half an hour or so. During that time, however, it makes its way speedily to the liver and many other cells in the body, inducing them to produce another hormone called insulin-like growth factor 1 (IGF-1). Almost every cell in the body is affected by IGF-1, especially muscle, bone, liver, kidney, skin, lung, and nerve cells. Commonly measured as a marker of growth hormone production, IGF-1 is the substance truly responsible for most of the restorative benefits we typically attribute to growth hormone.

The Perils of Low Growth Hormone

Only recently has growth hormone deficiency in adults been recognized as a serious health problem. Adults deficient in growth hormone suffer from the following:

- Premature cardiovascular disease
- Loss of bone density

- Abdominal obesity
- Decreased muscle mass, poor posture
- Thinning or sagging skin
- Depressed mood, anxiety
- Elevated levels of LDL cholesterol
- Slow wound healing
- Fatigue
- Low stamina for exercise
- Poor immune function

A study from the *Journal of Clinical Endocrinology and Metabolism* (April 2007) linked abdominal obesity in postmenopausal women with low growth hormone secretion, elevated inflammatory markers, and increased risk of cardiovascular disease. Test subjects who received supplementary growth hormone showed improvement in inflammatory markers. Researchers at Saint Louis University also found that obese people who received controlled doses of growth hormone lost weight and maintained the energy to exercise.

Even children who lack sufficient sleep are at risk of low growth hormone and obesity. According to data published in the *International Journal of Obesity* by researchers from Université Laval's Faculty of Medicine, the less a child sleeps, the more likely he or she is to become overweight. The risk of becoming overweight is 3.5 times higher for sleep-deprived children than for those who get the 9 to 10 hours of sleep they need.

Should We All Take Growth Hormone?

Boosting growth hormone certainly promises many exciting benefits, including less abdominal fat, more muscle mass, fewer wrinkles, increased bone mass, improved cholesterol levels, and stronger immune system function. But growth hormone supplementation is no panacea for health. Neither is it free of associated risks.

Abnormally high growth hormone can raise blood sugar, contribute to insulin resistance, increase the risk of type 2 diabetes, and cause abnormal bone growth. New research also suggests that elevated IGF-1 may be a risk factor for certain types of malignancies, especially prostate cancer.

3. THE HORMONES THAT CONTROL YOUR APPETITE AND FUEL FAT LOSS

Hormonal Imbalance 3—Low Serotonin
The Comfort of Sweet Serotonin

Though serotonin is typically recognized as a brain chemical, most of this neurotransmitter is produced in our digestive tract. Serotonin exerts powerful influence over mood, emotions, memory, cravings (especially for carbohydrates), self-esteem, pain tolerance, sleep habits, appetite, digestion, and body temperature regulation. Wow! When we're depressed or down, we naturally crave more sugars and starches to stimulate the production of serotonin. Also, when we're cold or surrounded by darkness, serotonin levels drop. Hey, maybe there is a reason for that dreaded winter weight gain after all!

Serotonin is often thought of as our "happy hormone," especially because its production increases

> **SEROTONIN STEPS UP DIGESTION**
> Because it is highly concentrated in the gut, serotonin also has positive effects on digestion. As a result, researchers have now developed serotonin-based medications to ease the painful symptoms of irritable bowel syndrome.
>
> HOT HORMONE FACT

when we're exposed to natural sunlight and when we focus on one thing rather than multitask. Production of serotonin is also closely linked to availability of vitamin B_6 and the amino acid tryptophan. So if our diet lacks sufficient protein or vitamins, we run a greater risk of serotonin deficiency. We may experience a dip in serotonin as a result of dieting, digestive disorders, and also stress, since high levels of the stress hormone cortisol rob us of serotonin.

What Happens with a Serotonin Imbalance?

A spike in serotonin rarely, if ever, occurs naturally. An elevated level of this hormone is usually a side effect of antidepressant medications specifically designed to boost serotonin. Too much serotonin can result in **serotonin syndrome**, a rare and life-threatening condition characterized by rapid pulse, headache, nausea, high blood pressure, decreased appetite, sweating, dilated pupils, an overall feeling of edginess, and, ultimately, unconsciousness. If you experience any of these symptoms while taking medications that influence your serotonin levels, see a doctor immediately.

Low serotonin is a far more common concern. In my professional opinion, serotonin deficiency has become an epidemic of equal proportion to obesity. I also believe this parallel is no coincidence.

HOT HORMONE TIP

ARE YOU SUFFERING FROM LOW SEROTONIN?
Perhaps your results of the Hormonal Health Profile have provided the first step in uncovering a potential serotonin imbalance. You can also use urinary neurotransmitter analysis to pinpoint your exact serotonin levels.

A FAT-PACKING HORMONAL IMBALANCE

HORMONAL IMBALANCE 3: LOW SEROTONIN
(Insomnia, Anxiety, and Depression)

According to the World Health Organization (WHO), depression is the leading cause of disability as measured by the Years Lost due to Disability (YLD). Both depression and anxiety are linked to elevated cortisol, coupled with an imbalance of our "feel good" hormones, including serotonin, dopamine, and noradrenaline. In some cases, low testosterone in men or decreased estrogen in women can also play a role.

WHY THE EPIDEMIC OF LOW SEROTONIN?

Plenty of sunlight; a healthful diet rich in protein, minerals, and vitamins; regular exercise; and good sleep support serotonin. When we measure our current lifestyle against all the elements necessary for the body's natural production of serotonin, the wide-ranging epidemic of low serotonin is certainly not surprising. Add in *chronic stress* and *multitasking*—two of the main causes of serotonin depletion—and it's a wonder any one of us has been left unaffected by low serotonin.

DEPRESSION, WEIGHT GAIN, AND HORMONAL IMBALANCE: A CODEPENDENT RELATIONSHIP

When you are depressed, your body naturally craves carbs in an attempt to raise serotonin. Of course, we all understand that excess carb consumption causes weight gain and possibly insulin and leptin resistance. Although antidepressant medications, such as selective serotonin reuptake inhibitors (SSRIs), are effective in raising serotonin in the short term, some evidence suggests these medications actually deplete serotonin in the long term. Plus, weight gain is one of the most common side effects of antidepressant drugs.

Serotonin is just one of a host of neurotransmitters secreted by the brain to regulate mood, attention, and energy levels. Ongoing stress, just like depression, can deplete our serotonin reserves, leading to intense food cravings, particularly for sugar and refined carbohydrates that tend to mimic the soothing effects of serotonin. Persistently low serotonin leads to sagging energy, bouts of depression, worrying, low self-esteem, difficulty making decisions, early morning waking, and compulsive eating.

Researchers from Tufts University have provided scientific support for the close link between anxiety disorders, depression, and higher risk of obesity. A study published in the March 2006 issue of the *Archives of Pediatrics and Adolescent Medicine* discusses the involvement of serotonin in both mood and appetite regulation. The data show that patients suffering from depression (and, therefore, low serotonin) often turn to food, particularly carbohydrates, to temporarily boost their levels.

In light of the clear link between obesity and depressed levels of serotonin (and dopamine, as you'll soon see), the likelihood is that many overweight and obese patients suffer from an imbalance of these hormones. To successfully initiate appetite control and weight loss, therefore, brain chemistry must be addressed along with blood sugar and insulin balance. The catch is that insulin resistance, often associated with obesity, also blocks the activity of serotonin in the brain. Successful treatment, then, must be aimed at restoring the body's response to insulin while also improving serotonin levels and activity within the brain.

Hormonal Imbalance 15—Low Melatonin
Marvelous Melatonin: The Secret to Restorative Sleep

Melatonin is released from the pineal gland and regulates your 24-hour body clock. It normally increases after darkness falls, making us feel drowsy. Acting as a hormone, melatonin influences nervous system function, as well as the endocrine and immune systems. Melatonin production typically peaks between 1 and 3 a.m., while you are asleep in the dark. Exposure to even small amounts of light from, say, the moon or your digital alarm clock, or to electromagnetic radiation from TVs, heating pads, or electric blankets, disrupts this process. Your melatonin production can also be compromised if you regularly take aspirin or ibuprofen, consume caffeinated products, drink alcohol, or smoke.

Because melatonin is a derivative of serotonin, its production is also dependent on adequate protein in your diet, which provides tryptophan, the amino acid building block of both melatonin and serotonin. Melatonin naturally tends to decline with age and menopause, which makes supplementation a helpful, natural option for people over 45 who experience sleep problems.

The Many Effects of Melatonin

Melatonin is a powerful antioxidant that maintains youthfulness, improves sleep, perks up libido, and boosts energy and resistance to infections. It affects your ability to fall asleep and stay asleep, as well as your sleep quality. It also indirectly influences your body composition through its relationship with growth hormone.

Melatonin aids in turning on the body's nighttime repair processes by allowing for a slight, but essential, dip in body temperature. Once the body has cooled sufficiently, growth hormone is released and begins to work its magic, repairing and rebuilding bone, skin, and muscle cells while we sleep. As an added bonus, melatonin decreases cortisol and protects us from the harmful effects of stress. Thanks to its dual effects on growth hormone and cortisol, melatonin helps our metabolic rate by preserving muscle tissue.

When melatonin goes up, serotonin goes down. For example, melatonin levels are known to rise in the winter, when we have less sunlight exposure. The correlative drop in serotonin is thought to be one of the main causes of seasonal depression, also known as seasonal affective disorder (SAD). Increased carbohydrate cravings and weight gain are common symptoms of SAD. Eating more carbs in turn causes the body to step up its production of serotonin. This technique can be an effective way to keep negative moods at bay, as long as it is used in moderation. Unfortunately, we tend to overeat comfort foods (such as chips, cookies, and candy) that pump up serotonin and leave us feeling fat, fuzzy, and even more depressed.

Hormonal Imbalance 2—Low Dopamine
Dopamine: The Pleasure "Rush"

If you are searching for stimulation or, as the song says, you just "can't get no satisfaction," you could probably use a good dose of dopamine. Dopamine is the neurotransmitter that's heavily involved in the pleasure center within the brain. It's released in high amounts during gratifying activities such as eating, sex, and other naturally enjoyable experiences. Being in love, fun social interactions, giving, exercise, and dancing are just a few of the activities that give you a pleasurable dopamine boost.

As a brain chemical, dopamine influences well-being, alertness, learning, creativity, attention, and concentration. Dopamine also controls motor functions and muscle tension, which explains why a deficiency of this hormone is linked to Parkinson's disease and restless leg syndrome (RLS), as well as cognitive changes such as depression, low libido, attention disorders, memory loss, and difficulties with problem solving.

While too little dopamine can leave us craving food, sex, or stimulation, too much can cause addictive behaviors. For instance, Parkinson's patients taking medications to support dopamine levels have been shown to become involved in gambling when their medications were increased. Paranoia or a suspicious personality may arise from too much dopamine, although more of this hormone in the frontal area of the brain relieves pain and boosts feelings of pleasure.

Dopamine isn't released only during pleasurable experiences, but also in the presence of high amounts of stress. So—pleasure and pain are closely related.

Dopamine and Addiction

Many researchers today agree that dopamine is one of the reasons why foods can be addictive. We also know stress stimulates the production of dopamine, which provides us with more energy, drive, and motivation, just as the addictive stimulants chocolate, caffeine (coffee, tea), sugar, and cigarettes can. This means we can become as addicted to stress as we can to stimulants simply because we are searching for a dopamine rush to beat fatigue.

Not surprisingly, almost all abusive drugs and addictive substances influence dopamine production. Alcohol, cocaine, nicotine, amphetamines, and even sugar can mess with our dopamine balance. According to Dr. Nora Volkow, director of the National Institute on Drug Abuse (NIDA), many smokers eat more when they are trying to quit because both food and nicotine share similar dopamine reward pathways. When less dopamine is stimulated as nicotine is reduced, food and sugar cravings naturally kick in to compensate. Fortunately, the Hormone Diet promotes strategies such as eating smaller amounts more frequently, enjoying more sex, not skipping meals, and increasing exercise, all of which can help provide the body with a natural dose of dopamine.

Dopamine for Weight Loss

Besides the many pleasures dopamine brings, this substance naturally suppresses appetite and aids weight loss. Antidepressant drugs such as bupropion (Wellbutrin or Zyban), which act on dopamine receptors in the brain, have been found to help with weight loss. A study at Duke University Medical Center showed weight loss occurred within just a few weeks and remained after a period of 2 years with bupropion use. Many of the study participants who took dopamine also reported feeling satisfied with smaller amounts of food.

Unfortunately, the body tends to work against us when it comes to dopamine production. Researchers at Princeton University found dopamine *decreased* in rats when they *lost weight* on restricted eating programs. With this drop in weight, *the rats' appetites increased and they began to eat more in an attempt to naturally restore dopamine levels.* How does this research translate for us? Supplements such as L-tyrosine, which increases the production of dopamine, may be beneficial to blunt the dopamine drop that occurs with weight loss and may ultimately allow us to sustain better appetite control.

Hormonal Imbalance 14—Low Acetylcholine
Aces for Acetylcholine

Acetylcholine is the neurotransmitter essential to the flow of communication between nerves and muscles. Movement, coordination, and muscle tone are influenced by acetylcholine because it is the messenger molecule that allows your muscles to contract.

The more we exercise, the more acetylcholine we use up. Athletes often have significant reductions in acetylcholine levels following strenuous activities such as running, cycling, and swimming. We can, however, use natural supplements that stimulate the production of choline, the building block of acetylcholine, to vastly improve stamina and even reduce post-exercise fatigue.

Keeping acetylcholine levels high is one of the secrets to maintaining strong, healthy, metabolically active muscle. Acetylcholine also stimulates growth hormone release, thereby improving tissue healing, promoting muscle growth, improving skin tone and bone density, and aiding fat loss (especially abdominal fat).

Besides muscle movement, REM sleep, memory, mental alertness, concentration, and learning are linked to acetylcholine. Healthy digestion and regularity are also controlled by the chemical message acetylcholine delivers to smooth muscle cells along the digestive tract. Acetylcholine declines naturally with aging. Combined with a decrease in physical activity, this drop could be a contributing factor to the constipation that plagues so many people later in life. This depletion is also thought to be one of the major culprits behind age-related memory loss, depression, mood changes, insomnia, and Alzheimer's disease.

Hormone Imbalance 4—Low Gaba
Get Mellow with GABA

Gamma-aminobutyric acid (GABA) is a naturally calming, inhibitory neurotransmitter involved in relaxation, healthy sleep, digestion, and the easing of muscle tension, pain, and anxiety. GABA appears to regulate the activity of our stimulating neurotransmitters dopamine, serotonin, and noradrenaline. It calms us down and indirectly helps with fat loss because of its beneficial effects on sleep, stress, tension reduction, and mood. Progesterone supports the activity of GABA, which may explain why many women using natural progesterone (orally or topically in creams) experience better sleep and less anxiety. And, of course, when your mood is better, you tend to make better food choices and take better care of yourself.

Leptin: Your Body Likes It Level

Leptin plays a key role in metabolism and the regulation of fatty tissue. It's released by your fat cells in amounts commensurate with overall body-fat stores. In other words, the more body fat you have, the higher your leptin will be. Leptin acts as a signal to the brain that allows us to determine when we are full or when we should continue eating—*when we respond to it properly.*

Gregory Morton, assistant research professor of medicine at Harborview Medical Center at the University of Washington, has investigated how leptin works on our hypothalamus to influence blood sugar metabolism and the stability of energy in the body. He found a direct relationship between insulin, leptin levels, and body fat stores. In fact, his work has shown that proper leptin signals in the brain effectively reduce our food intake, keep body weight down, and improve insulin sensitivity.

Because leptin levels naturally increase while we sleep, sleep deprivation can cause a significant drop in leptin. This depletion causes us to feel excessively hungry, which in turn leads to overeating.

Along with getting a good night's sleep, we can improve leptin production and our cellular sensitivity to leptin with regular exercise; sufficient caloric intake; consumption of healthy, unsaturated fats; and general weight loss. Good thing these activities are all covered in the Hormone Diet three-step plan!

The Benefits of Just the Right Amount of Leptin

- Lowers body weight
- Lowers percentage of body fat
- Reduces food intake
- Reduces blood sugar
- Reduces insulin
- Increases metabolic rate
- Increases body temperature (in fact, high leptin causes excessive sweating)
- Increases our activity level
- Inhibits the synthesis and release of appetite-stimulating neuropeptide Y (NPY)

Although balanced leptin offers many health-promoting, antiaging benefits, too much of this hormone is not a good thing. Excessive saturated fat and sugar intake and obesity can lead to soaring leptin levels and ultimately to **leptin resistance** (and insulin resistance—in truth, when we have one of these conditions, we most likely have the other, which is why I did not include leptin in the Hormone Health Profile). Under this condition, the brain no longer responds to leptin's appetite-suppressing signals. In the absence of leptin's controlling mechanism, appetite can surge, even when plenty of leptin is present. Leptin resistance is linked directly to obesity, insulin resistance, and inflammation, which means it must be addressed right at the outset of an effective treatment plan to allow for optimal weight-loss results. Unfortunately, the discovery of high leptin in obese individuals has dampened the hope of using leptin as a treatment for obesity, but researchers are still very focused on investigating this option.

Vital Vitamin D$_3$

Vitamin D is made from cholesterol with the help of the liver, kidneys, and skin when we're exposed to natural sunlight. In your body, vitamin D functions as a hormone. Production decreases with age, stress, sunscreen use, low cholesterol, and also when your liver or kidneys are not working well. Suboptimal vitamin D status is associated with bone disease (osteoporosis), diabetes, cancer, heart disease, inflammation, depression, and autoimmune disease. Some sources suggest muscle weakness, especially in the legs, is also a symptom of low vitamin D.

I have used vitamin D supplements for many years to treat seasonal affective disorder in my patients because it improves the action of serotonin in the brain. The Canadian Cancer Society recently recommended vitamin D supplementation as a protection against cancer of the breast, colon, and prostate. Vitamin D is also intricately involved with the regulation of insulin activity in the body, making it a very useful supplement for diabetics and those at risk of diabetes, including obese individuals. Vitamin D has been proven to improve immune system function and shows promise in the treatment of autoimmune diseases such as multiple sclerosis. All these findings have led me to recommend a daily dose of 2,000 to 5,000 IU of vitamin D to all my patients, even in the summer. It's a vital component of your basic supplement plan, outlined later in Step 2.

> **THE RIGHT FATS *HELP* YOU STAY SLIM!**
> Saturated fats, such as those in red meats and full-fat dairy products, increase our appetite by reducing the appetite-suppressing hormones leptin and CCK. Yes, you should limit your intake of these types of fats, but eliminating fat altogether is not the answer, either. Instead, choose healthy options such as avocado, olives, olive oil, walnuts, and almonds. These healthful, calorie-rich, nutrient-dense foods will actually keep your appetite in check and your cravings under control.

HOT HORMONE TIP

VITAMIN D₃ DEFICIENCY AND INSULIN RESISTANCE IN PREGNANCY

According to a study published in *Diabetes Metabolism Research and Review* (July 2007), more than 70 percent of pregnant women are deficient in vitamin D (< 25 nmol/L). Furthermore, the data reveal a positive relationship between vitamin D status and insulin sensitivity. Researchers now suggest that vitamin D deficiency could be used as a diagnostic indicator of insulin resistance.

Once again, you can sit back, relax, and take a deep breath.

Now that you have a handle on your hormones, the next logical step is to begin imagining the strong, fat-burning machine your body is going to become. You can do this much more easily once you have mastered the topic of the next chapter. It's all about your muscle and your fat.

CHAPTER 5

SKINNY OR FAT ISN'T WHERE IT'S AT: THE FACTS ABOUT BODY COMPOSITION

Here's what you will learn in this chapter:
- All about healthy body composition
- How to read your Hormone Body-Fat Map
- How fat fuels inflammation
- How fat is a hormonal hotbed
- All about marvelous muscle—hard bodies and hormonal wellness

Optimizing your muscle-to-fat ratio is one of the primary goals of the Hormone Diet. In this chapter, I'll explain why your fat and muscle determine a whole lot more than how you look in a tight T-shirt or how much you can bench press. Your balance of fat and muscle tissue dictates many facets of your health, including your hormonal stability, tendency toward inflammation, and potential for aging well. In fact, one of the best ways to slow the aging process is to maintain plenty of lean muscle and keep your body fat low.

Where's the Fat?
In general, fat's stored in two places in your body—as subcutaneous fat under the skin or as visceral fat in the abdominal cavity surrounding our organs.

Fat under your skin tends to accumulate in such lovely spots as the backs of your arms, the love handle above each hip, the sides of your back just under your shoulder blades, and on your belly, buttocks, and thighs. Women tend to have more subcutaneous fat and less visceral fat than men. More subcutaneous fat may be one of the reasons why women also tend to accumulate more cellulite.

Too much fat in any of these storage sites isn't good for us, but visceral fat is especially damaging to our health since it's linked to insulin resistance, heart disease, and diabetes. Fat in the abdominal region is a big red flag telling us the body is likely secreting excess insulin and is subject to inflammation.

Thousands of studies have documented the link between high insulin and abdominal fat. The sad truth is that the more visceral fat we have, the more insulin resistant we become, and the more abdominal fat we store. It's yet another vicious circle that leads to more and more ab fat accumulation.

Cynthia Buffington, director of research at US Bariatric, in an article called "Obesity Begets Obesity" states that "Various studies, including our own, have shown changes in the production (or clearance) of certain hormones in association with increasing body weight and regional fat distribution. Such hormonal changes may promote further weight gain and influence where the fat is distributed on the body," which sums up this concept nicely. The more overweight we become, the more likely our body is to develop its own agenda in order to cope. Packing on pound after pound is like tossing gasoline on the brushfire of hormonal imbalance.

Those of us with more visceral fat will experience more inflammation and higher amounts of the stress hormone cortisol. A study from the *Journal of Psychosomatic Medicine* (September/October 2000) completed by researchers at Yale University found that even slender women with high stress (and therefore cortisol) had more abdominal fat. So no matter what your body type, more cortisol, just like more insulin, equals more ab fat.

Research has also shown that our levels of precious, recuperative growth hormone tend to decrease as we accumulate more fat around the midsection.

Then there's the impact on testosterone. When more belly fat is present, this masculinizing hormone plummets in men and rises in women. Researchers from the University of Virginia Health System found high levels of androgens such as testosterone in obese girls in the early stages of puberty, which increases their risk of more severe health problems later in life.

So hormones can determine where you store fat, and fat stored in specific areas fuels hormonal imbalance—quite a quandary indeed. Of course, where your fat accumulates can have something to do with genetics, which is something we cannot change. But I believe our environment, daily habits, and hormones—factors we *can* control—have a much greater impact than our genetic predisposition. Studies involving twins growing up in different environments provide excellent support for this. If genetics was the determining factor, we would expect both twins to have similar health concerns regardless of their living arrangements, but this isn't the case. Clearly, healthy lifestyle habits are equally, if not more, important in the prevention of the expression of disease-causing genes.

Your Hormone Body-Fat Map

Where you store your fat says a lot about your hormonal state. Take a look at the following Hormone Body-Fat Map to see a clearer picture of the relationship between your hormonal imbalances and fat stores. These are the spots you should pay attention to once you start your three-step fix: Watch them change as you regain hormonal balance. Note that the same storage sites can reveal different information for men and women.

Fat-Storage Site	Hormonal Imbalance: Women	Hormonal Imbalance: Men
Belly or abdomen (apple shape)	Low/high estrogen High testosterone High cortisol High insulin Low growth hormone	High estrogen Low testosterone High cortisol High insulin Low growth hormone
Back of the arm (triceps)	High insulin Low DHEA	High insulin Low DHEA
Hips/buttocks/hamstrings (pear shape)	High estrogen Low progesterone	High estrogen
"Love handles" (above the hips)	Insulin and blood sugar imbalance	Insulin and blood sugar imbalance
Chest (over the pectoral muscles)	High estrogen	High estrogen (often coupled with high insulin and low testosterone)
Back ("bra fat")	High testosterone High insulin	High insulin
Thighs	Low growth hormone	Low growth hormone

Don't Be Frail or Fat—Be Fit!

Once you have a handle on your hormones, appetite, and where your fat is at, you need to form a clear picture of the body you are striving for. Guess what, it won't be the body of all those supermodels who say they never work out. Their oh-so-glam diet of caffeine, nicotine, and lettuce is not the solution for you.

You might be surprised to learn that many of the outwardly beautiful women we see in magazines may actually have a high percentage of body fat. And they could unknowingly be laying the groundwork for many chronic diseases associated with aging because they lack sufficient, healthy muscle.

Being superthin is very different from being superhealthy. The distinction lies in understanding body composition—the ratio of lean to fatty tissue that makes up your total body weight. Your body is composed of many tissues, including fat, bones, muscles, tendons, ligaments, and organs, and also plenty of water. Healthy body composition is determined not by the number on your scale or the size of your jeans but by your percentage of fat versus lean muscle. Keeping the percentage of fat *low* and lean muscle mass *high* is ideal for maximizing your strength, wellness, and hormonal balance.

Excess fat, bone loss, and muscle loss are all factors that can result in altered body composition. The "skinny-fat person" is someone who appears slim but has a high percentage of body fat. In this case, body composition is not altered by excess fat, but rather by an unhealthy deficiency of muscle. Let's look at an example of one of my real patients, since I haven't seen many supermodels in my clinic lately.

I had a 34-year-old male patient who, at 5 feet 10 inches, weighed only 132 pounds. I measured his body fat and the reading told me it was an unfavorable 22 percent. (The optimal percentage for men his age is 14 percent.) He was certainly not overweight, but he had an alarmingly low percentage of muscle. He had been vegan for over 12 years, which meant his diet probably lacked the protein needed to build and maintain muscle. Moreover, he had never done resistance training, only yoga. When I looked at his basal metabolic rate, I saw that it was a whopping 500 calories below the optimum for someone his age. Based on the rough estimate that to maintain 1 pound of muscle requires about 50 calories a day, he needed to safely gain at least 10 pounds of muscle to safely create a healthier body composition.

We worked together to balance his diet and recuperate his body from stress. Then he began the Hormone Diet exercise plan to build muscle—and his results were remarkable!

Obese versus Overweight

Obesity is a much more common form of altered body composition than the skinny-fat scenario. Not everyone who is overweight, however, is obese. Overweight individuals are classified as having 25 to 30 percent body fat. Obesity is clinically defined as a body fat percentage higher than 30, and although obesity is more common in women, men are more likely to be overweight.

Measuring Body Fat

Body composition is sometimes measured by body mass index (BMI), calculated by dividing weight by height. A BMI in the range of 25 to 29.9 is considered overweight, whereas 30 or more is considered clinically obese. A BMI of 40 or more is considered morbidly obese. These measurements can prove inaccurate for assessing body composition in people who are very short, very muscular, very tall, or who have edema (swelling and water retention). I don't use BMI charts very often, for these reasons.

Instead I use a professional bioimpedance analysis (BIA) machine in conjunction with waist circumference and waist-to-hip ratio measurements. The BIA has been used in thousands of clinical studies as a simple method to assess body fat percentage. It works by sending an electrical frequency through your body. This may sound spooky, but you feel nothing during the test. Different tissues conduct the signal at different rates, so the machine can provide a quick assessment of the amount of fat, water, and muscle in your body.

Typically, the electrical signal travels from your hand to your foot. This method is best because the signal zips through your whole body and can more accurately measure whether more fat is stored in your top or bottom half. The signal can also go from hand to hand via a handheld device or foot to foot while you stand barefoot on a specialized scale. Readings are most reliable first thing in the morning, after you have had some water but no food, since BIA readings are affected by hydration, electrolytes, eating, and exercise.

Although BIA testing is easier, calipers or skin-fold testing may be more accurate. Skin-fold testing is difficult to do on your own, so I recommend you invest in a BIA machine for home to use as an adjunct to your wellness plan. The BIA may not be 100 percent accurate, but it will be a great help in monitoring your progress over time. Check out www.tanita.com for more information on obtaining a BIA machine. Prices may range from $75 to $300.

Acceptable and Optimal Body-Fat Compositions for Men and Women				
	Men		Women	
Age Range	Acceptable % Range	Optimal %	Acceptable % Range	Optimal %
15–20	10–18	13	17–25	20
21–30	10–18	13	17–25	20
31–40	10–18	14	17–25	21
41–50	10–18	15	17–25	22
51–60	10–18	16	17–25	23
61–70	10–18	17	17–25	24
71–80	10–18	18	17–25	25
> 80	10–18	18	17–25	25

HEALTHY BODY FAT PERCENTAGES

Monitoring changes in body fat is especially valuable if you only have about 10 to 20 pounds to lose and you are doing resistance training. This is the method we use at Clear Medicine and it provides a wonderful source of motivation for our patients. In this scenario, the number on the scale may not change much, but you will be able to measure favorable changes in your body composition, such as muscle gain and fat loss.

Significant health problems are associated with obesity, including high blood pressure, osteoarthritis, heart disease, diabetes, stroke, sleep apnea, decreased quality of life, and premature death. Second only to smoking, obesity is a leading cause of preventable deaths.

Sadly, despite the known health risks, most of us are fat and getting fatter!

- According to figures published by the World Health Organization (WHO), by the year 2015 some 2.3 billion adults will be overweight and more than 700 million will suffer from obesity, a pathology seen in growing numbers of children.
- From 1980 to 2000, the percentage of obese Americans more than doubled, from 15 to 31 percent.
- Nearly 50 percent of adults in the developed world are overweight or outright obese.
- Africa has long been regarded as a continent plagued by famine, undernourishment, and starvation. However, as African populations have become increasingly Westernized, the number of overweight and obese people has skyrocketed. Once-undernourished populations have just as high an incidence of obesity as the United States, the current world leader in this condition. Today, more than 25 percent of Egyptians and 40 to 50 percent of South Africans are already obese.

Your Fat Sends Messages—The Hormones Produced by Fat

Over the last decade, scientists have made truly amazing discoveries about fat. Turns out it's not just an annoyance that hangs around making us feel unhappy about our appearance. Fat is now actually recognized as endocrine tissue that constantly sends and receives hormonal signals to regulate body weight, control inflammation, manage our appetite, direct blood clotting, and determine how our cells respond to insulin. Wow!

The worst part? *Fat fuels fat.* That's right—the more fat we accumulate, the greater our risk of obesity. With all the hormonal signals being sent and received from our fat, our fat actually controls how much more fat we store. As a result, we need to take charge of our fat cells to successfully initiate and maintain fat loss. The more fat we have, the more difficult this process; but taking charge is definitely doable and worth the effort.

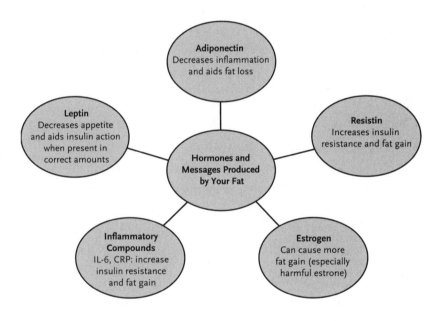

THE HORMONES AND ADIPOKINES PRODUCED BY FAT

In both men and women, fat tissue is a huge source of estrogen production because it contains the aromatase enzyme, which converts testosterone to estrogen. The links between estrogen dominance, obesity, and cancer are undeniable.

Other hormones produced in *and* sent out from your fat cells include leptin, resistin, and adiponectin.

The names may sound alien, but these tiny chemical signals (actually proteins produced by your fat cells) travel to your liver, brain, muscles, and other sites throughout your body. They're vital for keeping appetite under control and for shrinking your fat stores. Researchers have found that adiponectin *increases fat burning* and

SIMPLE, POWERFUL MEASUREMENT: WAIST CIRCUMFERENCE AND WAIST-TO-HIP RATIO

One of the quickest ways to determine whether you are hormonally imbalanced is to measure your waist-to-hip ratio (WHR). Calculating your WHR determines definitively whether the weight around your midsection exceeds that surrounding your hips and thighs.

Measure your waist just above your belly button, at the narrowest part of your waist. Measure your hips around the widest part of your buttocks, while standing with your feet together. A waist measurement of more than 35 inches for women or more than 40 inches for men is pushing into the unhealthy range. Next, calculate your WHR by dividing the measurement of your waist by the measurement of your hips.

If your WHR is greater than 0.9 for men or 0.8 for women, you are also at risk.

For example: Let's say Mary's waist measures 28 inches and her hips are 33 inches. Her waist-to-hip ratio would be calculated as follows: 28 ÷ 33 = 0.84. Because 0.8 is considered unsafe for women, Mary is at risk and needs to lose some belly fat. (I suppose she could also try gaining weight on her hips, but I have never had a patient go for this option!)

aids our insulin sensitivity. You can think of adiponectin as the fat factor that leads to its own demise. It's produced by your fat, yet helps to burn it up! Like leptin, adiponectin is definitely a fat-loss friend.

Adiponectin and leptin work in opposition to resistin, a hormone that contributes to fat gain by directly causing insulin resistance in the liver and muscle cells. While adiponectin aids fat burning, resistin actually fuels more fat from fat.

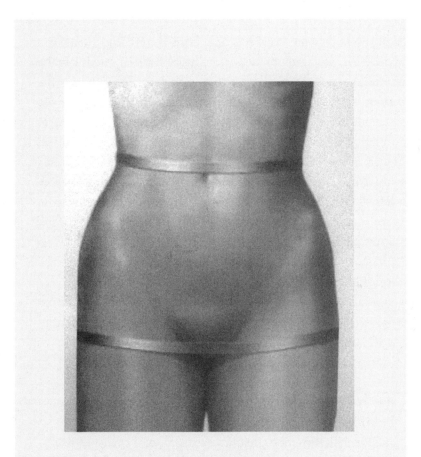

WAIST-TO-HIP MEASUREMENT

Adiponectin also offers us protection against inflammation caused by other compounds produced in the fat cells, called adipokines. Our fat tissues are now recognized as major culprits behind rampant inflammation, one of our major fat-loss foes. Pro-inflammatory compounds like TNF-alpha, IL-6, resistin, and C-reactive protein (CRP) arise from our fat cells and are also known to surge as both body fat and insulin resistance increase. These chemicals directly contribute to arterial damage, insulin resistance, leptin resistance, and heart disease and are typically about 30 percent *more prevalent* in obese people.

When you're fat, your body sets up a hormonal cascade that stimulates more fat, since adipokines create more fat cells, modulate the size of our fat deposits, contribute to inflammation, and influence the distribution of body fat. A 2000 study published in *Endocrine Review* showed abdominal fat in particular produced larger numbers of inflammatory mediators than other types of fat in the body—*ab fat truly is a fire in your belly.* The trouble is that attempting to lose fat while we are inflamed is something like trying to drain a sink with the stopper still in. The hormones that help us to get lean are blocked and fat loss becomes excruciatingly difficult. We absolutely must cool the fire of inflammation first to allow for successful fat loss.

Hormonal Messages Received by Our Fat

While our fat cells do plenty of communicating, they are also continuously receiving hormonal messages that can affect their size, number, distribution, and insulin sensitivity. Here's where the messages received by your fat cells come from.

- **Your fat-loss foes:** Hormones and conditions that increase the size, number, and distribution of your fat cells. These include inflammation, insulin, estrogen, and cortisol.
- **Your fat-loss friends:** The hormones that decrease the size,

number, and distribution of fat cells. These include growth hormone, thyroid hormone, glucagon, adrenaline, DHEA, progesterone, leptin, and testosterone. (Note: Estrogen, when properly balanced, aids fat loss.)

Fat is only one part of your body composition story. Let's talk about the magnificent impact of muscle.

Muscle Is Marvelous for Your Metabolism

Sure, hard bodies look great on the beach and at the gym. Strong, lean muscles are not only important for how you look and feel—they're vital for your enduring wellness. On the most basic level, good skeletal muscle strength and function give you the stability you need to move, walk, run, and avoid falling. Good muscle tone has many additional benefits, even when the body is completely at rest. These include:

- **A major metabolic boost:** With the help of your thyroid hormones, muscle tissue dictates your metabolic rate. Fat is far less metabolically active than muscle, which means the more muscle you have, the more calories your body burns and the fewer calories you need to maintain your weight. As a result, gaining unwanted weight is much easier when you have *less* muscle, simply because you are *less* likely to use all the calories you take in each day.
- **Aiding insulin sensitivity:** Muscle cells are important targets for insulin, since most of our insulin receptors are present within muscle tissue. As we age and naturally lose muscle, the risk of insulin resistance increases. When our cells lose their sensitivity to insulin, more of this hormone must be produced in order for it to do its job, and we become more prone to weight gain.

Use It or Lose It!

Research shows that muscle strength declines by 15 percent per decade after age 50 and 30 percent per decade after age 70. As you might expect, along with this decline in muscle mass comes a 5 percent decrease per decade in our metabolic rate. This process of losing muscle mass, strength, and function with aging is called **sarcopenia.** Scientists have found that sarcopenia occurs not only because we grow older, but also because we stop doing activities that utilize, build, and maintain muscle power. So, the old adage is true—*use it if you don't want to lose it.*

Is Exercise Enough to Keep You Strong?

Sadly, excercise is not enough. Strength peaks in our midtwenties and then begins to decrease. Data collected from over 20 years of studies show that muscle tissue degenerates *even* in people who maintain a high level of physical activity. These findings indicate that other factors besides inactivity contribute to muscle loss. I believe the major culprits are:

- **Poor nutrition:** Insufficient protein, vitamins, and minerals to build and maintain healthy muscle cells
- **Free radical damage:** Damage to muscle-cell mitochondria leads to cell death (less muscle) or dysfunction (weaker muscle)
- **Inflammation**
- **Increased stress hormone:** Can be caused by excessive cardiovascular exercise, excessive caloric restriction, and disease, and also by emotional, environmental, mental, and physical stress
- **Hormone imbalance:** Decline of hormones that maintain muscle mass and strength, including testosterone, DHEA-S, growth hormone, and acetylcholine

Fortunately, the loss of muscle due to aging is partially reversible with the Hormone Diet's three-step approach.

Your muscle restoration program includes strength training, good sleep habits, inflammation control, stress management, glycemically balanced eating, natural hormone replacement (if necessary), and professional-strength supplements.

Lasting Fat Loss Means *Safe* Fat Loss

It appears that the most successful way to slow the aging process is to maintain healthy muscle mass and to eat a highly nutritious, low-calorie diet. But your diet should never involve extreme caloric restriction, no matter what the latest headlines say. *New York* magazine promoted one particular diet as "The Diet to End All Diets" (October 30, 2006) because it promised "the fewest calories your body can stand." Starving is not without its repercussions, as this type of caloric restriction can ravage both your hormonal balance and your metabolism. A weight-loss program that compromises muscle while you lose fat is metabolically harmful and only serves to speed the aging process. Not what you're looking for, I'm sure.

I tell my patients this: Your health reserves lie within your muscles. When faced with an illness, surgery, or other stressful event, your body will naturally tap into muscle tissue for energy to support you during the experience. Always do your best to make sure your reserves are full.

Safe fat loss means losing *only* fat while preserving muscle. A healthy, long-term solution avoids severe caloric restrictions or fad-diet approaches that are unsustainable and always result in hormonally driven rebound weight gain.

Remember, your body and your hormones are programmed to work against you by increasing your appetite and slowing your metabolic rate when you reduce your caloric intake. With a slowed metabolism, you gain weight and feel tired and sluggish. Conversely, using the correct weight-loss techniques will give your metabolism an energizing boost that leaves you feeling brighter and looking your best.

Study after study proves that many of the health complications associated with obesity improve with weight loss. But Dr. Samuel Klein, a professor at the Washington University School of Medicine, raised an important issue in his paper "Outcome Success in Obesity" published in the journal *Obesity Research* in 2001. Although Klein begins by stating that many health improvements kick in after only 5 to 10 percent of initial body weight is lost, he goes on to add: "There is no conclusive evidence that weight loss decreases mortality in obese people." Even though overweight people effectively lower their health risks when they shed pounds, Klein shows that *they still do not appear to live any longer.* Now, you might be thinking, Great, if I'm overweight, I might as well just stay this way. Not so. Klein's study does not tell us that losing weight is pointless; it instead provides us with valuable insight into why the *way* we lose weight is extremely important.

> ## HOT WEIGHT-LOSS FACT
>
> **UNSAFE FAT LOSS CAN BE DEADLY**
>
> A 1999 study of obese men showed that intentionally losing 20 pounds did not increase mortality in those with obesity-related illnesses, but it did boost the number of cancer-related deaths. Could this increase in cancer-related mortality be associated with the release of toxins from fat cells during weight loss? Just one more reason why detox before and after weight loss is so critical.

Dr. Klein notes that "Dietary intervention is the cornerstone of weight-loss therapy." Although I agree diet is important, it's just one facet of an effective program. Hormonal balance through sleep, detoxification, supplements, a toxin-free lifestyle, stress management, exercise, and conquering inflammation are just as important as your nutrition habits for safe and lasting weight loss. Finally, safe fat loss means completing a detox at the beginning of your weight-loss journey and again after the first few months, because *the majority of toxins in your body are stored within the fat cells.* While detox takes time and commitment, reducing the negative impact of toxins released during fat loss is critical to your health and your long-term weight-loss success.

You've reached the end of Part One. At this point your brain is surely chock-full with everything you'll ever need to know about your hormones, your muscle, your fat, and your metabolism. Now we're moving on to Part Two, The Three-Step Fix.

PART TWO

THE THREE-STEP FIX

Live in rooms full of light
Avoid heavy food
Be moderate in the drinking of wine
Take massage, baths, exercise, and gymnastics
Fight insomnia with gentle rocking or the sound of running water
Change surroundings and take long journeys
Strictly avoid frightening ideas
Indulge in cheerful conversation and amusements
Listen to music.

AULUS CORNELIUS CELSUS,
Roman encyclopedist, ca. 25 BC–ca. AD 50

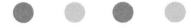

INTRODUCING THE THREE-STEP FIX

Winning the War Against Fat

Imagine all the things you do and think in a day. From your smallest tasks to your biggest worries, all your habits, thoughts, and activities influence your hormones and, ultimately, your ability to lose fat. Naturally, the next question is, *What can you do to achieve and maintain the balance you need for the healthy body you want?*

The answer is all laid out for you here in my three-step fix. This three-step plan not only brings back the hormonal balance you need to accelerate fat loss, but it also addresses all potential causes of weight gain that prevent you from achieving your weight-loss goals, including:

- Hormonal imbalance
- Sleep deprivation or poor sleep habits
- Compromised digestion
- Toxicity or inadequate liver function
- pH imbalance (excess body acidity)
- Nasty nutrition and nutrient deficiencies
- Lack of exercise
- Lack of sex
- Toxic body-care products
- Inadequate body temperature regulation

Quite a list of offenders! I hope you now realize that if you haven't been successful at reaching or maintaining your fat-loss goals before, the problem may not be lack of discipline on your part.

The Hormone Diet Three-Step Fix

Because our hormones are so delicately intertwined, this plan is structured to allow each balancing step to set the stage for the next. To achieve optimal results that last, follow the guidelines in the order I have presented them, and move through each stage one at a time.

In the introduction of this book I told you that the Hormone Diet will offer you amazing results because of the precise way it helps you identify and effectively overcome the major fat-packing factors that accelerate weight gain and prevent fat loss. This program enables you to determine why you haven't been able to beat those last stubborn pounds. It then guarantees that you can reap the rewards of your hard work in the gym and discipline in the kitchen.

Now you can put all the science and philosophy you've learned into action. With the help of your Hormonal Health Profile results and the recommendations to come, implementing your action plan and accomplishing your health and weight-loss goals will be easier than you ever imagined.

Tips for the Three-Step Fix

First of all, don't rush. If you invest your efforts wisely now, you'll put an end to yo-yo dieting for good. Also, don't be concerned that I haven't included exercise, beyond walking, until the fourth week of your program (though you can continue working out if you are already doing so). The first two steps build your foundation for enduring, optimal results and prepare your body for the metabolic boost exercise offers.

You have the rest of your life to be lean, fit, strong, healthy, and vibrant. Imagine: After these 6 weeks, you'll never have to search out another "get-skinny-quick" approach again.

At the end of your three steps you can expect wonderful and lasting results such as these:

- Improved digestion
- Less pain and inflammation
- Restorative sleep
- Safe fat loss and increased muscle mass
- Improved strength and stability
- Glowing skin, healthier looking hair
- Better appetite control
- Increased energy and stress recuperation
- Stronger libido, sexual enjoyment, and increased fertility
- Metabolic revival
- Better mood, memory, and concentration
- Protection from many of the diseases of aging
- Slowed aging and illness prevention through maximized immunity and antioxidant defense

Before you begin, I encourage you to focus on achieving great health, feeling good, gaining strength, and building muscle, and *not* on attaining Hollywood's perception of the perfect body. Recall our discussion from Chapter 5. Your goal should be a healthy body that's strong and full of vitality. And remember, healthy weight loss means losing fat—not muscle.

Good luck with your three steps! I hope you find this process as enjoyable and rewarding as so many of my patients have.

CHAPTER 6

LAYING THE GROUNDWORK:
GETTING PREPPED FOR THE THREE STEPS

Here's what you can expect to complete by the end of this chapter:

- Your Best Body Assessment
- A kitchen mini-makeover
- Shopping for your detox

This chapter will give you the guidance needed to fully assess your body and risk factors for hormonal imbalance before embarking on your journey to optimal wellness. You'll also establish benchmarks—besides your weight—that will help you to monitor your health improvements and fat loss. First, you'll establish a quantifiable framework for hormonal balance, safe fat loss, and enduring wellness with your Best Body Assessment. The system that follows will provide you with the basic tools needed to manage your risk factors.

So many factors come together to create your total health picture. Your sleep, energy level, tolerance for exercise, memory, outlook on life, self-esteem, ability to laugh, sex life, quality of friendships, family role, connection to nature, spirituality, and coping skills are all factors that influence your overall health. Changes or disruptions in any of these areas are early warning signs of hormonal, and health, imbalances. You have to pay attention to and be aware of what's going on in your body and life. I've treated far too many patients who dismissed their feelings of fatigue or lack of libido for years. Believe me, taking charge of your health will always result in a better quality of life.

I also encourage you to believe you *are* healthy. Refuse to continue in an unhealthy environment, relationship, or job. Refuse to spend time worrying about your health—worry is simply praying to your fears. Make the choice, take action, and refuse to accept habits and circumstances that prevent you from achieving optimal health. You deserve to be happy and well!

Your Best Body Assessment

As discussed in Chapter 5, establishing your *body composition* and full range of body benchmarks will help you monitor your progress (and keep you motivated) far better than the number on your scale alone. Most of these variables can be measured easily at home with the right tools. The blood test, of course, will require a visit to your doctor's office. (I recommend you ask your family physician for a complete panel of blood tests at least once a year to continually monitor possible risk factors for disease.)

These are the tools you will need to successfully complete your Best Body Assessment.

1. A daily or weekly journal to record your efforts outside of this book. (I recommend this. It's better to record your habits and assessments more often than at the start and end of your 6 weeks.)
2. Litmus paper pH testing strips from your local health food store.
3. A flexible tape measure.
4. A scale.
5. A watch or heart rate monitor.

6. A bioimpedance analysis (BIA) machine is optional, but you can purchase a scale with a BIA built in. Visit www.tanita.com for information on obtaining a BIA for home use. If you can't afford one, don't worry; the rest of the Best Body Assessment measurements still provide a very good indication of your overall health. You can also visit an integrated doctor (MD, ND, or DC) or even a local health club for a body composition test.

7. If you have high blood pressure, I strongly suggest investing in a BP monitor to use at home daily. Check your local pharmacy.

When you have all the tools you need, complete your Best Body Assessment.

Your Best Body Assessment
1. Determine your body composition.

- Weigh yourself first thing in the morning on an empty stomach and record your body weight
  Start date: _____ End of 6 weeks: _____

- Waist measurement (Remember, this measurement should be < 40 inches for men; < 35 inches for women. Refer to page 120 for a refresher on how to take your waist and hip measurements properly.)
  Start date: _____ End of 6 weeks: _____

- Hip measurement
  Start date: _____ End of 6 weeks: _____

- Calculate your waist-to-hip ratio by dividing your waist measurement by your hip measurement (ideal waist-to-hip ratio is < 0.9 for men; < 0.8 for women)
  Start date: _____ End of 6 weeks: _____

- If possible, measure your body fat percentage via bio-impedance analysis either at home or at a local health club first thing in the morning on an empty stomach. (You may drink water beforehand.)

  Start date: _____ End of 6 weeks: _____

2. Check your body pH.

Acidity in the whole body (outside the stomach) is a major cause of hormonal imbalance. The measure of the acidity or alkalinity of a substance is its pH. The pH scale runs from 0 to 14. A lower pH number means higher acidity, and generally less oxygen is present. A higher pH indicates more alkalinity. A solution is considered neutral, neither acid nor alkaline, when it has a pH of 7. Our body continuously strives to maintain its normal, slightly alkaline pH balance of about 7.0 to 7.4. We experience health problems when the pH of our bodily fluids and tissues is pushed out of its comfortable neutral zone.

Understanding pH

Although the stomach should contain plenty of acid to do its job effectively, a slightly alkaline environment is optimal everywhere else to allow the body's metabolic, enzymatic, immunologic, and repair mechanisms to function at their best. The most common form of pH imbalance outside the stomach is *excess acidity*. This condition has become prevalent today because poor diet, insufficient or excessive exercise, and chronic stress can lead to excess acid in our internal environment. High-protein foods, processed cereals and flours, sugar, coffee, tea, and alcohol are acidifying, whereas vegetables, millet, soy, almonds, and wild rice are alkalinizing.

> **HOT HORMONE FACT**
>
> **REDUCE EXCESS BODY ALKALINITY**
>
> Excess alkalinity in the body is rare but requires treatment with supplements of calcium-magnesium and green food. It can be an indication of insufficient protein intake or endocrine imbalance.

When our body becomes acidic, minerals such as potassium, sodium, magnesium, and calcium may be stolen from our vital organs and bones to combat or buffer the acid. If these mineral losses and metabolic abnormalities continue, we increase our risk of developing a number of conditions, including:

- Obesity, slow metabolism, weight gain, and inability to lose weight
- Chronic inflammation
- High blood pressure
- Diabetes
- Bladder and kidney conditions, including kidney stones
- Weakened immunity
- Premature aging
- Osteoporosis: weak, brittle bones; fractures; and bone spurs
- Joint pain, aching muscles, and lactic acid buildup
- Low energy and chronic fatigue
- Mood swings
- Slow digestion and elimination
- Yeast/fungal overgrowth

These problems are not surprising, since excess acid also interferes with our hormones. For example, in an acidic environment, as much as twice the amount of estrogen may be needed to exert its effects in the body, and neither thyroid nor growth hormone will work at their best.

If you have a health problem, you are likely a walking acid trip. No matter what type of therapy you choose to treat your condition, resolution will not come until your pH balance is restored.

You will enjoy the most dramatic results from the three-step system when your body is slightly alkaline. Acidity decreases your body's ability to absorb the vitamins and minerals from your foods and supplements, interferes with your ability to detoxify, disrupts your metabolism, and makes you more prone to fatigue and mood changes. For all these reasons, I have included pH testing as part of your Best Body Assessment.

Test your saliva or urine using litmus paper strips purchased from your local health food store or from www.thehormonediet.com.

WHEN?
Test your pH first thing in the morning or 1 hour before a meal or 2 hours after eating.

HOW?
Saliva: *Before* brushing your teeth, fill your mouth with saliva and swallow; repeat; *spit directly on* the pH test strip. This three-step process will ensure a clean saliva sample. Measure your saliva pH in the same manner again later in the day, at least 2 hours after eating.

Urine: Collect a small sample of your first morning urine in a clean glass container; dip the pH strip into the container.

In either case, match your strip to the associated color on the package of pH papers to determine your pH.

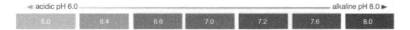
◄ acidic pH 6.0 — alkaline pH 8.0 ►

| 6.0 | 6.4 | 6.6 | 7.0 | 7.2 | 7.6 | 8.0 |

Record your pH measurement here:
  Start date: _____ End of 6 weeks: _____

WHAT'S NORMAL?
If the pH of your saliva stays between 7.0 and 7.4 all day, your body is functioning within a healthy range. If your urinary pH fluctuates

between 6.0 and 6.5 in the morning and 6.5 and 7.0 in the evening, your body is within a healthy pH range. First morning urine should be slightly more acidic, as you eliminate waste accumulated throughout the night.

Continue to measure your pH daily if your values are abnormal; otherwise, testing once a week will suffice.

TIPS TO REDUCE EXCESS BODY ACIDITY

- Most fruits and vegetables are highly alkalinizing. If you follow the Hormone Diet as presented and ensure two-thirds of your plate is occupied by veggies at lunch and dinner, you will get a minimum of 8 to 10 servings a day.
- A nice mug of warm lemon water upon rising and/or prior to meals can cleanse your liver, stimulate the flow of digestive juices, and reduce body acidity.
- Have a daily helping of alkalinizing greens, such as 1 cup of spinach, kale, collards, mustard greens, rapini, watercress, or bok choy.
- Choose millet and quinoa to replace acid-forming grains such as wheat and rye.
- Use either a juicer or a blender to make your own alkaline juices and smoothies at home. Powdered green-food supplements are also very helpful. I use one first thing each morning on an empty stomach. Make blender drinks using alkaline juices, green powdered supplements, and fruits.
- Use olive oil, which is less acid-forming than other vegetable oils.
- Use buffered vitamin C to alkalinize the system and increase your absorption of magnesium.
- The sleep and stress tips that make up Step 1 of your three-step program (especially your breathing/meditation exercise) will improve acid balance and promote alkalinity. Your exercise plan

also helps because of its stress-reducing properties.
- If the above suggestions do not restore your body's pH balance, purchase an alkalinizing product such as Tri-Alkali Powder from Pure Encapsulations or Basictabs from BioMed and take as directed. (See www.clearmedicinestore.com.)

3. Measure your blood pressure.

If you don't have a blood pressure (BP) monitor at home, check it at your local pharmacy or your doctor's office. Optimal BP is 110/70 and shouldn't increase with age. When I find readings of 125/80 or higher with my patients, I begin mild hypotensive therapy, which includes salt restriction and supplementation with potassium and magnesium and the amino acid L-arginine, in addition to the three steps.

Monitor your blood pressure daily if you currently have high blood pressure or are at risk.

Start date: _____ End of 6 weeks: _____

4. Measure your resting heart rate.

You may do this by recording your pulse as soon as you awaken, *before you get out of bed*. Measure your pulse for 15 seconds, then multiply the number by 4 to calculate your number of heartbeats per minute. Note that if your pulse increases from one week to the next, you may be overexercising.

Start date: _____ End of 6 weeks: _____

5. Visit your doctor and request one blood test.

To achieve maximal fat loss, we must identify all the invisible, internal factors that can interfere with metabolism. We also want to get a baseline for *early* identification of disease risk factors. I can't stress enough the importance of annual blood testing—it can mean the difference between life and death.

For the purposes of this fat-loss program, however, I suggest a blood test that will assess your *insulin sensitivity*. Although the Hormonal Health Profile helps to identify many signs of insulin resistance, the blood work will provide definitive proof. We can also use the results of these tests as a major marker to monitor your progress. I recommend taking the test and repeating it after you have completed your three steps and are living your new lifestyle.

Don't stress if you can't get to the doctor or don't want to have your blood drawn. Your waist-to-hip ratio and Hormonal Health Profile (the group of signs/symptoms for Hormonal Imbalance 1) will still provide good insight into your insulin sensitivity. But please make sure that you still keep up with your regular blood tests at your annual physical.

THE BLOOD TEST YOU NEED
- Your *fasting* blood glucose and insulin
  and
- A *2-hour pp* blood glucose and insulin test (This is basically the same glucose and insulin test repeated 2 hours after you have eaten.)

HOW IT'S DONE:
You'll go to the lab first thing in the morning with an empty stomach. The technician will draw a sample of your blood to test your glucose and insulin. You'll then leave the lab and eat a big breakfast (e.g., orange juice, toast, pancakes, etc.). Brace yourself—the perfect meal may actually be a McDonald's breakfast of hot cakes with syrup and orange juice! You'll wait and then return to the lab to have your blood drawn again to test your glucose and insulin levels 2 hours later. Do not exercise during this time span.

This test will reveal exactly what's happening with your glucose and insulin in both the fasting and fed states.

If your insulin is elevated at any point, your risk of diabetes is greater. *In fact, if your insulin is elevated you are considered to be a hyperinsulin secretor, displaying signs of insulin resistance.* More specifically, *abnormal* findings are indicated by the following test results:

Fasting insulin: >7 IU/mL

2 hours after eating insulin: >60 IU/mL

Fasting glucose: >86 mg/dL

2 hours after eating glucose: >100 mg/dL

If you are indeed insulin resistant (or heading in that direction), you're more prone to abdominal fat gain and will benefit most from a Glyci-Med dietary approach such as the Hormone Diet. This two-part blood test will also allow you to be much more proactive about your health, since measuring fasting glucose alone (the typical practice) picks up insulin resistance in the late stage of disease, when diabetes is already full-blown. Insulin is often the first imbalance to present itself; high blood sugar is last.

In my clinical practice, I perform many more tests on each patient (see Appendix A for a summary of the tests). But because a glucose/insulin imbalance can appear with any one of the fat-packing hormonal imbalances, this one simple test is the best starting point to determine how well your diet will work, as well as being a strong indication of your overall wellness.

WHAT IF YOUR BLOOD TEST RESULTS ARE ABNORMAL?
If you find your blood insulin is high after fasting or after eating, you can take extra steps now to enhance your fat-loss results.

Although *all* three steps work to improve your insulin response, you may want to add a supplement to improve your insulin response and accelerate fat loss. Your options are outlined in Chapter 13, under Hormonal Imbalance 1.

Give Your Kitchen a Mini-Makeover!

Before you embark on your detox in Step 1, you may want to take some time to clear your cupboards of foods that impair healthy hormonal balance. The list below covers foods you should never eat—I recommend you remove them from your kitchen immediately to prevent further hormonal disruption. Other nasty foods you have in stock, such as low-fat packaged foods, should be gradually phased out of your home.

CHECK LABELS IN YOUR CUPBOARDS, FRIDGE, AND FREEZER AND IMMEDIATELY REMOVE THE FOLLOWING:

- Products containing artificial sweeteners (aspartame, Splenda, etc.)
- Products containing high-fructose corn syrup
- Vegetable oil, palm oil, shortening, margarine, and cottonseed oil; anything containing partially hydrogenated oils; products containing trans fats
- Processed and packaged foods that contain preservatives and lack nutrients, e.g., prepared pasta side dishes
- Packaged products such as sliced meats that contain sulfites and nitrites

PITCH PLASTICS!

The next step in your mini-makeover is to replace all your plastic food storage containers with glass. Gradually phase out condiments and foods in plastic bottles (or recycle them all now) and try to purchase only products in glass.

Always choose metal, glass, or wood instead of plastic for storing, reheating, and serving foods. Use paper wraps instead of plastic, and never microwave your food covered by plastic wrap or in plastic containers or Styrofoam. Potentially harmful or cancer-causing, estrogenlike chemicals called dioxins can leach into your foods and drinks, especially when heated or frozen.

Avoid water in plastic bottles as much as you can, and never drink water bottled in plastic if it has been heated or frozen in your car. Do *not* refill plastic bottles. Purchase all types of drinks in glass bottles as often as possible, or choose stainless steel as a travel-friendly option.

Shop Before You Detox

At this point, you may want to stock up on the body-cleansing, hormone-enhancing foods you'll be eating while you complete your detox. Don't worry! I guarantee you'll have plenty of tasty choices that will leave you feeling energized and satisfied. Your shopping list is provided on page 442.

We have covered all the prep steps you need to get started. You've completed your Best Body Assessment, rid your kitchen of hormone hazards, and created a detox shopping list. Are you pumped? You're now set for the three-step fix.

STEP 1
RENEW AND REVITALIZE

YOUR FIRST 2 WEEKS

I am seeking, I am striving, I am in it with all my heart.

VINCENT VAN GOGH

CHAPTER 7

SUPERB SLEEP FOR
HORMONAL BALANCE

These are the hormonal benefits you can expect to enjoy from superb sleep:

- Tamed cortisol and a calm nervous system
- Replenished DHEA, the antiaging hormone
- Reduced insulin and subdued inflammation
- Increased GABA and serotonin, the relaxation and feel-good hormones
- Better testosterone status and protection from the harmful effects of excess estrogen
- Increased melatonin and growth hormone for greater nighttime repair and fat-burning benefits
- Increased thyroid hormone to maximize your metabolism
- Enhanced appetite control through increased leptin and suppression of the appetite-stimulating hormones ghrelin and NPY
- More acetylcholine to keep your muscles moving and your mind and memory sharp

Hectic schedules. Bigger workloads. More hours in front of the computer and TV. There are more reasons why we lack sleep than there are hours in a day. *Along with managing stress, ensuring you routinely get a good night's rest is the most important factor for restoring hormonal balance.* Great quality sleep is absolutely vital for fat-loss success. If you've failed at dieting before, chances are that insufficient or improper sleep was a contributing factor.

According to recent statistics, sleep deprivation affects more than 70 million North Americans. In fact, we're spending $24 billion a year just trying to fall asleep. But that's still only a fraction of the $100 billion we spend annually in our attempts to lose weight.

Are You Sleep Deprived?

Ask yourself the following questions:

- Do you fall asleep as soon as your head hits the pillow?
- Do you rely on an alarm to wake you up?
- Do you feel tired during the day?
- Do you tend to sleep more on the weekends?

If you answered yes to any of the above, you are probably sleep deprived.

Sleep and Your Hormones

Sleep deprivation perpetuates a vicious circle of excess stress hormones, reduced sleep-inducing melatonin, and low growth hormone. Your hormonal state also influences your ability to sleep. For instance, hormonal imbalances, such as the low progesterone often associated with PMS or the low serotonin common with depression, can lead to many frustrating nights of tossing and turning or repeatedly waking in the wee morning hours.

Sleep to Stay Slim

Sleep is an absolutely fascinating innate function that depends on the intricate interplay of environmental signals and various structures and chemicals within your body, beginning with the hypothalamus gland. The hypothalamus regulates your internal clock, also known as the circadian rhythm, which dictates your natural sleep-wake cycle. This gland gathers information about body temperature and light exposure to influence our normal sleep habits and hormone-release patterns.

Body temperature is directly linked to our level of wakefulness arousal—believe it or not, the warmer we are, the more alert we become.

Once melatonin is released, it causes your body to cool down and sink into deeper sleep, which is when growth hormone is released. At this point, more cell reproduction takes place and protein breakdown slows substantially. Essentially, your body rebuilds itself during deep sleep, especially your bones and skin and muscle cells. Since proteins are the building blocks needed for cell growth and for repair from the damaging effects of factors such as stress and ultraviolet rays, deep sleep may truly be "beauty sleep." And remember, the release of growth hormone is also encouraging for fat loss.

Growth hormone naturally declines as we age, but poor-quality sleep and low melatonin can cause its production to drop off even further. Without sufficient melatonin, we lose the rejuvenating and fat-burning benefits of growth hormone and become susceptible to abdominal weight gain.

Sleep and Stress

Not surprisingly, sleep has profound effects on your nervous system. Throughout most of the sleep cycle, the sympathetic nervous system (fight or flight) relaxes while the parasympathetic nervous system (rest and digest) is stimulated. (The reverse is true during the REM, or dreaming, phase of sleep.) Activity also *decreases* in the parts of your brain that control your emotions, decision-making processes, and social interactions.

In addition to calming the fight-or-flight nervous system, sufficient rest and recuperation effectively reduce cortisol. A recent study published in *The Lancet* supports these claims, as it showed sleep deprivation caused stress hormones to rise in the evening and heightened the stress response during waking hours. Meanwhile, another study published in the *Journal of Clinical Endocrinology & Metabolism* in 2001 was one of the first to show that chronic insomnia leads to high cortisol and hyperactivity of our stress-response pathway in the brain.

We know high cortisol fuels appetite and makes us feel hungry, particularly for sugary and carb-laden treats, even when we have eaten enough, causing our blood sugars to spike, our insulin to soar, and, eventually, more unwanted fat to collect around the abdomen. After only a few nights of sleep deprivation, otherwise healthy people appear prediabetic on glucose tolerance tests, in that regulating blood sugar after a high-carbohydrate meal can take up to 40 percent longer than normal. Besides making us feel lousy, even short-term sleep debt can make us fat!

Sleep and Appetite

Sleep helps you to lose weight by influencing the hormones that control your appetite and increase your metabolism. A 2004 study at the University of Chicago was the first to show sleep as a major regulator of appetite-controlling hormones and also to link the extent of hormonal variations with the degree of hunger change. More specifically, researchers found *appetite-enhancing ghrelin increased* by 28 percent, whereas *appetite-curbing and metabolism-enhancing leptin decreased* by 18 percent among subjects who were sleep deprived. Appetite was not the only factor found to increase with lack of sleep. The desire for high-calorie, high-sugar foods also jumped with insufficient slumber.

In the same year, researchers at the Stanford School of Medicine found that subjects who had only 5 hours of sleep per night had less leptin, more ghrelin, and experienced an increase in their BMI, *regardless of diet and exercise.* Boy, even the most committed dieters are clearly fighting a losing battle if they do not get the rest they need.

HOT HORMONE FACT

WHY MEALS MAKE US SLEEPY
Scientists at the University of Manchester were the first to discover that the brain neurons that keep us awake and alert are turned off after we eat. It appears the sugar in the foods we eat tells the brain to stop producing orexin, the peptide that increases both appetite and wakefulness. This insight into the activity of orexin may explain why we tend to crave a nap after a big meal and also why we may have a tough time sleeping if we are hungry.

This is precisely why I have included sleep as the first of the three steps in your program for hormonal health and weight loss.

The Hormone Diet Sleep Solution: Four Steps for Hormone-Balancing Sleep

I love sleep. My life has the tendency to fall apart when I'm awake, you know?

—ERNEST HEMINGWAY

Let's face it, no one feels good after endless nights of tossing, turning, or staring at the ceiling. But besides leaving you feeling less than your best, poor sleep interferes with your hormonal balance, appetite control, and fat loss, *even when* your dietary and exercise routines are right on track. Lack of sleep also contributes to inflammation.

Real lasting changes in your body will occur only when you make total lifestyle adjustments. Correcting sleep problems is the first of these vital adjustments. So, try my simple, four-step plan for a lifetime of sweet slumber—although you may find that you require only the first two steps.

Step 1: Create the Ideal Environment for Hormone-Balancing Sleep

The look, feel, temperature, lighting, and sounds in your bedroom can either help or hinder your sleep. So before you ever hit the pillow, you have to make sure your space is set up to promote healthy sleep.

- **Make your room as dark as possible.** When you hit the hay, you should not be able to see your hand in front of your face. If you must use an alarm clock, turn it away from you. I use blackout curtains and recommend my patients do the same. Your children should also sleep in the dark. If they're afraid of the dark, try turning off the night light after they've drifted off to sleep. Why make your room a den of darkness?

When light hits your skin, it disrupts the circadian rhythm of the pineal gland and, as a result, hinders the production of melatonin. Studies have shown that even a small amount of light can cause a decrease in melatonin levels, which affects sleep, interferes with weight loss, and may increase your risk of cancer.

- **Use low lighting in your bedroom.** Once you settle into bed, avoid using overhead lights and lamps with high-wattage bulbs. My husband and I have replaced our overhead light fixture with a ceiling fan, and we each use our own clip-on or handheld book lights for reading. These are great for lighting only the page, rather than shining in your eyes or illuminating the entire room, which can potentially interfere with your sleep or your partner's.

- **Be aware of electromagnetic fields (EMFs) in your bedroom.** These can disrupt the pineal gland and the production of melatonin and serotonin. They may have additional negative effects, including increased risk of cancer. EMFs are emitted from digital alarm clocks and other electrical devices. If you must use these items, try to keep them as far away from the bed as possible—at least 3 feet away.

- **Turn off the TV, turn on your love life.** A television is another source of hormone-disrupting EMFs. Studies show that you will enjoy better sleep and more of it without a TV in the bedroom. Besides, you're also likely to have more sex when you ban the tube from your sleep space. The reasons why sex is so important for your hormonal balance, appetite control, and weight loss are explained in greater detail in Chapter 14, but basically, the more sex you have, the better your hormonal health. And the better your hormonal health, the more often you will have enjoyable sex. If you must have a TV simply to turn your mind off at the end of the day, use the timer function to make sure the set goes off if you fall asleep. That way you'll never wake from the noise or light from the TV. Also, keep the television at least 6 feet from the bed.

- **Use your bed for sleeping and sex only.** If you have kids, you know how easily your bedroom can become grand central station for the entire family. You should definitely avoid engaging in any other activities in bed, as you may start to associate the bedroom with sleep-robbing chores and tasks, rather than relaxing sleep and intimacy with your partner. Above all, *never* work in bed.

- **Create bedroom "Zen."** In my last two homes, I painted the bedroom in calming, dark, earthy tones. Shades like these help make the bedroom a relaxing place. Over the years I've also realized that clutter is a state of mind. Keeping your bedroom neat and clutter-free can be challenging, especially if you live in a small space. Just remember, the primary purposes of the bedroom are sleep and sex. You'll be amazed how much better both will be if you try to keep your bedside tables and dresser tops clear of clutter.

- **Choose comfortable, soothing bedding.** Several companies now offer organic cotton bedding lines that are free of harmful dyes and toxins. These can be a great investment if you have sensitive skin or simply care about the impact of heavy pesticide use on the environment. Personally, I find all-white bedding very soothing and welcoming after a long day of sensory overload. Whatever your taste dictates, select bedding that pleases your eye and feels good on your skin. You should also make sure your bedding keeps you warm but doesn't overheat you. In winter, you may wish to use a light duvet, whereas a thin blanket with a sheet might suffice for summer. Small changes like these will help create a calming, comfortable environment conducive to restful sleep.

- **Keep your bedroom cool but not cold.** No matter how chilly the weather gets outside, your bedroom temperature should be no warmer than 70°F for sleeping. Remember, your body needs to cool slightly at night to ensure the proper release of your sleep-inducing hormone, melatonin. At the same time, make sure your air conditioner is not blasting all night long in the summer. Research shows that over–air conditioning can cause weight gain.
- **Consider purchasing a white-noise device.** If you live in an apartment building or noisy neighborhood, you're probably familiar with the aggravation of being wakened by sounds. You may even wake when your partner walks around at night or snores. If you find you are easily wakened by sounds, the hum of a white-noise machine or a household fan may help. You can also try wearing earplugs to block out sleep-disrupting sounds.
- **Avoid using a loud alarm clock.** Waking up suddenly to the blaring wail of an alarm clock can be a shock to your body; you'll also find you feel groggier when you are roused in the middle of a sleep cycle. Getting enough sleep on a regular basis should make your alarm clock unnecessary. Sleeping through an alarm or relying on an alarm daily may indicate that you are sleep deprived. If you do use an alarm, you should awaken just before it goes off. If you must use one, I recommend the Bose alarm. It starts off at a moderate volume and slowly gets louder, so you aren't jarred out of your sleep. You can also investigate a sunrise alarm, an alarm clock with a natural light built in that simulates a sunrise. This method of waking has the added bonus of improving your mood and increasing your energy throughout the day.
- **If you go to the bathroom during the night, keep the lights off.** Even brief exposure to light can shut down the melatonin

production that's so crucial for good sleep. If you absolutely must use a light in the bathroom, try a flashlight or night light instead of the bright overhead light. Another option is to use a dimmer switch or a night light fitted with a red bulb, since red light exposure at night appears to have less of a negative impact.

- **Invest in a comfortable mattress.** Your mattress should be comfortable for you and your partner, not too hard or too soft. When my mom starting having hip and shoulder pain, we looked at a number of factors and finally came to the conclusion that her mattress was too hard. As soon as she changed it to a pillow-top mattress, the problem was solved. The right degree of firmness or softness is a personal thing, and your preference may change with age (just like my mom's did). If you need to shop for a new mattress, you may wish to consider the recommendations I've provided in Appendix B to reduce your exposure to toxins through your mattress.
- **Don't sleep with your pets or children.** Doing so may disrupt your precious sleep. Have them sleep in their own beds, instead.

Step 2: Implement the Hormone Diet Sleep-Right Rules

Once you've turned your bedroom into a healthy, sleep-inducing oasis, the next critical step is to start sleeping correctly. You may not have known that there is actually a proper way and time to sleep. It's true!

When, how, and how much we sleep is important. Failing to follow these recommendations can impede the fat-burning and hormone-balancing benefits you should gain from sleep each and every night.

Here are the Hormone Diet guidelines for hormone-enhancing sleep.

- **Sleep in complete darkness.** Again, even a small amount of light can hamper your sleep.
- **Sleep nude** (or at least with loose-fitting nightclothes—but nude is better). Do not sleep in tight undergarments (bras, girdles, briefs, etc.). Tight clothing will increase your body temperature and interfere with melatonin release while you sleep.
- **Establish regular sleeping hours.** Try to get up each morning and go to bed every night at roughly the same time. Oversleeping can be as detrimental as sleep deprivation. How you feel each day is an important indication of how much sleep is right for you.
- **Get to bed by 11 p.m.** Since the invention of electricity (not to mention television and computers), we have begun staying up later and later. This change has resulted in a largely sleep-deprived society. Our stress glands, the adrenals, recharge or recover most between 11 p.m. and 1 a.m. Going to bed before 11 p.m. (in fact, 10 p.m. is even better) is optimal for rebuilding your adrenal reserves. I know this can be difficult to achieve, so I recommend my patients start going to bed 15 minutes earlier each week until they reach their new target time.
- **Sleep 7 to 9 hours each night.** The American Cancer Society has found higher incidences of cancer in individuals who consistently sleep fewer than 6 hours or more than 9 hours nightly. Oversleeping is just as harmful as sleep deprivation. Consistently needing more than 9 hours of sleep every night warrants a visit to your doctor for further investigation, as this may indicate an underlying medical condition such as hypothyroidism or depression, or a deficiency of iron, folic acid, or vitamin B_{12} (though some of us simply require more or less sleep than others). If you awaken without an alarm and feel rested, you're likely getting the right amount of sleep for you.

- **See the light first thing in the morning.** Daylight and morning sounds are key signals that help waken your brain. Turning on the lights or opening the blinds is the proper way to reset your body clock and ensure that your melatonin levels drop back to "awake" mode until the evening. Exposure to morning light has also been proven to be one of the simplest ways to increase your energy for the entire day. It's also been shown to boost testosterone in men and fertility in women by stimulating luteinizing hormone release from the pituitary gland. Enhance this action further by exposing yourself to sunlight and by getting outside during the day. I can't say enough about the benefits of getting outside, even for 10 to 20 minutes in the morning light.
- **Keep household lighting dim from dinnertime until you go to sleep.** Believe it or not, this simple step not only prepares your body and hormones for sleep, but it also helps your digestion.

Step 3: Use These Tips If You Have Difficulty Falling or Staying Asleep

After many years of doing things the same old way, many of us tend to develop and grow accustomed to poor sleep habits. As with any bad habit, you must break the cycle by *retraining* your body and mind to sleep again. Whether you have problems falling asleep, wake up frequently throughout the night, wake too early, or experience poor-quality sleep overall, implement as many of these lifestyle modifications as possible. If your sleep disruption is severe or chronic, you may also want to begin using one or more of the natural sleep aids I have suggested as the fourth step.

- **Avoid stimulating activities before bed, such as watching TV or using the computer.** Computer use in the evening raises dopamine and noradrenaline, our brain-stimulating hormones that should naturally be higher during the daytime. In the evening, engage in calming activities or those that involve focusing on one thing, such as reading or meditation, which make you more serotonin dominant. Choose relaxing reading materials that have nothing to do with your work or career. Stop all your work-related activities at least 2 hours before bed. Allow yourself some downtime. Watching television can also be too stimulating for some people; if you suspect this is true for you, break your bedtime TV habit!

- **Develop a calming bedtime routine.** Breaking bad habits often requires cultivating good ones. Reading something spiritual or listening to soft music can become cues that help train your body and mind to relax. Choose your nighttime reading carefully—if it's too enticing, you may stay up too late reading; if it's upsetting or emotional, you may find falling asleep more difficult. Select books, music, or other soothing stimuli that make you feel good and help take your mind *off* the stresses of daily life.

- **If you cannot sleep, get out of bed and do something else until you feel the urge to sleep.** Tossing and turning in bed only leaves you feeling frustrated. Try getting up for a while, but keep the lights low and the TV and computer off. Staring at the clock will also make your sleepless situation worse, so remove the clock from view while you are in bed.

- **Make a to-do list or try writing in a journal.** If you find you often lie awake in bed with endless thoughts of what you must do or things you have done churning through your head, get out of bed and write down your feelings. You'll be surprised by how much relief this process can provide.

- **Exercise at the right time.** Exercising fewer than 3 hours before bedtime may be too stimulating and can impede your ability to fall asleep. Yoga and strength training are exceptions, as these activities are often less stimulating than cardiovascular exercise. Working out 3 to 6 hours before bed, on the other hand, will help you maximize the benefits of exercise on sleep, since the body actually increases deep sleep to compensate for the physical stress of your workout. Exercise also promotes healthy sleep patterns because of its positive effect on body temperature. After a workout, your body gradually cools down, which naturally makes you sleepy. To relax your muscles and trigger the sleep response after exercise, try a hot bath with Epsom salts. Soak in water as hot as you can stand with 1 to 2 cups of Epsom salts for at least 20 minutes. Place a cold towel around your neck if you feel too warm while in the bath.

- **Exercise your mind, too.** Try the daily crossword or Sudoku. People who are intellectually and mentally stimulated during the day feel an increased need to sleep to maintain their performance. Uninterested or bored people do not sleep as well.

- **Take a hot bath, shower, or sauna before bed.** As it does with exercise, your body will naturally cool down after a hot bath or shower, making you feel sleepier. Take a hot bath about 2 hours before bedtime, keeping the water hot for at least 25 minutes to stimulate the drop in body temperature that makes us tired. Again, add Epsom salts to detoxify your body and relax your muscles. An

> **INFRARED SAUNA FOR DETOX**
> Infrared radiation penetrates about $1/2$ inch into the skin to heat the body without significantly heating the air or our core body temperature. The skin is the largest organ in your body and one of the main detoxification pathways. Deeply heating the skin and subcutaneous fat, and the good sweat that comes with it, is one of the most effective ways to reduce toxin accumulation, eliminate harmful heavy metals, aid weight loss, stimulate circulation, curb cellulite, and enhance health. We have one of these at Clear Medicine clinic, and you can also check the resource section if you are interested in an infrared sauna.

HOT HORMONE FACT

infrared sauna is also a great option for detox, weight loss, and aiding sleep. See the resource section for your options.

- **Avoid napping.** If you are getting enough sleep at night, you shouldn't feel tired during the day. Craving a snooze in the afternoon is a good indication that you are sleep deprived, and in reality, napping will not make the situation better. Staying awake until nighttime is best, but if you have to catch a nap during the day, keep it to a maximum of 30 minutes.

- **Avoid caffeine at any time of the day.** Caffeine may be metabolized at different rates in different people. A dose of caffeine usually takes 15 to 30 minutes to take effect and lasts for 4 to 5 hours. In some people, it may last much longer, making caffeine use in the afternoon a bad idea. If you must have caffeine, limit it to small amounts in the morning only. Caffeine may also negatively affect the natural release cycle of cortisol, which is generally highest in the morning and lowest in the evening. Cortisol release rises slightly at 2 a.m. and 4 a.m., then hits its peak around 6 a.m. If this pattern is disrupted, you may awaken at these times and find you are unable to fall back asleep. Although this may sound inconceivable, cutting out caffeine has amazing effects on your energy—within only a week or two!

- **Avoid bedtime snacks that are high in sugar or simple carbohydrates.** Carbohydrate-rich snacks such as breads, cereals, muffins, cookies, and other baked goods prompt a short-term spike in blood sugar, followed by a sugar crash later on. When blood sugar drops, adrenaline, glucagon, cortisol, and growth hormone are released to regulate blood glucose levels. These hormones can stimulate the brain, causing you to awaken and possibly stay awake. Try to avoid eating for at least 2 hours before going to bed. If you do need to eat something, reach for a protein-rich, high-fiber snack, such as a few almonds and half an apple. Protein provides the amino acid tryptophan. The body converts tryptophan to serotonin and melatonin, hormones that are important for sleep. The sugars from the fruit may also help the tryptophan reach your brain and take effect more readily.

- **Try to avoid fluids in the 2 hours before bedtime.** Keeping drinks to a minimum before bed will reduce the likelihood—or frequency—of sleep-sabotaging trips to the bathroom. Remember, if you must answer the call of nature during the night, try to keep the lights off or as dim as possible. Men experiencing frequent trips to the bathroom due to a prostate concern may benefit from Bell Prostate Ezee Flow Tea, available at most health food stores.

- **Go easy on the alcohol.** Yes, a few drinks can make you feel drowsy, but the effect is short-lived. The body metabolizes alcohol as you sleep, which can result in sleep interruption. Alcohol may cause sleep disorders because it appears to affect brain chemicals that influence sleep. It may alter the amount of time it takes to fall asleep, shorten total sleep time, and possibly prevent you from falling into the deeper stages of sleep—the stages in which your body does most of its healing. One glass of wine with dinner isn't likely to affect your sleep, since it takes about 90 minutes to metabolize 1 ounce of alcohol. One ounce or more within 2 hours of bedtime, however, may unpleasantly disrupt your sleep.

- **Complete your meditation or visualizations (further described in Chapter 9) in the evening.** These are highly effective techniques to reduce or eliminate body tension and anxiety. They can help calm your mind, relax your muscles, and allow restful sleep to ensue. Much like a physical workout, exercise that involves deep breathing or progressive relaxation, such as yoga and meditation, is excellent not only for your sleep, but also for your life.

Step 4: Use Natural Sleep Aids to Ease Sleep Disruptions

When taken properly and for the right reasons, natural supplements can be very effective at improving the quality and quantity of your sleep, with few—if any—side effects. If you have followed all my hormone-balancing sleep tips for 2 weeks and still do not see an improvement in your sleep, natural sleep aids are your next best option.

The most important step in selecting a natural sleep aid is to first determine the cause of your sleep disruption, because different supplements can be more effective than others for specific sleep-robbing conditions. Difficulty falling or staying asleep may result from stress, vitamin or mineral deficiency, excess caffeine intake, certain medications, menopause, anxiety, depression, low melatonin, muscle tension, pain, and a whole host of other reasons too numerous to list. Fortunately, many herbal remedies, vitamins, minerals, amino acids, and hormones are available to assist you in your quest for a good night's rest.

Understand that finding the right sleep remedy for you may be a trial-and-error process. You may also wish to combine a few products to create the perfect "sleep cocktail" for your needs. My favorite sleep remedy is two tablets of a calcium-magnesium combination (about 300 to 500 mg of each in a citrate base for better absorption) and two or three capsules of a product called Seditol (available through my Web site and some health food stores, it's a patented herbal blend of extracts of *Magnolia officinalis* and *Ziziphus spinosa*). Taken at bedtime, it works like a charm to combat the most common cause of sleep disruption—stress! But here's a list of other options you can choose from.

GABA: A FAVORITE CHOICE FOR RELIEVING TENSION, ANXIETY, AND PAIN WITH SLEEP DISRUPTION

GABA is an inhibitory neurotransmitter—a brain chemical that has a calming effect. It's well suited for individuals who experience anxiety, muscle tension, or pain.

Take 500 to 1,000 mg before bed. Alternatively, take GABA 10 to 20 minutes before meals, beginning with your evening meal. The standard dose of 200 mg four times daily can be increased to a maximum of 500 mg four times daily, if needed. The latter dosage should not be exceeded, and you should reduce the dose if you experience loose stools.

TAURINE

Taurine is an amino acid that plays a major role in the brain as an inhibitory neurotransmitter. Comparable in structure and function with GABA, taurine provides a similar antianxiety effect that helps calm or stabilize an excited mind. Taurine has many other uses, including treating migraines, insomnia, agitation, restlessness, irritability, alcoholism, obsessions, depression, and even hypomania/mania—the "high" phase of bipolar disorder or manic depression.

By inhibiting the release of adrenaline, taurine also protects us from anxiety and other adverse effects of stress. It even helps control high blood pressure and improves the action of insulin. You may have noticed it as an ingredient in some of the energizing, high-caffeine soft drinks, as it is used to soften overstimulation.

Take 500 to 1,000 mg a day. Taking the last dose right before bed is often most helpful. Taurine should be taken without food.

TRYPTOPHAN

Tryptophan is an amino acid that is the building block of serotonin. Remember, serotonin is our "happy hormone," essential to mood, sleep, memory, and appetite. Tryptophan is effective for insomnia related to depression or to a deficiency of serotonin.

Take 500 to 1,000 mg at bedtime. Note that tryptophan supplements are available by prescription only and should be taken with 50 mg of vitamin B_6. It's most effective when taken on an empty stomach or with a piece of fruit.

5-HTP: A FAVORITE CHOICE FOR DEPRESSION, ANXIETY, EATING DISORDERS, AND CONDITIONS ASSOCIATED WITH PAIN

A derivative of tryptophan that's also used to create serotonin, 5-HTP has been found to be more effective than tryptophan for treating sleep loss related to depression, anxiety, and fibromyalgia. And 5-HTP appears to increase REM sleep. It also decreases the amount of time required to fall asleep and the number of nighttime awakenings.

Take 50 to 400 mg a day, divided into doses throughout the day and before bed. Take it with food if you experience nausea.

MELATONIN: A FAVORITE CHOICE FOR AGES 50+ (ESPECIALLY THOSE WITH HIGH BLOOD PRESSURE) AND SHIFT WORKERS

Melatonin decreases as we age, as well as during times of stress and depression. New research shows it may also be useful for reducing high blood pressure. Supplements are usually only effective for insomnia in people younger than 45 to 50 when melatonin levels are low. To determine if your levels are deficient, I suggest a saliva test for melatonin. You can request a test kit from www.thehormonediet.com.

Take 0.5 to 3 mg at bedtime. Try opening up capsules and pouring them under your tongue. You can also purchase melatonin in sublingual form for ready absorption.

L-THEANINE: A FAVORITE CHOICE FOR REDUCING ANXIETY AND BOOSTING DAYTIME ENERGY

L-theanine is your best choice for relaxation and tension relief throughout the *day*. A calming amino acid naturally found in green tea, it's known to support relaxation without causing drowsiness. L-theanine works by increasing the production of GABA in the brain. Similar to the effects of meditation, it also stimulates alpha brain waves naturally associated with deep states of relaxation and enhanced mental clarity. L-theanine may increase learning, attention, and sensations of pleasure as well. These effects are likely due to the natural dopamine boost brought on by L-theanine.

Take 50 to 200 mg of L-theanine without food. In very high-stress situations, 100 mg to a maximum of 600 mg can be taken every 6 hours.

MILK PROTEIN HYDROLYSATE CONCENTRATE (CASEIN TRYPTIC HYDROLYSATE OR CASEIN HYDROLYSATE): A FAVORITE CHOICE FOR ANY SLEEP OR STRESS CONDITION

Regardless of whether the stress you experience is physical, emotional, psychological, or environmental, milk protein hydrolysate is documented to prevent the associated rise in cortisol by calming your brain's stress pathway. This product can be used to address all types of sleep disruption and to reduce the harmful effects of sleep deprivation, stress, anxiety, or depression. It's safe to say that this product got me through writing this book!

Take 75 to 300 mg a day. Try opening the capsules and pouring the contents under your tongue for rapid sleep or stress relief.

ASHWAGANDHA: A FAVORITE CHOICE FOR BUSY EXECUTIVES OR PATIENTS WITH UNDERACTIVE THYROID

Ayurvedic medicine practitioners use this dietary supplement to enhance mental and physical performance, improve learning ability, and decrease stress and fatigue. Ashwagandha is a general tonic that can be used in stressful situations, especially insomnia, restlessness, or when you are feeling overworked. Studies have indicated that ashwagandha offers anti-inflammatory, anticancer, antistress, antioxidant, immune-modulating, and rejuvenating properties.

The typical dosage is 500 to 1,000 mg twice daily. Capsules should be standardized to 1.5 percent withanolides per dose.

RELORA: A FAVORITE CHOICE FOR ALL TYPES OF STRESS, DEPRESSION, AND ANXIETY

A mixture of the herbal extracts *Magnolia officinalis* and *Phellodendron amurense*, Relora is medically proven to reduce stress and anxiety. This natural sleep aid is my favorite choice for patients who tend to wake up throughout the night, for highly stressed individuals, and for menopausal women with hot flashes that cause sleep disruption. It can significantly reduce cortisol and raise DHEA within only 2 weeks of use.

In a study published by University of Mississippi professor Dr. Walter Chamblis in the *Journal of Psychopharmacology* (2001), 78 percent of participants reported greater feelings of relaxation and well-being when taking Relora. Seventy-four percent said they experienced better sleep when using the supplement.

Relora can be used to prevent the health conditions associated with stress, including poor immunity, high blood pressure, insomnia, sleep disruption, loss of vitality, and weight gain, especially in relation to metabolic syndrome.

Take two 250 mg capsules at bedtime and one upon rising. It is best taken without food. I find the most effective formula contains a mixture of B vitamins and folic acid as well.

PASSIONFLOWER

Passionflower is the herb of choice for insomnia. It aids the transition into restful sleep without the narcotic hangover sometimes associated with pharmaceutical sleep aids. As an antispasmodic, it is helpful in treating tension and stress. It can also be effective in the treatment of nerve pain such as neuralgia and the viral infection shingles.

Passionflower extracts have been studied for their potential ability to decrease anxiety and prolong sleeping time. They have also been tested in combination with other sedative and antianxiety herbs such as valerian. Findings suggest that passionflower may enhance the effectiveness of these other treatments, and together with valerian it may reduce the stress hormone NPY. It may also reduce muscle spasms and decrease pain in some instances.

Take a 100 mg capsule (standardized extract) twice daily to alleviate anxiety.

VITAMIN B6

Vitamin B$_6$ is useful to help correct abnormally high cortisol release throughout the night. Those who wake frequently, particularly at about 2, 4, and 6 a.m., will benefit most from this supplement.

Take 50 to 100 mg before bed.

PHOSPHATIDYLSERINE

Phosphatidylserine is ideal for nighttime worrying, as it influences the inappropriate release of stress hormones and protects the brain from the negative effects of cortisol.

Take 100 to 300 mg before bed.

SPECIFICALLY FOR RESTLESS LEG SYNDROME (RLS)

RLS is a neurological disorder characterized by severe, uncomfortable sensations in the legs, especially prevalent while lying down. Supplements of folic acid, iron, magnesium, and vitamin E may provide some relief from the unpleasant, sleep-disrupting symptoms of RLS. Supplements such as phenylalanine and L-tyrosine that increase dopamine, involved in motor function and muscle tension, can also be of benefit, but these are best taken in the morning or during the early afternoon rather than at nighttime because they are energy enhancing.

CHAPTER 8

YOUR ANTI-INFLAMMATORY DETOX:
LOOK AND FEEL BETTER IN JUST 2 WEEKS

These are the hormonal benefits you will enjoy from the Anti-Inflammatory Detox:

- Improved hormonal balance and fat burning with better liver function
- Relief from the effects of harmful excess estrogen
- Reduced insulin and less inflammation
- Restored serotonin activity and enhanced mood, memory, and focus
- Maximized activity of thyroid hormone, our metabolic master
- Support of the breakdown and clearance of cortisol from the body
- Better appetite control, freedom from cravings, and enhanced fat burning through improved leptin levels

Now that you have worked on establishing better habits for sound, restorative sleep, you're ready for the next process in the Hormone Diet plan—ridding your body of hormone-disrupting toxins and fat-packing inflammation.

Toxins Make Us Fat!

Whether we realize it or not, we are constantly exposed to toxins. Potentially harmful compounds enter our bodies in the form of pesticides, fertilizers, hormone-based food additives, prescription and over-the-counter drugs, air pollution, fumes, heavy metals, and even the skin-care products we use every day. Toxins are also naturally found in our body as the end products of the metabolic process and bacterial waste.

No matter whether we consume them via our foods, inhale them from our surroundings, or absorb them through our skin, toxins can pile up in our systems, especially when our natural toxin-elimination mechanisms are not functioning optimally. Even worse, an accumulation of toxins in the body can interfere with our hormones, neurotransmitters, and nervous system activity, resulting in weight gain and a host of health problems.

Toxins affect many of the hormones that influence our body composition and ability to lose weight, including thyroid hormone, testosterone, estrogen, insulin, cortisol, and leptin. Some toxins can mimic particular hormones, causing abnormal activity. Like a stranger finding your house key and letting himself in, other toxins can sneak in and take the place of our hormones in their normal receptor sites. In this case, the stranger puts his own key in your lock, but cannot open it because the key does not fit. But as long as the wrong key is stuck in the lock, the correct key cannot get in to open the door.

Tons of Toxins

Over 80,000 industrial chemicals have been developed in the past 75 years, including heavy metals, solvents, phthalates, polychlorinated bisphenols, and organophosphates. Exposure to industrial chemicals such as pesticides, dyes, perfumes, flavorings, and plastics, even in *extremely small quantities,* has been shown to significantly increase the body mass of mice—and men, too! Many of these chemicals are endocrine blockers that disrupt our hormones and increase fat storage. I could dedicate an entire book to the full list of chemical offenders, but I've narrowed my discussion here to two of the biggies: bisphenol and phthalates.

Bisphenol-A (BPA)

Research has shown that bisphenol, a chemical commonly found in most plastics (including water bottles), alters fat cells when it interacts with insulin. Bisphenol has been found to spark and accelerate two of the biological mechanisms underlying obesity: an increase in the number of fat cells in the body and the enhancement of their fat-storing capabilities. So the presence of this chemical can influence not only the production of more fat cells, but also their increase in size!

Phthalates

Phthalates are a group of chemical compounds used in many household items, including water bottles, soaps, shampoos, and cosmetics, plastic containers, toys, pipes, and even medicines. Current estimates suggest that more than 75 percent of North Americans have significant levels of phthalates in their urine.

Phthalates offer a fascinating, yet frightening, example of the interrelationship of hormonal balance, reproductive health, and obesity. High exposure to this and other toxins can lead to compromised ovarian function, inhibited sperm motility, and the early onset of puberty. Phthalates, in particular, have been connected to reproductive problems in baby boys, smaller penis sizes, testicular problems in adolescents, and poor semen and testosterone production in men. Researchers at the University of Rochester Medical Center have now linked this phthalate-induced reduction in testosterone to abdominal obesity, insulin resistance, and the onset of type 2 diabetes in men. The study, published in *Environmental Health Perspectives* (March 2007), showed that the highest levels of phthalate metabolites appeared in the urine of men with abdominal obesity and insulin resistance.

We Are Terribly Estrogen Toxic, Too

In Chapter 3, I discussed estrogen dominance as one of the main causes of hormonal imbalance and obesity. Besides the estrogen we produce naturally, we tend to accumulate even more of it in our lifetime, thanks to an abundance of estrogen and estrogenlike compounds in our environment. Because of mounting health concerns, the World Health Organization (WHO) has sanctioned a review of endocrine-disrupting chemicals, especially those with estrogenic activity linked to prostate and breast cancer. A study published in the *Journal of Environmental Health Perspectives* by researchers at the University of Texas showed that even minuscule concentrations of estrogen-upsetting chemicals in our environment are capable of causing endocrine disruption within just 30 seconds of exposure.

Canadian and British researchers have discovered a disturbing proliferation of hermaphrodite fish in the Great Lakes due to the presence of estrogens in the water. These hormones have made their way into the lakes in the form of industrial chemicals, oral contraceptives, hormone replacement therapy drugs, and raw sewage from women who use these products. Scientists initially noticed that certain species of male fish were developing eggs. Just 2 years later, the same fish population was almost completely wiped out because their reproductive capabilities were ravaged. Scary.

On an even more chilling note, what happens to us when we drink this water or eat these fish? Researchers from the University of Pittsburgh School of Medicine may have some insight. They treated cultured breast cancer cells with extracts from the estrogen-laden fish. Once exposed to the fish extracts, the cancer cells grew more rapidly!

Your Body's Natural Toxin-Cleansing Team

Our liver, kidneys, and small intestine are the body's natural cleaning team, working together to package toxic compounds for removal. Over time, the function of these organs, especially the liver, can be compromised by illness, poor nutrition, stress, pollution, or toxic lifestyle habits (e.g., using drugs, alcohol, or tobacco).

When the cleanup process is not being carried out as it should, toxic byproducts cannot be properly neutralized. As a result, toxic compounds from the liver are reabsorbed and stored in the fatty tissues of the body rather than excreted. As you would expect, this toxic buildup leads to a dramatic increase in long-term health risks—and it doesn't leave us feeling our best in the short term, either. Complaints such as headaches, weight gain, acne, PMS, infertility, and poor memory often arise when our detox organs are in need of some support.

Let's talk about *how* the Hormone Diet detox actually works to restore your body balance before delving into the details of your action plan. It tackles toxins and inflammation via the five keys to healthy digestion and by supporting healthy liver function.

The Five Keys to Healthy Digestion

KEY 1: REDUCE INFLAMMATION BY REMOVING FOOD SENSITIVITIES

Heartburn, headaches, difficulty getting out of bed in the morning, feeling and looking tired even after sufficient sleep, an inability to lose weight, bloating, and relentless water retention can all be related to food sensitivities or intolerances. Because the connection between the symptom and a specific food can be difficult to pinpoint, those who suffer these discomforts often go on feeling worse and worse as their immune system takes a constant beating.

Many of us with food sensitivities don't even realize how bad we feel until the problematic foods are removed from our diet. Then suddenly getting out of bed becomes easier; our energy, mood, and concentration improve; and joint pain, headaches, and sinus congestion disappear.

During your anti-inflammatory detox, you'll take the most allergenic foods out of your diet for a specific period of time to give your body a break and a chance to calm down and detoxify. Slowly reintroducing each food after a 10-day break can allow you to connect particular symptoms with your food choices.

All that experimenting with different foods may sound like a major inconvenience, but the results can be invaluable. For example, I see little point in eating cottage cheese as a source of low-fat protein if it contributes to chronic sinusitis, abdominal cramping, acne, or digestive upset. Why not go for an alternative source of protein that's just as effective for fat loss, but that still allows you to look and feel great?

Perhaps the possibility of reducing the appearance of cellulite might provide you with more encouragement. Did you ever think that those pesky pockets of cellulite could actually be caused by an allergic reaction? Well, the immune response to food proteins may indirectly contribute to increased amounts of cellulite. A delayed allergic reaction to foods may occur within blood vessels, causing inflammation in the vessel walls and subsequently triggering clotting mechanisms. This increased inflammation in the arteries and capillaries may contribute to poor circulation, a known cause of cellulite and reduced lymphatic drainage. Believe it or not, avoiding food intolerances (and following the other recommendations outlined in later steps of the Hormone Diet) may diminish the appearance of cellulite and stop its formation for good.

The results we have seen at Clear Medicine with patients who have discovered their food sensitivities are remarkable. I recall one patient who had suffered with headaches for 20 years—they were gone after just 2 weeks of avoiding wheat. Another woman had bleeding from the bowel for 2 years—it was gone after a single week on a dairy-free diet. A flight attendant who complained of water retention and swelling so bad that she was unable to wear her shoes at the end of the day shed 14 pounds and her water-retention problem after only 4 weeks of eliminating corn and wheat.

Uncovering food sensitivities is a powerful process that I encourage all of my patients to explore. But what you do with the information is up to you. Once you have determined the effects of particular foods on your health, *you* have to decide whether you want to continue eating them.

An estimated 30 percent of North Americans have low stomach acidity. Natural aging, a poor diet, and chronic use of certain medications such as corticosteroids, antibiotics, and antacids can impair your stomach's ability to produce acid. Certain medical conditions are also commonly associated with low stomach acid, including hypothyroidism, asthma, eczema, allergies, acne rosacea, adrenal dysfunction, osteoporosis, autoimmune disease, psoriasis, and chronic hives.

The signs and symptoms of low acidity in the stomach or digestive enzymes include the following:

- Bloating, belching, and gas, especially after meals
- Indigestion
- Constipation
- Heartburn or reflux
- Multiple food allergies
- Feeling nauseated after taking supplements
- Weak, peeling, and cracked fingernails
- Redness or dilated blood vessels in the cheeks and nose
- Adult acne
- Hair loss in women
- Iron deficiency
- Undigested food in the stools
- Chronic yeast infections

Even though the removal of allergenic foods during a detox is often all that's needed to eliminate uncomfortable bloating or gas, it's not always the solution. If you continue to wake with a flat stomach but look as if you're 5 months pregnant by the end of the day, take animal- or plant-based enzymes with your meals. And if you're searching for a simple way to check for low stomach acidity, look at your fingernails. Chances are your stomach acid levels are low if you see lengthwise (not sideways) ridges. I, however, recommend a more specific test that's easy to do at home: the HCl challenge. Visit www.thehormonediet.com for instructions on how to complete this simple test that can help you to determine whether you have the appropriate level of hydrochloric acid (HCl) in your stomach for optimal digestion. But don't do this test if you have ulcers.

KEY 3: REESTABLISH HEALTHY BACTERIAL BALANCE
The maintenance and protection of our healthy digestive-tract bacteria through proper nutrition and, if necessary, supplementation, is very important to good health. Under normal circumstances, friendly bacteria found in our digestive system live with us in symbiotic harmony, but factors such as poor diet and medications such as birth control pills, antibiotics, and corticosteroids can upset this balance and lead to a host of difficulties.

We now know these live microorganisms are cancer protective, immune enhancing, and anti-inflammatory. Other documented benefits of probiotics include the following:

1. **Relief of all types of digestive system upset.** This includes diarrhea, constipation, gas, bloating, etc.
2. **Less fat storage.** Research completed at the Department of Genomic Sciences at the University of Washington found increased fat storage in rats lacking probiotics.
3. **Hormonal balance.** Bacteria in the digestive tract play a hugely important role in the breakdown of excess estrogen. If you are taking the birth control pill, be sure to use a probiotic supplement regularly to avoid the unfavorable symptoms of excess estrogen including weight gain, especially around the hips and thighs.
4. **Vitamin production and nutrient absorption.** This includes vitamins K, B_{12}, and B_5, as well as biotin.

5. **Prevention of yeast infections.** If you're a woman with recurrent yeast infections, the bacterial balance in your large intestine is compromised and you would likely benefit from a probiotic supplement.
6. **Elimination of bad breath.** Eating plain organic yogurt or taking probiotic supplements for 6 weeks or more can help fight certain chemicals in the mouth that contribute to bad breath and gingivitis.
7. **Inflammation control.** Probiotics are proven to be beneficial for relieving symptoms of inflammation, including arthritis, ulcerative colitis, and Crohn's disease.
8. **Allergy relief.** Allergy-based symptoms such as eczema, seasonal allergies, asthma, and hives have been found to improve with probiotic supplements.
9. **Prevention of colds and flus.** Daycare- and school-age children who take supplements of acidophilus and bifidus are sick less often. Supplementing with beneficial bacteria also stimulates immunity in adults, strengthening our resistance to bacterial and viral infections.

KEY 4: RESOLVE INFLAMMATION AND POOR IMMUNITY
BY REPAIRING THE DIGESTIVE-TRACT WALL

The competency of the entire wall of the digestive tract is dependent on healthy food choices, bacterial balance, sufficient enzymes and acid levels, and inflammation control. An imbalance in any one of these important factors may result in an irritation of the digestive-tract wall. When that happens, tiny holes may form, allowing partially digested material, toxins, or bacteria to pass through. In the short term, this problem, also known as *leaky gut syndrome*, causes symptoms of digestive upset, gas, bloating, pain, weakened immunity, and allergic symptoms. In the long term, a compromised digestive tract wall can lead to toxic weight gain, obesity, allergies, depressed immunity, autoimmune disease, attention-deficit/hyperactivity disorder (ADHD), depression, and joint inflammation or disease.

Several supplements can help repair a damaged digestive-tract wall. These include glutamine, deglycyrrhizinated licorice (DGL), aloe vera, plantain, and marshmallow. With the exception of glutamine, these products are known as demulcents because they help coat and heal the digestive-tract wall. Most, if not all, of us can use help to repair our gut wall, which is why I have recommended a gut-healing and detoxifying fiber supplement as part of your detox protocol.

KEY 5: REDUCE NEGATIVE EFFECTS OF STRESS ON DIGESTION
Your digestive system has as many nerves as your spinal cord. (So when you get a gut instinct, go with it!) Unfortunately, this design leaves our digestive system susceptible to the effects of stress. When the "fight-or-flight" nervous system is stimulated, digestive function effectively shuts down, as bloodflow to the area is redirected to our limbs. Chronic stress is known to bring on symptoms of irritable bowel syndrome, such as constipation or diarrhea, and to exacerbate symptoms of inflammatory bowel diseases.

In a study published in the *British Medical Journal* (February 2007), researchers found that irritable bowel syndrome (IBS) patients were significantly more likely to report high levels of stress and anxiety. They were also prone to be driven individuals who would carry on *regardless* of their level of discomfort until they were forced to rest— a pattern of behavior known to worsen and prolong the condition.

Determining which comes first, the emotional state or the digestive symptoms, can be difficult. Those of us who suffer from IBS may learn as children to cope with stressful situations by developing digestive symptoms. Other research suggests that IBS sufferers have difficulty adapting to life situations in general, though that is tough to assess.

One of my favorite supplements for patients experiencing stress or anxiety along with digestive issues is the amino acid 5-hydroxytryptophan (5-HTP). As a precursor to serotonin, 5-HTP can help alleviate both concerns since most of this "happy hormone" is produced by cells around your digestive tract and not, as you might have guessed, in your brain. This connection has prompted researchers to develop new medications that influence serotonin for the purpose of treating irritable bowel syndrome.

The Lasting Benefits of the Five Keys to Great Digestion

The first 2 weeks of the Hormone Diet center on optimizing your sleep, enhancing immunity, reducing stress, conquering inflammation, and improving digestion—all at once. This is good news, considering the astounding number of people who are plagued by these health problems. The steps outlined here offer many other positive benefits as well, including more energy, glowing skin, stronger mental focus, less joint pain and stiffness, and, of course, fat loss.

Moving on from the digestive system, we should now discuss the other primary organ responsible for ridding us of toxins, aiding fat burning, and clearing the body of waste—the liver. Your liver is also a major player in achieving hormonal balance because it controls the production of certain hormones, such as your fat-burning friend T3 thyroid hormone, and the breakdown of others, such as the fat-burning foe cortisol.

An Unhappy Liver Hinders Detoxification and Fat Loss

Similar to the way it does in our muscles, fat burning in the liver occurs through a complex pathway involving our PPARs (peroxisome proliferator-activated receptors). A 2006 study published in the *American Journal of Physiology—Gastroenterology and Liver Physiology* reported that toxins, including drugs and alcohol, can cause abnormalities in the fat-burning pathways of the liver. This causes less fat burning, and leads to increased storage of fat in the body and possibly *in* our liver cells, too. Over time, excess fat stored in liver cells can be harmful to liver structure and impair its function. In the past, a fatty liver was most often associated with excess alcohol intake. However, rising rates of obesity, diabetes, insulin resistance, high cholesterol, high blood pressure, and elevated triglycerides are now the main culprits behind the greater prevalence of fatty liver disease. According to research from the Mayo Clinic, this condition may affect as many as one-third of American adults. More recently, as of September 2008, experts think that as much as 10 percent of overweight children and half of those who are obese may suffer from fatty liver.

Is It Time for a Detox?

Besides all of these larger issues, there is a very basic reason why I suggest beginning your health restoration and fat-loss program with a liver and bowel detox. The signs and symptoms of hormonal imbalance and ill health are often completely resolved when body detoxification is supported. No more symptoms, no need for further, unnecessary treatment. What could be better?

But here are a few questions you can ask yourself to determine your detox need:

- Do you feel tired or lethargic?
- Do you have difficulty concentrating or staying focused?
- Do you experience frequent colds or flus?
- Do you have joint pain or stiffness?
- Do you have frequent headaches?
- Have you had a change in body odor or taste in your mouth?
- Do you have dark circles under your eyes?
- Does your skin lack luster?
- Are you overweight?
- Do you have acne, eczema, or psoriasis?
- Do you have constipation (less than one bowel movement per day)?
- Do you have gas, bloating, or indigestion?

- Do you look puffy or bloated?
- Do you have high cholesterol or fatty liver disease?

The more yes responses you have, the greater your need for a natural, anti-inflammatory detox!

By following the nutrition and supplement guidelines presented in this chapter, you will successfully complete your body detox in just 2 weeks. I recommend going through this body detox process at least twice a year, preferably in the spring and fall. Your health is absolutely worth the investment. (At this stage, you may also want to refer to Appendix B to discover ways you can detoxify your space.)

Getting Started with Your Body Detox

Stick to this anti-inflammatory diet for 14 days. If you're currently experiencing symptoms (fatigue, headaches, gas, bloating, heartburn, acne, eczema, etc.) and find that they are still present at the end of the 2-week period, you *can* extend your cleanse up to 6 weeks before moving on. Otherwise, on Day 11, you'll begin reintroducing some of the foods you've temporarily removed from your diet.

Before you get started, you should eat up (or get rid of) your current supplies of the foods that aren't allowed during your detox. This will help you to avoid cheating or falling off the wagon. Plan your meals according to the detox rules. Shop for specific foods and supplements, and make sure all of your social commitments involving alcohol are out of the way before you begin.

Since the focus is determining food sensitivities and reducing inflammation during these 14 days, caloric intake is not the crucial matter. You should, however, consume at least three meals per day that contain a detox-friendly protein source (egg, turkey, chicken, etc.). Snacks are optional on the Hormone Diet plan, though at least one is recommended in the afternoon, before strength training, or after a workout. You should also consume a serving of grain products (such as rice, gluten-free bread, millet, or quinoa) or sweet potatoes a maximum of once a day, with each serving no larger than the size of your fist. Limit soy and nuts to one serving a day. Then just make sure you avoid the forbidden foods. Please remember *not* to restrict your calories. If you cut your food intake too much, you'll simply hamper your metabolism by creating (or aggravating) imbalances in your stress and blood sugar hormones.

Foods to Eat, Foods to Avoid

The following food groups *must be removed from your diet* during your body detox because they are inflammatory or allergenic:

- **Dairy products.** Yogurt, cheese, milk, cream, sour cream, cottage cheese, casein, whey protein concentrate. One daily serving of 100 percent pure whey protein isolate or sheep and goat milk cheeses is *allowed.*
- **All grains that contain gluten.** Wheat, spelt, rye, kamut, barley. Note that most breads, bagels, muffins, pastries, cakes, pasta, durum semolina, couscous, cookies, flour, and cereals are off-limits, *unless they are gluten free.* Oatmeal, although gluten free, is *not* allowed on the detox.
- **Corn.** Popcorn, corn chips, corn breads or muffins, fresh corn, canned or frozen niblets.
- **Oils:** Hydrogenated oils, palm kernel oil, trans fatty acids, soybean oil, corn oil, cottonseed oil, vegetable oil, shortening, and margarine. Limit your intake of safflower and sunflower oil.
- **Alcohol and caffeine.** During your detox I recommend you cut these out completely. Too much of either one will elevate stress hormones and contribute to hormonal imbalance.
- **Peanuts and peanut-containing products.** Peanut butter, peanuts in the shell, trail mix containing peanuts, etc. Check labels carefully, as many products list peanuts as ingredients.

- **Sugar and artificial sweeteners.** Table sugar (sucrose) and all products with sugar added must be cut out completely. Foods to avoid include maple syrup, honey (except for the small amount in your homemade salad dressings), rice syrup, foods and drinks containing high-fructose corn syrup, packaged foods, candies, soda, juice, etc., as well as all diet products containing aspartame, etc.
- **Citrus fruit.** Oranges, tangerines, and grapefruit. Lemons are okay.
- **Red meats.** Pork, beef, lamb, all types of cold cuts, bacon, and all types of sausages.

The following anti-inflammatory and immune-enhancing foods are *permissible* during your detox program:

- **Gluten-free grains and starchy grains.** Millet, quinoa, rice, buckwheat, rice pasta, rice cakes, rice crackers, sweet potatoes, squash, potatoes, amaranth. Have just one serving per day (the size of your fist).
- **Vegetables.** Unlimited amounts of all vegetables except corn.
- **Fruits.** All fruits *except* oranges, tangerines, grapefruit, canned fruits, raisins, dates, and other nonorganic dried fruits.
- **Beans.** All beans are allowed.
- **Nuts and seeds.** All nuts except for peanuts; all seeds are fine. Maximum serving is one small handful per day.
- **Fish and meat.** All poultry (chicken, turkey, duck, etc.), fish, and seafood are fine.
- **Dairy.** Feta cheese (made from sheep's or goat's milk), goat cheese (1 tablespoon maximum per day), small amounts of butter (1 teaspoon maximum per day).
- **Oils.** Canola oil, flaxseed oil, hemp oil, avocado oil, small amounts of butter, and extra-virgin olive oil are the only oils you should consume.

- **Eggs.** Both yolks and whites are okay.
- **Milks.** Oat, almond, rice, and soy milks are fine, but avoid those with sugar added.
- **Soy products.** All soy products are allowed unless you have noticed digestive upset (gas, bloating, or other symptoms of indigestion) when you have eaten these products in the past. Selections include tofu, tempeh, soy nuts, soy milk, and whole soybeans. Keep soy consumption to one serving a day at most.

Don't worry—I've outlined a detox diet meal plan later on in this chapter, and I've included recipes in Appendix C.

Your Detox Supplement Plan

While you are on the detox diet, you should also include the supplements outlined in this section. Although they're not a mandatory part of your program, I strongly recommend including them in order to enhance your liver detox. These supplements will boost:

- The breakdown and elimination of hormones in the liver and digestive system
- Antioxidant protection
- Your energy and metabolic rate

The Clear Detox products, originally formulated for use by patients at my clinic, are now easily available through www.thehormonediet.com. These products specifically enhance the breakdown and elimination of excess hormones that are our fat-burning foes. I have also recommended other brands here, but don't feel you have to purchase these exact items. Those with similar ingredients should be fine, provided they are from a reputable company. Ask the staff at your local health food store for advice.

1. **A probiotic supplement.** Recall that replacing healthy bacterial balance in the gut is one of the five keys to healthy digestion.

Yogurt naturally contains probiotics, but supplements are more effective as a concentrated source. All probiotic supplements should be refrigerated. During your detox, I recommend a probiotic with at least 10 to 15 billion cells per capsule, while a good maintenance dose is 1 to 2 billion of both lactobacilli and bifidobacteria once a day, without food.

You can also alternate the use of probiotic supplements—1 month on, 1 month off—after your detox. In most cases, daily supplementation is not necessary unless you are taking a medication that affects bacterial balance. For example, during antibiotic therapy you should take increased doses of probiotic supplements 3 hours before or after your medication and continue to take them for twice the length of time of your antibiotic treatment. Take a probiotic supplement daily if you are on the birth control pill, corticosteroids, or HRT.

Some people experience bloating when they first begin taking probiotic supplements. If you're bothered by this, simply reduce the dosage and slowly increase it as your body adapts.

Recommended brands include the following:
- Ultra Flora Plus (Metagenics): 1 or 2 capsules per day on an empty stomach
- HMF Forte (Genestra): 1 or 2 capsules per day with food
- Smooth Food 2 or All-Flora (New Chapter): 2 capsules per day on an empty stomach
- Clear Flora (Clear Medicine)

2. **An herbal cleansing formula for the liver and/or bowels that contains milk thistle, dandelion, turmeric, artichoke, and/or beet leaf.** These herbs improve the flow of bile, aid liver function, reduce inflammation, improve estrogen and cortisol metabolism, and reduce fatty liver, a factor known to accelerate aging.

Recommended brands include the following:

- Clear Detox—Hormonal Health (Clear Medicine)
- Lipo-Gen (Metagenics)
- Liver-G.I. Detox (Pure Encapsulations)

3. **One serving per day of a bowel-cleansing formula containing fiber.** Choices include glucomannan, apple, beet, or flax fibers; glutamine; the herbal formula triphala and preferably herbs to coat and heal the digestive tract wall, such as deglycyrrhizinated licorice (DGL), aloe, and/or marshmallow. This type of product will promote healthier, more frequent bowel movements while you detox your liver and digestive system. It will also help maintain the integrity of your digestive tract wall, thereby reducing inflammation and leaky gut syndrome.

Triphala is a standardized blend of three fruit extracts—*Terminalia chebula, Terminalia belerica,* and *Emblica officinalis*—in equal proportions. It is an Ayurvedic herbal blend commonly used for supporting intestinal detoxification, occasional constipation, and overall colon health.

Soluble fiber is fermented in your large intestines by your intestinal microflora and will help create an intestinal environment that allows beneficial bacteria to thrive. When taken with appropriate amounts of water, soluble fiber also bulks up the stool to support larger, softer stools and healthy bowel movements. As the bulk moves through your intestine, it helps to collect and eliminate other waste and toxins from your intestinal walls.

Recommended brands include the following:
- Clear Detox—Digestive Health (Clear Medicine)
- G.I. Fortify (Pure Encapsulations): one serving of the powder per day mixed in, or followed by, 1 cup of water

Note that as a cheaper, although somewhat less effective, alternative to these bowel-cleansing products you can add $1/4$ cup aloe vera juice or gel and 2 tablespoons of ground flaxseeds per day to your smoothies.

4. **You may include supplements to reduce inflammation** (see page 283 for your options). My first choice for treating inflammation is a supplement of omega-3 fish oils. Take 4 to 6 g per day with food. Wobenzym, turmeric, or resveratrol are my second-line interventions. I recommend picking resveratrol if you want to kick-start your weight loss. It's touted to be the French Paradox in a bottle, which means that in addition to its anti-inflammatory effects, it may allow you to eat more without experiencing weight gain.

The products listed here are necessary only during your detox, though you can certainly finish your bottles should they happen to last longer than 2 weeks. The exception is the supplements added to reduce inflammation. You should continue these as long as your signs or symptoms of inflammation persist. Fish oils and resveratrol may be taken for a lifetime—I say they should be used this long!

Coming Off the Detox

Once you have avoided certain foods for the first 10 days of your detox, you'll slowly reintroduce them. Often it's the end of a detox that's the most important part because it allows you to make the connection between certain foods and how they make you feel.

Reintroduce each food one by one, one day at a time as I outline in your menu plan on page 194. You will try the least allergenic foods first, followed by the foods with the greatest tendency to cause problems. You won't eat each test food again until you have introduced all the other foods. For example, test rye on Day 11 with 100 percent rye bread or Ryvita crackers. Then you'll stop eating rye again and introduce plain organic yogurt on Day 12. On Day 13, yogurt is avoided again and you'll try low-fat cheese. On the last day of your detox, cut out the cheese again and try wheat by having some whole-wheat pasta or bread.

I recommend you test rye, dairy, and wheat first because they are permitted in the next step of your diet, as long as your body likes them. When you reintroduce these foods, be on the lookout for symptoms that point to an allergy or intolerance. Check the chart I have provided below to see the most common reactions to certain foods. Keeping a food diary at this point can certainly be helpful.

As you move on to the next step in the Hormone Diet, you may, for your own enjoyment, continue adding other foods you've been avoiding since the start of your detox, though I normally do not include sugar, alcohol, or caffeine in the reintroduction process. My feeling is that most of us will continue to consume these foods on our cheat days—regardless of their potential negative effect. But I do recommend avoiding them until you are done with the reintroduction process, and longer, if you wish to continue losing weight.

COMMON REACTIONS WITH REINTRODUCTION OF FOODS AFTER DETOX THAT CAN INDICATE A FOOD SENSITIVITY

Food	Typical Reactions
Rye (try 100% rye crackers or bread)	Gas, bloating, constipation, fatigue immediately after eating the food, fatigue on waking the next day, irritability, anxiety, headaches, water retention (e.g., can't get your rings off, puffiness under the eyes), dark circles under the eyes on waking the next day. You may also notice a gradual decline in your energy over a period of time once you have put rye back into your diet.
Plain organic yogurt	Gas, bloating, constipation, diarrhea, sinus congestion, postnasal drip, constant need to clear your throat; allergies (especially environmental) may worsen.
Low-fat cheese	Gas, bloating, constipation, diarrhea, sinus congestion, postnasal drip, constant need to clear your throat; allergies (especially environmental) may worsen.
Spelt (try 100% spelt bread or pasta)	Similar to rye.
Wheat (try 100% whole-wheat bread or pasta)	Similar to rye.
Red meats (try lean cuts of pork and beef on separate days)	Joint pain or stiffness, constipation, indigestion, upset stomach.

Detox Q and A: A Few Common Questions Answered

What can I expect to feel while I am cleansing?

Headaches, fatigue, irritability, and general malaise are common for as many as 4 or 5 days into the diet, as your body is doing a lot of housecleaning. *Allow yourself time to rest if you feel sluggish.* Drink lots of water and take extra vitamin C to reduce detox symptoms. By the third or fourth day, you should feel your energy increasing and mental focus improving. If you typically drink a lot of coffee (more than 4 cups per day), decrease the amounts you consume slowly throughout the first few days to minimize the effects of caffeine withdrawal. Also, drink at least 2 liters of water per day. Reverse osmosis water is best; spring water should be your second choice. Distilled water should be avoided because it may leach minerals out of your body.

If you need encouragement and motivation to keep you on track, remember this: *The more severe your detox reactions, the more you really needed it!*

Will I begin to lose weight during the detox?

I have already mentioned that the very act of eating helps maintain our metabolic rate because of the thermogenic effects of food. Eating is a physical process that requires energy to support digestion and absorption. Of all the macronutrients, protein requires the most energy to digest and absorb. Both Step 1 (the detox) and Step 2 (the Glyci-Med approach) promote the consumption of protein with every meal. When you combine the benefits of protein with reduced water retention and bloating commonly experienced with a detox diet, your weight loss will be off to a good start.

Can I exercise during the detox?

If you usually exercise, continue with your current routine but be aware that headaches, fatigue, or feelings of malaise are common during the first few days of a detox. If you experience these symptoms, allow your body to rest, and select less-intense forms of exercise such as yoga, walking, or Pilates. And be sure to keep drinking plenty of water.

If you are not exercising at this point, now is not the time to dive into an intensive workout regimen. You'll have enough to think about already, so don't try to do too much at once. We'll get you exercising once you reach Chapter 15 at the 4-week mark—when your metabolism will be primed for a shake-up. For now, I would like you to go for a walk after dinner, if only for 15 or 20 minutes.

Can I eat out when doing the detox?

Yes, you can still eat out. Japanese food, seafood, dairy-free risotto, Chinese food, salads, grilled chicken, fish, turkey, vegetables, and potatoes are all fine, but keep an eye out for hidden sugars and unhealthy oils in sauces, soups, and dressings. Don't be afraid to ask your server for specific details about what you're ordering. You should absolutely avoid fast-food restaurants unless you are picking up a salad.

What should I do if I experience constipation (less than one bowel movement per day) during the detox?

Keeping your bowels moving regularly is critical at all times, but especially during your detox, to avoid accumulation and reabsorption of toxins in the bowels. On occasion, dietary changes or reduced intake of fibrous grains can cause constipation. Try one or more of these solutions to help things "move along" if you find you need some help.

- **Increase your intake of flaxseeds**. Add 1 or 2 tablespoons daily to your smoothies, salads, or water. Whether you purchase them ground or grind your own, flaxseeds should be kept in the freezer for maximum freshness. You can also supplement with a nonirritating, psyllium-free fiber powder or capsules such as MetaFiber (Metagenics), G.I. Fortify (Pure Encapsulations), or Gentle Fibers (Jarrow).

- **Increase vitamin C.** Take 3 to 8 g of vitamin C (spread out throughout the day, not all at once). Vitamin C is a great natural laxative in higher doses.
- **Take magnesium citrate.** This supplement can encourage bowel movements because it's a natural muscle relaxant. Take 200 to 800 mg per day. Start with a low dose and increase it gradually. (As with vitamin C, don't take your magnesium all at once.) Magnesium and vitamin C are present in the Clear Detox products, not only to encourage regular bowel movements, but also for their antioxidant and hormone balancing benefits.
- **Take essential fatty acids to help lubricate the bowels.** If you choose a liquid form, 1 tablespoon per day is plenty. Good brands include Nordic Naturals fish oils, Carlson fish oils, Opti EPA (Douglas Labs), or Balanced EPA-DHA liquid (Metagenics). All of these come in liquid form and most are also available in capsules. Liquid forms should be kept in the fridge or freezer. If you choose capsules, take 2 to 4 capsules once or twice a day with food. If you find that fish oil "repeats," put the bottle in the freezer and take it with food, or purchase an enteric-coated formula.

More Tips to Help Your Detox

I have compiled a few tips over the years to help patients get through their detox. The good news is that over 99 percent of people feel better after they've completed this health-promoting process.

Don't be shocked if your emotions run high when you embark on your detox. Food is an emotional thing, heavily tied to many of our social and family activities. Don't get down or beat yourself up if you fall off track. Simply do your best and remember that you are doing this as a favor to yourself. If you manage to cut out *even two* potential offenders during your detox, you'll do your body a lot of good. Maybe next time you'll succeed in cutting out a few more problematic foods.

In the meantime, try these helpful detox tips.

- **Check your dates or clear your calendar.** If you have a party or special event planned, wait until *after* these activities to start your detox. Your liver will probably need the detox even more at that point.
- **Stock your kitchen.** Make sure your fridge and cupboards are filled with detox-friendly foods to make snacking and meal prep easier.
- **Fess up.** Let everyone know you are detoxifying. You'll be surprised by how many people will be interested in what you are doing—they may even want to join you. After your detox, you'll look good and feel even better. Don't be surprised when everyone starts asking you what you have been up to.
- **Recruit other detoxers.** Like any difficult undertaking, detox can be easier when you have a friend or two on board with you from the get-go. A friend of mine detoxes with me every time.
- **Record your feelings.** Get yourself a journal and write down how you feel as you detox. This process will help you notice improvements and can help you track your reactions to certain foods.
- **Pamper yourself.** I encourage you to designate 30 minutes to an hour daily as *your time* on an ongoing basis. But during your detox, try to think of one fantastic thing to do each day and do it—a massage, a facial, a sauna, a day at a pool, a stay at a fancy hotel in your area, a manicure and pedicure (toxin free, of course), a bubble bath, a hike, a yoga class—whatever you need to do to reward yourself for getting healthy.

Walk!

From this point onward, walking should be part of your life. Even a short stroll can be a simple and highly beneficial way to avoid cheating or falling off track with your diet, and to lessen the harmful effects of stress and fatty foods on your body. Studies prove that walking after an unhealthy meal can curb the effects of stress by reducing the amounts of fatty acids, sugars, and stress hormones that are released into the bloodstream and subsequently stored as fat. This gentle form of exercise strengthens nearly every aspect of your body. Numerous studies have shown that heading out for even just a leisurely walk can prevent heart disease and offers excellent stress-reducing effects. Exercise also promotes wakefulness and relaxation and improves the quality of your sleep.

Your Detox Sample Menu Plan

Days 1 to 10

On Days 1 through 10 of your detox, pick and choose from any of the meal suggestions in Appendix C marked "detox friendly" by the symbols ✿☺. But I have outlined menus for the designated days for the reintroduction of specific foods here.

Day 11: Reintroducing Rye

SUGGESTED MEALS

Breakfast: 2 slices 100 percent rye bread with ⅓ of an avocado spread on the bread and 1 whole boiled egg plus 2 more egg whites. Pay attention to how you feel after you have eaten this meal, and the next, containing rye.

Lunch: Sweet Potato, Squash, and Ginger Soup (page 419). (Remove the cheese to make it a ✿☺ meal option.) 3 Wasa crackers

Snack: Your choice

Dinner: Your choice

Day 12: Reintroducing Yogurt

SUGGESTED MEALS

Breakfast: Organic apple with 1 cup plain yogurt. Pay attention to how you feel after you have consumed the yogurt.

Lunch: Your choice

Snack: ½ cup plain yogurt and 10 almonds. Pay attention to how you feel after your snack containing yogurt.

Dinner: Your choice

Day 13: Reintroducing Cheese

SUGGESTED MEALS

Breakfast: Organic apple with 1 cup low-fat cottage or ricotta cheese. Pay attention to how you feel after you have eaten this meal.

Lunch: Your choice

Snack: 2 slices of low-fat Swiss cheese and veggies. Again, pay attention to how you feel.

Dinner: Your choice

Day 14: Reintroducing Wheat

SUGGESTED MEALS

Breakfast: Kashi GOLEAN cereal with soy milk and blueberries. Pay attention to how you feel after you have eaten this cereal containing wheat.

Lunch: Your choice

Snack: Your choice

Dinner: Quick-and-Easy Pasta with Tomato Sauce (page 434). Note: Use the version with ground turkey and *not* the one with cheese during Day 14 of your detox. Pay attention to how you feel after you have eaten this whole-wheat pasta.

Although I haven't specifically included them, you may introduce lean cuts of red meat back into your diet on Days 15 and 16. Definitely introduce beef and pork one at a time on separate days, and pay attention to how you feel after you eat these meats again. Moving forward, you should limit your red meat intake to a few times a month because it's high in inflammatory saturated fats.

While I always encourage you to follow your detox diet as closely as possible, *don't fret if you break the rules a few times.* In most cases, if you're sensitive to the food, you'll still notice some sort of reaction when you reintroduce it into your diet.

Once you've completed your detox and learned how to manage stress as outlined in the next chapter, you'll be ready for the lifelong nutrition plan that will wipe out food allergies, restore hormonal balance, and promote fat loss. Now that's a powerful combination for better health!

THE HORMONE DIET 14-DAY DETOX

Review of Suggested Servings and Allowed Foods Step 1: Anti-Inflammatory Detox	
BENEFITS	Calm Inflammation Reduce Allergies Reduce Bloating and Water Retention Lose Weight Increase Energy Improve Sleep Improve Skin and Digestion

Foods to enjoy	Foods to avoid
Grains and starchy vegetables—one serving the size of your fist daily: Millet; buckwheat; rice and rice products, such as rice pasta, rice cakes, and rice crackers; sweet potatoes; amaranth; quinoa; squash; and potatoes.	**All grains that contain gluten:** Wheat, spelt, rye, kamut, amaranth, and barley. Cut out oatmeal, bread, bagels, muffins, pastries, cakes, pasta, durum semolina, couscous, cookies, flour, and cereals.
Vegetables: All vegetables except for corn.	**Corn:** Popcorn, corn chips, fresh corn, canned corn, etc.
Fruits: All fruits except for oranges, tangerines, grapefruit, raisins, dates, and non-organic dried fruit.	**Citrus and processed fruits:** Oranges, grapefruit, tangerines, canned fruits, and nonorganic dried fruits.
Nuts and seeds—one serving per day: All nuts and seeds are fine except for peanuts. Choices include cashews, walnuts, Brazil nuts, sesame seeds, pumpkin seeds, sunflower seeds, pecans, etc.	**Peanuts:** Peanut butter and any products containing peanuts. Also avoid pistachios.

Foods to enjoy (continued)	Foods to avoid (continued)
Fish and meat: All poultry (chicken, turkey, duck, etc.). Fish and seafood are fine.	**Red meats:** Beef, pork, luncheon meats, cold cuts, sausage, bacon, and lamb.
Dairy–1 tablespoon daily: Feta (made from sheep's or goat's milk), goat cheese. Replace dairy milks with oat, almond, rice, or soy milk.	**Dairy:** Cow's milk cheeses, milk, yogurt, sour cream, and soups and sauces containing dairy.
Soy products: All soy products are fine unless you have noticed digestive upset (gas, bloating, indigestion, or other symptoms) when you have eaten these products in the past. Choices include tofu, tempeh, soy nuts, soy milk, and whole soybeans. Limit soy to one serving per day.	**Alcohol and caffeine:** Coffee, nonherbal tea, sodas, and all alcoholic beverages.
Sweeteners: Stevia, maple syrup, and honey are allowed in small amounts in salad dressing mix only.	**Sugar and artificial sweeteners:** Table sugar, any product with sugar added, rice syrup, maple syrup, high-fructose corn syrup, packaged foods, candies, soda, juice, etc.
Oils: Canola oil, avocado oil, flaxseed oil, butter, and extra-virgin olive oil are the only oils you should consume.	**Oils:** Hydrogenated oils, trans fatty acids, palm oil, soy oil, corn oil, cottonseed oil, vegetable oil, shortening, and margarine. Limit your intake of safflower and sunflower oils.
Eggs: Yolks and whites are fine.	
All beans: Chickpeas, lentils, black beans, etc.	

THE HORMONE DIET 14-DAY DETOX SUPPLEMENT PLAN

When and How to Take It	Supplement
On rising (no food)	Probiotic supplement
	Liver-cleansing formula (Clear Detox—Hormonal Health)
	If needed: anti-inflammatory supplements
With breakfast/dinner	**Optional:** Multivitamin and omega-3 fish oils with breakfast and dinner
Before bed (no food)	Probiotic supplement
	Bowel-cleansing high-fiber formula (Clear Detox—Digestive Health)
	If needed: anti-inflammatory supplement

You may wish to use the following chart (or if you don't like to write in this book, print it from www.thehormonediet.com) to track possible reactions when reintroducing specific foods back into your diet:

FOOD REACTIONS TO WATCH FOR

Food	Reactions to Watch For	Symptoms Noted (if any)
Rye (try 100% rye crackers or rye bread) on Day 11	Gas, bloating, constipation, fatigue immediately after eating the food, fatigue on waking the next day, irritability, anxiety, headaches, water retention (can't get your rings off, puffiness under your eyes the next day), dark circles under your eyes on waking the next day. Or you may notice a gradual decline in your energy over a period of time once you have put the rye back into your diet.	
Plain organic yogurt on Day 12	Gas, bloating, constipation, diarrhea, sinus congestion, postnasal drip, constant need to clear your throat. Allergies (especially environmental) may worsen.	
Low-fat cheese on Day 13	Similar to yogurt.	
Wheat (try 100% whole-wheat bread or pasta) on Day 14	Similar to rye.	
Red meats (try lean pork or beef, introduced on separate days) on Days 15 and 16	Joint pain or stiffness, constipation, indigestion, upset stomach.	

HEAVY METALS

Are heavy metals weighing you down?

Just as acidic body pH has a widespread influence on most bodily processes and your overall wellness, the presence of heavy metals can disrupt your hormones and compromise your health. So investigating your risk of heavy metal toxicity is definitely a worthwhile addition to your body detox program.

What are heavy metals?

Antimony, arsenic, aluminum, bismuth, cadmium, cerium, cobalt, copper, gallium, gold, iron, lead, manganese, mercury, nickel, platinum, silver, tellurium, thallium, tin, uranium, vanadium, and zinc are examples of minerals and metals that are harmful when an overload is present in your body. A priority list called "Top 20 Hazardous Substances," compiled by the Agency for Toxic Substances and Disease Registry (ATSDR www.atsdr.cdc.gov/), includes the heavy metals arsenic (1), lead (2), mercury (3), and cadmium (7) high on the list.

Where do we get them from?

Heavy metals accumulate in our soft tissues, brain, bones, and fat. We can be exposed to them at work, at home, or outdoors through occupational contact, food, or water. Acute exposure may come from inhalation of fumes or skin contact with heavy metal dust, usually in the workplace. Exposure can also happen slowly over time from sources such as old plumbing pipes, lead paint, smoking, dental amalgams (fillings), cookware, a tainted water supply, or consumption of ocean fish and seafood. Heavy metals may also be present in personal-care products. For example, certain lipsticks are known to contain lead, and aluminum is an ingredient in most antiperspirants. As evidenced by recent headlines, even some imported children's toys are a cause for concern.

What happens when we have heavy metal toxicity?

Certain heavy metals interfere with our hormones and, consequently, our metabolism. For instance, mercury, which is often present in large ocean fish, inhibits thyroid hormone and growth hormone. Heavy metal toxicity is also very damaging to our nervous system, cognition, lungs, kidneys, liver, eyes, and other vital organs. Long-term exposure may result in slowly progressing, muscular and neurological degeneration that mimics signs of Alzheimer's disease, Parkinson's disease, muscular dystrophy, and multiple sclerosis.

How do you know if you have heavy metal toxicity?

The best way to assess your risk of heavy metal toxicity is through a stool or urine test, available through Doctor's Data, Inc. You may want to consult an integrated-health practitioner in your area or visit www.thehormonediet.com and look under testing recommendations for more information.

What can you do if you have heavy metal toxicity?

You must seek professional medical attention in any case of heavy metal toxicity, especially since treatment options vary depending on the type of metal toxicity you experience. However, there are a number of herbs and supplements that you may use to support your body's own natural chelation (metal removal) mechanisms.

The two most common metal toxicities I have seen in my practice to date involve mercury and lead. My treatment recommendations include oral chelation with DMSA (also known as

2,3-dimercaptosuccinic acid), which has a strong affinity for removing both mercury and lead. Rectal suppositories of ethylene-diaminetetraacetic acid (EDTA) have a strong affinity for lead, but also remove all other metals. EDTA was one of the first chelators developed. Visit www.detoxamin.com or the resource section of www.thehormonediet.com for more information. If you're taking prescription medications or if you have a specific medical condition, consult your doctor before using either of these products.

In conjunction with products designed to remove heavy metals, antioxidants and detoxifying agents should be used. A full heavy metal protocol may include whey protein, vitamin C, chlorella, selenium, zinc, cilantro, a high-potency multivitamin, and a blend of essential amino acids. Fiber supplements and liver support (milk thistle, MSM, and turmeric) should also be used to aid elimination. Regular sessions in an infrared sauna are an excellent complement to any heavy metal detoxification protocol, especially for mercury toxicity.

If you suspect you have heavy metal toxicity, don't try to take care of it on your own. Consult a licensed health-care provider to help assess your situation and, if necessary, supervise detoxification.

CHAPTER 9

STRATEGIES FOR STRESS SURVIVAL

These are the hormonal benefits you can expect to enjoy from subduing stress:

- Controlled cortisol and a calm nervous system
- Replenished DHEA, the antiaging hormone
- Reduced insulin, better craving control, and increased ab fat loss
- Increased GABA, dopamine, and serotonin, our relaxation and feel-good hormones
- Topped-up testosterone and protection from the harmful effects of excess estrogen through balanced progesterone
- More melatonin and growth hormone to work metabolic magic on night-time repair and fat burning
- Maximized effects of thyroid hormone, the metabolic master
- Better appetite control via increased leptin and suppressed appetite-stimulating hormones, ghrelin and NPY

Sleeping well and cooling inflammation through detoxification are critical components in the first of your three steps to hormonal health. But Step 1 would be incomplete without tackling one more major lifestyle change. To achieve true hormonal harmony and create the foundation for lasting fat loss, you absolutely must bring your stress hormones under control. The high levels of cortisol associated with excessive stress interfere with almost every other hormone involved in metabolism regulation, appetite control, and fat burning.

You might think stress isn't a problem for you. If so, hey, that's amazing. Though to really assess the role stress plays in your life, you need to fully understand the various ways in which stress can present itself. It can be immediate and short lived, such as narrowly missing a crash on the highway. Or it can be chronic, lasting days to weeks to months to years as we're faced with a divorce, an illness, loss of a job, or a death in the family. I conducted my own research into stress and discovered a few interesting and often overlooked examples that may surprise you.

The Stress of Loneliness

A powerful study completed by researchers at Northwestern University in 2006 showed just how strongly our social and emotional experiences affect our hormonal balance and overall health. Subjects who went to bed feeling lonely, sad, or overwhelmed exhibited high levels of cortisol and a low mood the next day. This study was the first to prove that experiences influence stress hormones just as stress hormones influence experiences. Interestingly, individuals who got out of bed with low cortisol reported fatigue throughout the day. We need cortisol, just not too much.

PLUG YOUR EARS AND CUT CORTISOL?
New York City receives over 350,000 noise-related complaints each year! In fact, noise is the number-one complaint called in to the city's 311 citizen service hotline. Loud noises stress us. This may be a first for a diet plan, but nonetheless I recommend wearing earplugs or noise-cancelling earphones to cut cortisol spikes caused by noise. Taking this small extra precaution can give you a surprising leg-up on stress. You'll be amazed how much better you will feel at the end of an airline flight or after a day's work without the added stress of sounds hammering in your ears.

HOT HORMONE TIP

The Stress of Commuting

Millions of North Americans commute to work every weekday. If you're one of them, did you ever imagine your daily commute could be contributing to your ab fat—and not just because of all that sitting? Researchers from Cornell University have found a link between a longer commute to work, whether by car or by train, and greater feelings of frustration, irritation, and stress. The research team measured the salivary cortisol of 208 commuters taking trains from New Jersey to Manhattan. All of the subjects had routinely high cortisol readings, proving that commuting is a stressful aspect of work for many people. For some, commuting can be *the* most stressful aspect. Certainly we need to consider commuting stress to be an important, although often overlooked, part of environmental health.

The Stress of Overexercising

Whether we engage in strength training or aerobic activity, cortisol is released during exercise in proportion to the intensity of our effort. Both high-intensity and prolonged exercise cause increases in cortisol, which can remain elevated for hours following a workout. Numerous studies have proven that this rise in cortisol tends to occur with very strenuous exercise and when we exercise for longer than 40 to 45 minutes. Performing repeated strenuous workouts without appropriate rest between sessions also results in chronically elevated cortisol.

You may already be aware of the adverse effects of high cortisol on your health, mood, body composition, and performance. Chronically high cortisol, which is commonly associated with a decrease in muscle-enhancing growth hormone, DHEA, and testosterone, can cause muscle breakdown and suppress our immune function. Researchers at the University of North Carolina have also linked strenuous, fatiguing exercise to higher cortisol and lower thyroid hormones. Remember, thyroid hormones stimulate your metabolism, so depletion is definitely not a desired effect of exercise! The same study found thyroid hormones remained suppressed even 24 hours after recovery, whereas cortisol levels remained high throughout the same period.

Overexercising can lead to loss of muscle, frequent colds and flus, poor recovery after exercise, and slower gains from your workout efforts. Plus, your risk of illness and injury increases as your metabolic rate slows. Certainly these are not the effects you are looking for when you join a gym.

Poor diet, inadequate supplementation, and lack of rest play a key role in excess cortisol secretion. Experiments measuring cortisol in trained athletes on carb-restricted, high-protein diets found that these athletes had *higher* cortisol. When researchers had the athletes take sugar supplements during their workouts, the cortisol and immune-suppression responses to exercise were lessened.

Bear in mind that most athletes are better conditioned to the stress of exercise than the rest of us—these effects would be worse in someone who's not physically fit to begin with. My point is, if you try to lose weight by slashing your calorie intake, eliminating carbs, and going crazy on the cardio machines, you will do more harm than good. Rather than getting fit and losing weight, you'll crank up your cortisol and damage your metabolism. I cringe when I hear a stressed-out patient mention plans to complete a marathon. The added stress of training for such an event can have disastrous effects.

The Stress of Marital "Bliss"

Professor Janice Kiecolt-Glaser from Ohio State University has made some interesting discoveries about stress hormones and (supposedly) happily married couples. She analyzed cortisol in newlywed couples after they had a 30-minute conversation about a few areas of disagreement in their marriage. The results showed high cortisol and weakened immune-system markers. After a transition period, Kiecolt-Glaser had the couples talk about how they met, what attracted them to each other, and other positive aspects of their relationship. The cortisol levels fell, as expected, in 75 percent of the participants. In the remaining 25 percent, cortisol went up or stayed the same. Even more interesting, when the researchers followed up with the women after the study, those who showed higher cortisol levels were twice as likely to end up divorced. The body does not lie, even when the mind does.

Repair versus Protection Mode

All stress responses require energy from storage sites in your body, whether that energy comes from fat in your fat cells or sugar stored in your muscles and liver. This fuel supports the increase in heart rate, blood pressure, and breathing, as nutrients and oxygen are transported to your vital organs or muscles at greater rates to cope with stress. While your body is busy handling these stress-induced tasks, all nonessential, long-term processes are put on hold.

Basically, our bodies can exist in one of two states: growth, repair, and rebuilding mode or protection mode. The longer the body remains in protection mode, the less time and energy is left over for renewal and regrowth. This redirection of energy makes a lot of sense when we are facing a bear—digestion, immune activity, and reproduction become much less important in moments of life-versus-imminent-death. But what happens when the bear is long gone, yet the high-stress response lingers? We become chronically imbalanced, which leads to muscle wasting, premature aging, fat gain, disease, and even death. Do you need more reason to start ridding your body of stress?

We can't control the infinite number of stressors that surround us every day, but we can control our perceptions and responses. Each one of us has a unique set of physical and mental responses to stress, and these can change over time. I've seen some patients suddenly develop anxiety so severe that they lost the ability to drive and had to take a leave of absence from work. Others have come into my office with physical symptoms of hives, palpitations, or insomnia. Stress always shows its nasty face in one way or another. The trick is to recognize it and refuse to let it take over.

Stress is most often related to feeling out of control. I also strongly believe anxiety is a sign that we are *not making decisions that are in accordance with our values*. It can also be a sign that we are *failing to do something we know in our hearts we should be doing.* For example, I commonly see health-related anxiety in busy executives who go for months or even years without making proper eating and rest a priority. There are three books that I highly recommend to help you gain a stronger understanding of the powerful connection between your emotions, stress, and the origins of illness.

1. *Women's Bodies, Women's Wisdom* by Christiane Northrup, MD (Bantam Books, 2002)
2. *When the Body Says No: The Cost of Hidden Stress* by Gabor Maté, MD (Vintage Canada, 2004)
3. *Anatomy of the Spirit: The Seven Stages of Power and Healing* by Caroline Myss, PhD (Three Rivers Press, 1997)

Adrenal Gland Burnout: Another Consequence of Chronic Stress

If you always feel tense or anxious, your body will remain in a constant state of heightened arousal. Constantly overproducing cortisol and adrenaline day after day because of ongoing stress, multitasking, skipping meals, excessive calorie restriction, insufficient carbohydrate intake, too much protein consumption, lack of sleep, or too much coffee will lead to adrenal gland burnout. At this point, your adrenal glands can't keep up with the constant stimulation and outrageous demands for adrenaline and cortisol production, and they simply shut down.

When your adrenal glands go on strike, cortisol levels plummet, resulting in chronic fatigue, lack of stamina for exercise, more allergy symptoms, sleep disruption, blood sugar imbalances, depression, increased cravings, and weakened immunity. In the presence of these damaging conditions, your risk of autoimmune diseases such as rheumatoid arthritis and lupus also skyrockets.

If your adrenals are "shot," the Hormone Diet will recuperate you. When you reach Step 3, which involves exercise for hormonal balance, stick to yoga and strength training rather than cardio until you have come out of your depleted state. You will also need extra supplements to restore your adrenal gland function. Check out your options in Chapter 13 for advanced supplements to aid cortisol balance (Hormonal Imbalance 5).

The Hormone Diet Stress Solution:
The Four Elements to Conquer Stress

Being a type A personality, a natural-born worrier, and someone who has developed three hormonal conditions—hypothyroidism, depression, and polycystic ovarian syndrome—after highly stressful periods in my life, I've had my struggles with stress management. I certainly understand how stress makes us sick. (How ironic that I'm now writing a book that touches on how to handle the problem!) I do, however, feel my experiences have helped me be a better caregiver, especially in clinical practice. I hope sharing this information will help you, too.

I've chosen to include stress relief as part of Step 1 because it is such an important factor in the Hormone Diet program. Besides, making stress management a priority now will allow you to start dealing with it sooner rather than later. The recommendations I present in this chapter will take longer than 2 weeks to implement, and even longer to become lifelong habits. Just make sure you practice, practice, practice as often as you can and know that your efforts *will* make a difference.

There are four elements to conquering stress, no matter what the source.

1. RELIEVING STRESS NOW: Identify activities you can do or habits you can adopt to immediately lessen stress and its negative effects on your health. These include deep breathing, meditating, exercising, sleeping well, eating healthfully, getting massages, and even laughing.

2. SETTING YOUR GOALS: You need to develop a sense of *where you are* in your life right now and *where you want to be*. Lack of direction can create chaos and lead to anxiety or stress. If you find you're drifting, you need to set goals (even small ones) and create the concrete roadmap that will take you where you want to go.

3. VISUALIZING SUCCESS: Once you've created your map, you can use visualization techniques to help reduce stress and turn your goals and dreams into reality.

4. HARNESSING THE POWER OF POSITIVE BELIEF: What you believe ultimately dictates how you think, feel, and experience all aspects of your life. This requires the ability to be positive, express gratitude, gain wisdom, and appreciate the good and the not-so-good in life. Arguably, this is the most important aspect of successfully handling stress and *dis-ease*.

All four elements require commitment, but the first element—involving the actions you can take to reduce stress—is often easier than the second and third. The fourth is by far the most difficult, especially if you aren't naturally a positive person. All of the elements involve personal evaluation, growth, and development, which can feel uncomfortable at first but pay wonderful dividends later on. As the Greek philosopher Socrates put it, a life unexamined is a life not worth living.

Stress-Reducing Element #1: Relieving Stress Now

Poor lifestyle choices can crank up your stress pathway and increase cortisol, even if you aren't actually "stressing" about something. Making sure you don't worsen your stress response by skipping meals, skimping on sleep, drinking more alcohol than is healthy, or eating unhealthy foods is extremely important, yet we all tend to do exactly these things.

When we are stressed, we certainly eat more sweets and fatty foods than normal. Sometimes figuring out which comes first, the lifestyle or the stress, is difficult. Every step of your Hormone Diet system provides you with new tools and habits to help you bust out of the stress cycle for good. Great sleep, balanced nutrition, exercise, supplements to reduce stress (see the supplement options for excess cortisol in Chapter 13) and basic supplements to protect your body from stress (the Hormone Diet supplement plan in Chapter 12) are all essential stress-fighting routines extensively covered elsewhere in this book. Here, I will suggest three specific stress-reducing tools to complement your healthy lifestyle habits: meditation, massage, and laughter.

Meditate

The word may conjure up images of flowing white robes, chanting, or bare-chested yogis, but you can actually leave the crystals, candles, and incense at the door. Meditation is as easy as listening to the sound of your breath or repeating a word or phrase for 10 minutes each day. We now know that meditation may actually reshape the brain, modify our responses to daily situations, and train the mind. Meditation works. It's often recommended by doctors as an essential component of any wellness program.

> *In terms of aging, the most significant conclusion [about meditation] is that the hormonal imbalance associated with stress—and known to speed up the aging process—is reversed. This in turn slows or even reverses the aging process, as measured by various biological changes associated with growing old. From my experience with studies on people using Transcendental Meditation, it has been established that long-term meditators can have a biological age between 5 to 12 years younger than their chronological age . . . Meditation alters the frame of reference that gives the person his experience of time. At a quantum level, physical events in space-time such as heartbeat and hormone levels can be affected simply by taking the mind into a reality where time does not have such a powerful hold.*
> —DEEPAK CHOPRA, a leader in mind-body medicine,
> from *Ageless Body, Timeless Mind*

Meditation also has amazing effects on your hormones. It lowers the stress hormones cortisol and adrenaline and raises our anti-aging, antistress hormones DHEA and serotonin. Meditation isn't difficult to learn and do, but it does require commitment, patience, and practice.

Think of meditation as the cheapest and easiest sport to play. The only requirement is discipline and the ability to comfortably spend a few moments alone without distractions. Ultimately, blocking off this chunk of time for introspection is the greatest challenge, as many of us would rather spend it zoning out with an episode of *Survivor* than practicing conscious awareness of our internal environment. All too often we attempt to avoid or distort reality rather than embrace it. But once you incorporate meditating into your daily routine, you'll find the journey to enlightenment is accompanied by endless physical, emotional, and spiritual benefits.

HOW TO MEDITATE IN FIVE SIMPLE STEPS

1. **Get comfortable.** Sit or lie in a comfortable, quiet place where you will not be interrupted or distracted. You may want to designate a space at home for this.
2. **Clear your mind.** Close your eyes, rest, and *do nothing*.
3. **Concentrate on your breath.** Focus on the sound of your breathing and how it feels flowing in and out of the edge of your nostrils. I find it useful to imagine my breath washing in and out like waves on the beach. You can also pick a word or a phrase that is soothing or meaningful to you. One patient of mine, an extremely tense 85-year-old man with high blood pressure, picked the word "quiet," which I thought was a great choice. Repeat the word or phrase to yourself each time you exhale.
4. **Practice body awareness.** Check for tension, especially in your jaw, scalp, forehead, shoulders, lower back, and hips—all the way down to your toes—by consciously examining that body part. Relax the areas that feel tight as you continue breathing.

5. **Stay in tune with your breathing or the repetition of your word or phrase.** You'll be amazed at how often thoughts start creeping into your mind. Just acknowledge them and return your focus to your breathing. With practice, the amount of time you'll be able to sit without your mind wandering will lengthen, and you may even find that solutions you've been searching for will appear.

Some forms of meditation may actually involve physical, repetitive motions such as running or cycling. If you want to meditate while engaging in these activities, practice staying focused on your breathing and allow thoughts to flow freely. Using this form of meditation is very helpful for people who have a difficult time sitting still.

Meditation can help you prepare for the second element in coping with stress—realizing and setting your goals. I often find clear ideas come to me after meditating, just after waking up and during or after exercise—moments when my mind is free of chatter. The shower is another time when ideas seem to flow. Who knows, maybe the sound of the water calms my brain waves enough to let me hear my inner thoughts. No matter where they happen for you, these moments can be a rich source of wisdom and clarity about where you need to head next.

Get a Massage

We know that the cortisol and adrenaline we produce when we're under stress are destructive to our body tissues, immune system, and adrenal glands when they are present in high amounts for long periods of time. One of the functions of the liver is to break down stress hormones and sex hormones. Massage, which assists the bloodflow and lymphatic delivery of hormonal waste to the liver, expedites this breakdown process, thereby helping to relieve stress in the body.

A study from the *International Journal of Neuroscience* (October

2005) found that massage therapy decreases cortisol and increases levels of serotonin and dopamine. It also increases endorphin release, which is excellent for treating pain, depression, and anxiety. Massage helps ease activity in the sympathetic nervous system (fight or flight) and increases our parasympathetic response (rest and relax). I've had patients report that their memory is better for 2 to 3 days after a massage. I suspect the improvement can be linked to the reduction of cortisol after a massage, since we know cortisol is rough on our brain cells, especially those involved in memory.

Remember, anything that reduces our fight-or-flight response can help improve weight loss, lessen water retention, and improve appetite control. So beyond simply feeling good while you are on the table, massage has definite physiological benefits.

Laugh

Professor Lee S. Berk of Loma Linda University in California has found that the mere anticipation of laughter has significant hormonal effects. In a recent study, one group of subjects was told they were about to watch a funny movie, while the second group was told that they would be reading magazines for an hour. Those who were told about the movie had 27 percent more beta-endorphins and 87 percent more human growth hormone. In previous studies, Berk found that laughter reduced cortisol and adrenaline and enhanced the immune system for 12 to 24 hours. Watch funny movies and make time for laughter in your life—or just think about doing it!

I once prescribed the movie *Planes, Trains, and Automobiles* to a 65-year-old woman constantly worried about her health and told a diabetic man of 35, "Don't come back here unless you've done something *fun*." I kid you not.

Stress-Reducing Element #2: Setting Your Goals

Whatever you are meant to do, move toward it and it will come to you.
—GLORIA DUNN

Until I reached the ripe old age of 30, I wasn't able to write about my goals. It seemed too overwhelming because I felt I had no idea what my goals were. I've had many conversations about this topic with a wise friend, Paul. He provided the first simple tip to guide me toward identifying my goals and putting them down on paper. Paul sits down at the beginning of every year and draws a circle. Within the circle he draws a hexagon. Each side of the hexagon drawn in the circle corresponds to a section of life.

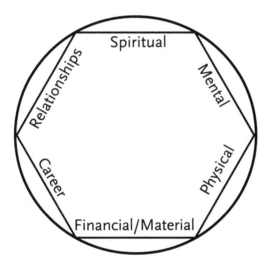

Paul thinks life should be full and well rounded, like the circle. When it is, the "wheel" rolls along smoothly. When one area is not as full, that side of the circle becomes flattened, like the edge of a hexagon, and the circle of life won't roll. It becomes imbalanced when we fail to equally allocate our focus to all six important areas of our lives. It's a simple visual and it works for me.

So I broke down my goals into these categories and thought about *what I would like to achieve* in each area. Next to each goal I wrote *the benefit of achieving the goal, how I expect to reach it,* and *the disadvantage of not achieving this goal.* For example:

Spiritual

GOAL: TO MEDITATE FOR 10 MINUTES AT THE END OF EACH DAY.

- **Benefit of achieving this goal:** Greater clarity, mental focus, relaxation, improved health, less anxiety.
- **Drawback of not achieving this goal:** Continued anxiety, decreased body awareness, lack of creativity, and more stress.
- **How will I reach this goal?** I will create a small space in my house, free of televisions, phones, computers, and other distractions. This will be my space for calming and centering my thoughts. I will spend 10 minutes in this space before bedtime each day.
- **When will I complete this goal?** By July 30, 2012.

Eventually I was able to write down both short-term and long-term goals. I highly recommend you do the same. Try writing your goals when you go away on vacation or at different milestones during the year, such as New Year's, a birthday, the beginning of a new season, or any time you feel motivated to focus, create a plan, and make changes. You may or may not be able to create goals in all areas, and that's okay. The most important thing is that you just start doing it.

I suggest you get a journal to keep by your bedside or write your goals on a page that you can post in a visible spot in your home. When you write your goals, use positive language. Instead of "I will stop nagging," try "I will provide support and encouragement." I'm no expert in goal setting, but this process has worked well for me and the patients I have shared it with.

A SIMPLE, BUT INFLUENTIAL RELATIONSHIP EXERCISE

Since relationships can be a major source of stress (recall the example of cortisol levels in "happily" married people earlier in this chapter), maintaining awareness of the people in your life is very important. One exercise I find very useful is to write down qualities that *describe the relationships you need or wish to have*—at work, with your partner, or even with your friends. This exercise can be great for couples because it eliminates the need for "mind reading" when it comes to understanding each other's needs and desires within the relationship, thereby helping to eliminate resentment or unfulfilled expectations. The exercise can also provide opportunities for clear reflection on the relationships you currently have, as well as creating a template for the people and connections you would like to draw into your life.

Stress-Reducing Element #3: Visualizing Your Success

There are some people who live in a dream world, and there are some who face reality; and then there are those who turn one into the other.

—DOUGLAS EVERETT

I think Shakti Gawain, author of *Creative Visualization*, is the best author to teach you about visualization. She defines creative visualization as the technique of using your imagination to create what you want in your life. She goes on to explain that the energy of your thoughts and feelings attracts energy of the same frequency. Whatever we spend the most time thinking about is exactly what we will attract into our lives.

MUSIC TO TRAIN YOUR BRAIN
Listen to music to increase alpha brain waves when you visualize. An alpha brain wave state, associated with deep relaxation, has been found to be much more effective than a beta brain wave state, which is more prevalent when we're busy with work or tasks. You can also stimulate more alpha waves by meditating right before you do your visualization exercises.

This is the Law of Attraction, and it's the key message delivered in *The Secret* by Rhonda Burns and *The Law of Attraction* and *Ask and It Is Given* by Esther and Jerry Hicks. No matter the author you choose, they all communicate a similar philosophy: We have to imagine the way we want our lives to manifest.

If we are negative or fearful that a particular event may befall us, that event may be exactly what we attract into our lives. I'll take this a step further and suggest that *when our hormones are balanced, we have a much better chance of achieving the physical and mental state that allows us to think, feel, and be positive. Likewise, being positive sets the groundwork that allows for achievement of hormonal balance.* This approach to living with good health and happy hormones is the very essence of the Hormone Diet.

How to Visualize

1. **Set your goal.**
   For example: I want to be strong, lean, and healthy.
2. **Create a clear picture or idea.**
   Believe you are already strong, lean, and healthy.
   Include as many details as you can; envision yourself moving freely and feeling energized; *see* your flat stomach, strong arms, and toned legs!
3. **Focus on these images often.**

HOT HORMONE TIP

In quiet meditative periods and casually throughout the day, focus on these images clearly, but in a light, gentle way, so they become integrated into your life.

4. **Give it positive energy.**
Make strong, positive statements to yourself. See yourself achieving your goal. Try to suspend doubt and disbelief.

5. **Don't forget to breathe.**
Breathe calmly and deeply.

So you now have two very good stress-relief options: meditation and visualization. One involves trying to think of nothing, and the other involves visualizing everything you would like to achieve, have, feel, or experience in as much detail as possible. Cool.

You're free to choose the option that resonates with you, or you may want to incorporate both. Visualizing your success first thing in the morning and meditating to quiet your mind in the evening are wonderful ways to bookend your day. I know we are all busy, and finding time to do both can be challenging. But I fit in my visualizations when I go to bed at night—just 5 to 10 minutes per night. I fit in my meditation when I'm walking the dog in the morning—while I get my daily dose of serotonin-boosting sunlight, too!

Right now I am using the healing visualizations from "Adam" described in his book *The Path of the DreamHealer* (Penguin, 2006). I highly recommend his books and DVDs for health-promoting visualization exercises that you can use for yourself or a loved one. I also suggest going to one of his group healing presentations. (Visit www.dreamhealer.com for details.)

I have seen for myself the incredible benefits that come from regularly doing these simple but powerful mind exercises. I have witnessed them many times with my patients and see them with my mom, who is living with liver cancer as I write this book.

Stress-Reducing Element #4: Harnessing the Power of Positive Belief

He who has a why to live for can bear with almost any how.
—FRIEDRICH NIETZSCHE

The most powerful example I can share with you about this element comes from one of my patients whose mother was diagnosed with lung cancer. Four weeks after her diagnosis, before her treatment even started, she suddenly developed difficulty breathing and died just a day later. My patient told me the situation had probably worked out for the best because his mother didn't want to go through the process of being ill. What a positive way to look at a truly traumatic event in one's life.

Another patient, a 36-year-old man I was treating for a rare blood-clotting disease that caused his lungs to fill with fluid, provided me with an inspiring example of positive thinking. He was awaiting a lung transplant, constantly struggling for air because of his disease. His lips were often bluish because of the poor oxygen exchange in his body. One fall day, I was giving him acupuncture treatments and looked out the window while he was resting on the table. I sighed, "Ah, soon we're going to look out and there'll be no more leaves on the trees." To which he replied, *"Yes, but then we can see farther."*

This approach to life is by far the most important determinant of your well-being. Believing that everything happens for a reason and trusting that you will be taken care of by the universe, God, or whatever higher power you feel most comfortable with will work wonders to reduce your stress and anxiety. Powerful beliefs will also help you adapt to life and all it has to offer.

No matter what happens—or doesn't happen—to you, you can always take heart in believing the outcome is for a greater good: to teach you a lesson, provide an opportunity for growth, help you gain inner strength, or perhaps allow you to form a special connection with someone.

There are many good sources for ideas on stress-reducing element #4, but I'll limit my recommendations to these top choices:

1. *A New Earth* by Eckhart Tolle (Penguin reprint, 2008)
2. *The Four Agreements* by Don Miguel Ruiz (Amber-Allen Publishing, 2001)
3. *The Seven Spiritual Laws of Success* by Deepak Chopra (New World Library, 1994)

Summary of Instructions for Step 1: Strategies for Stress Survival

Implement the elements for conquering stress that you feel will work for you.

1. RELIEVE STRESS NOW. Meditate and/or visualize for at least 10 minutes each day in conjunction with the recommendations outlined in upcoming steps of the Hormone Diet plan. Get a massage at least once per month.
2. SET GOALS. Write your goals in the six categories: spiritual, mental, physical, financial/material, career, and relationships.
3. VISUALIZE. Spend a few moments each day imagining your success in as much detail as possible.
4. BELIEVE IN THE POSITIVE. Understand the power of positive thinking and the Law of Attraction. You'll naturally be more positive when your hormones are balanced. When you are in a positive state, hormonal balance flows.
5. USE SUPPORTIVE SUPPLEMENTS when necessary to restore your hormonal balance and stress recuperation (see Chapter 13).

STEP 2

REPLENISH YOUR BODY AND BALANCE YOUR HORMONES

YOUR SECOND 2 WEEKS

*A man's health can be judged by which he takes
two at a time—pills or stairs.*

JOAN WELSH

CHAPTER 10

NASTY NUTRITION: EATING HABITS
THAT DISRUPT OUR HORMONES

In the end, the biggest risk to the culture may be the inevitable false or misleading low-carb claims and influx of products that ladle on heapings of calories in exchange for carbs. If enough people are seduced by these foods and fail to lose weight, low carbs will go the way of low fat: a strategy that works when you stick to the rules but fails when marketers rush in with promises no one can keep.
"THE LOW-CARB FOOD CRAZE,"
Time magazine, May 3, 2004

Here's what you will learn in this chapter:
- The nutritional habits that instantly cause hormonal imbalance and result in weight gain
- What, when, and how we eat are all important for good health and fat loss

A discussion of the nasty nutrition no-nos will help you before you jump into the specifics of the Hormone Diet nutrition plan in the next chapter. In today's fast-paced, overprocessed, obesity-plagued society, our failure to pay attention to our food choices is a widespread and serious problem. Every day, we reach for inflammatory foods, fast foods, foods containing high-fructose corn syrup and added sweeteners, hormone-infused foods, and fat- and sugar-free foods—all major culprits of perpetuating hormonal imbalance. We also tend to consume too much alcohol and not enough fiber. In the end, we are left feeling fuzzy, flabby, and fatigued. And then, to make matters worse, our poor food choices at mealtimes are compounded by when or how we choose to eat.

Let's talk about each of these hormone-harming habits one by one. Armed with this information, you can start making changes and feeling better by your very next meal.

Foods That Fan the Flames

I've told you plenty about the perils of inflammation and its serious effects on hormones, health, and weight loss. Well, proinflammatory foods increase inflammation and contribute to your risk of chronic illness, including heart disease, diabetes, and Alzheimer's disease. Here are the foods you should avoid to help keep inflammation in check.

- **Refined sugars and grains.** Foods such as white flour, white rice, and table sugar (sucrose) can trigger inflammation by raising blood sugar and insulin. Junk foods, high-fat meats, sugary treats, and fast foods all increase inflammation in your body. (Many of these foods also contain unhealthy fats that further exacerbate the problem.)
- **Foods containing trans fats.** Margarine; foods made with partially hydrogenated oils.
- **Processed meats.** Lunch meats, hot dogs, and sausages contain nitrites and sulphites that are associated with increased inflammation.
- **Excess saturated fats.** These fats, naturally found in meats, shellfish, egg yolks, and dairy products, can promote inflammation. These foods also contain a fatty acid called arachidonic acid. Although some arachidonic acid is essential for your health, too much of it in your diet will contribute to

inflammation. Choosing omega-3 eggs, low-fat milk and cheese, and lean cuts of meat will lessen the inflammatory fallout.

- **Foods that cause allergies.** Most people with true food anaphylactic allergies are aware of them and make a point to steer clear of the offending food. Those of us with food sensitivities or intolerances, however, may not realize that certain foods cause inflammation, faulty digestion, and even compromised immunity. Another reason why experimenting with the removal and slow reintroduction of foods that commonly cause sensitivities from your diet can be a valuable exercise.

- **Too much omega-6 fatty acid.** Omega-6 and omega-3 are essential fatty acids that cannot be produced in the body. Sixty years ago the average American diet included a 1:2 ratio of omega-6 to omega-3. Today, the ratio is estimated at about 25:1. The optimal ratio is 1:1. We obtain much of our omega-6 from safflower, corn, and sunflower oils, which are commonly used in baked goods and packaged items. (Now they are also commonly used in place of trans fats in trans fat–free products.) Too much of these oils in our diet can turn on the hormonal signals involved in inflammation and even stimulate abnormal cell growth. Studies have shown that breast cancer, colon cancer, and prostate cancer cells grow at a much faster rate in the presence of these oils.

In Chapter 1, you got the scoop on inflammation as a cause of hormonal imbalance. There you saw a study by Dr. Paresh Dandona and his team, from the State University of New York, who found that overconsumption of *any macronutrient*—protein, carbohydrate, or fat—can contribute to inflammation. Well, their study even went as far as to link specific, brand-name foods with immediate inflammatory effects:

A 930-calorie meal consisting of an Egg McMuffin or a Sausage McMuffin and two McDonald's hash browns appears to trigger inflammation within arteries "within an hour."

Fast Food: A Fast Track to Fat

These days, we can barely drive around the block without spotting those famous golden arches. We know it's not so good for us but we, as a society, love our burgers, fries, and sodas. Here are some truly amazing fast food facts.

- Each day, 1 in 4 North Americans visits a fast-food restaurant.
- Americans spent $134 billion on fast food in 2005.
- French fries are the most eaten vegetable in America; tomatoes are the most commonly eaten fruit simply because they are the main ingredient in ketchup.
- The fast-food industry in the United Kingdom is estimated to have grown by 14 percent between 2003 and 2007; the industry is now worth more than $15 billion. The United Kingdom also happens to be the most overweight nation in Europe and has the highest rate of childhood obesity.

Fast foods are highly processed, loaded with fat and sugar, and low in the essential nutrients necessary to support your body's own natural production of the hormones involved in repair, growth, mood, mental function, and metabolism. Fast foods also promote inflammation and insulin resistance because they are practically devoid of fiber.

If you haven't done so already, I recommend you check out two very interesting resources on the dangers of fast food: the book *Fast Food Nation: The Dark Side of the All-American Meal,* by Eric Schlosser, and the documentary *Supersize Me,* by Morgan Spurlock.

We're Already Sweet Enough

Our seemingly insatiable desire for sugar and sweeteners can also take some of the blame for making us fatter. We consume roughly 100 pounds of sweetener per person per year. The average adult consumes about 10 to 14 teaspoons of sugar every day!

Sweeteners come in many forms: table sugar, honey, high-fructose corn syrup (HFCS), fruit juice concentrates, artificial sweeteners, and sugar alcohols (like xylitol). Sometimes we know we're eating them, but many times we don't. Sweeteners are used in the obvious places—cookies, cakes, jams, coffee drinks, juices, sodas—the list is endless. They're hiding out in many other products we use daily: salad dressings, breads, pasta sauces, sports drinks, energy bars, "healthy" breakfast cereals, and more. Table sugar, honey, maple syrup, and corn syrup are all sources of carbohydrates. They also contain calories many of us forget to include when measuring our daily carbohydrate intake, especially when we drink them. Naturally, our insulin surges after consuming these products.

HFCS foods (sports drinks, sodas, and many fat-free foods, such as salad dressings) are particularly troublesome because they influence the hunger and appetite-controlling hormones ghrelin and leptin. Remember, ghrelin tells us we are hungry by stimulating NPY in the brain, and leptin tells our brain we're full. HFCS has been shown to lower leptin secretion *so we never get the message that we're full.* HFCS also fails to shut off ghrelin production the way food should. As a result, ghrelin stimulates more NPY in the brain, causing us to feel hungry even though we have food in our stomach. Furthermore, HFCS foods tend to pack a whole lot of calories into a small serving, resulting in tons of extra calories that end up being stored as fat. The long-term effects of consuming too many HFCS foods or drinks are weight gain and a much greater risk of the signs of metabolic syndrome, including high blood pressure, obesity, and eventually diabetes.

Frequently drinking fructose-sweetened beverages increases the production of fat in your liver, causes fat accumulation, and contributes to fatty liver, while also blocking your fat-burning genes (PPARs). These beverages essentially overload your body with so many calories that it cannot adapt.

WATCH YOUR DRINK CHOICES!
We all know we should limit sugary sodas. But even so-called healthy drinks can give us an unexpected sugar blast.
(Note: 1 teaspoon = 5 grams)
* Hype (8 ounces): 64 grams
* Minute Maid Cranberry Grape (8 ounces): 38 grams
* Tropicana Twister Soda (Orange) (8 ounces): 35 grams
* Sunkist Orange Soda (8 ounces): 35 grams
* Fanta Orange (8 ounces): 34.3 grams
* Sun Drop (8 ounces): 33 grams
* SoBe Adrenaline Rush (8 ounces): 33 grams
† Starbucks Dulce de Leche Frappuccino Blended Crème (16 ounces; Grande): 85 grams
† Starbucks Caffè Vanilla Frappuccino Blended Coffee without whip (16 ounces; Grande): 67 grams

Sources:
*www.energyfiend.com/sugar-in-drinks/
†www.starbucks.com

Harmful Hormones in Our Foods

Hormones are often used in farming to make animals grow more quickly or to increase milk production in cattle. There are six steroid hormones currently approved by the USFDA for use in food production: estradiol, progesterone, testosterone, zeranol, trenbolone acetate, and melengestrol acetate. Zeranol, trenbolone acetate, and melengesterol acetate are synthetic growth hormones used to make animals grow faster. Current federal regulations allow the use of these hormones on growing cattle and sheep but not on poultry (chickens, turkeys, and ducks) or pigs. Much of the controversy surrounds beef, since hormones are given to more than 90 percent of beef cattle in the United States.

The FDA also allows the use of the protein hormone rBGH (recombinant bovine growth hormone) to increase milk production in dairy cattle. This substance is not approved for use in dairy cattle in Canada and Europe, however, due to concerns for both animal welfare and human health.

The use of rBGH increases insulin-like growth factor 1 (IGF-1) in the milk of treated cows by as much as tenfold. Though IGF-1 naturally occurs in humans and cows, higher than normal levels of this substance have recently been linked to breast and prostate cancers in humans. To date, no studies show that drinking milk with high IGF-1 causes levels of this hormone to increase in humans, but researchers do know IGF-1 can be absorbed into the bloodstream from our digestive tract. Who wants to take the chance?

To make matters worse, heavy milking can make hormone-treated cows more prone to mastitis, a bacterial inflammation of the udder. Residues from the antibiotics used to treat the cows then end up in the milk we drink. You've already learned about the importance of healthy bacterial balance in your gut as part of your detox. Well, antibiotic residues from cow's milk can definitely disrupt this delicate balance in your GI tract.

Our children are more at risk from the effects of growth hormone and other substances in dairy products because they tend to drink a lot more milk per unit of body weight. Many health experts, including Lindsey Berkson, author of *Hormone Deception,* worry that hormones in our food supply could be at least partly responsible for a growing trend toward early puberty.

As mentioned earlier, steroid hormones are also problematic additions to our foods. Both estradiol and progesterone are considered probable carcinogens by the National Toxicology Program at the National Institutes of Health. Even though the FDA has concluded that the amount of hormone residue in food is negligible compared with the amount the body produces naturally, many health experts agree that *any* excess is too much. Estrogen has been linked with breast cancer in women, and testosterone with prostate cancer in men. Progesterone has been found to increase the growth of ovarian, breast, and uterine tumors. Rather than taking chances with our health, we can certainly opt for hormone-free organic meat and dairy products instead.

In 1989, the European Union issued a ban on all meat from animals treated with steroid and growth hormones—a ban that is still in effect today.

The Fat-Free Fake-Out

Have you ever wondered why obesity rates soared just when all those fat-free products started hitting the supermarket shelves? The words "fat free" definitely make for enticing packaging, but we now know they're by no means our golden ticket to weight loss. In most fat-free foods, the fat calories are simply replaced with loads of sugar. So while we thought we were watching fat and cutting calories, we were packing on pounds and sending our insulin through the roof.

Besides getting an insulin surge from fat-free products, we also run the risk of eating and eating until we are truly stuffed. Remember, *fats help us feel full* and actually prevent overeating by stimulating the release of leptin and CCK. Both hormones work on the satiety center in the brain to tell us when we are full. If our meals are devoid of fat, our brains take much longer to get the stop signal. One of my favorite examples of fat-free offenders to avoid is fat-free, fruit-flavored yogurt. Next time you are in the grocery store, check its carb content. Then put it back on the shelf!

I encourage you to carefully look at portion sizes and nutrition labels when considering fat-free products. For example, some foods may be considered fat-free in tiny portions, but if you eat a larger amount, even that small bit of fat per serving adds up. In other cases, the full-fat version and the low-fat alternative contain almost the same number of calories. Low-fat ice cream, for example, has 80 calories per scoop, whereas the full-fat version is only 95 calories. Companies simply add sugar and vegetable gums to low-fat ice creams to make up for the lack of taste and volume.

The Skinny on Artificial Sweeteners

The number of Americans who regularly consume sugar-free products increased from fewer than 70 million in 1987 to more than 160 million in 2000. During the same period, the consumption of regular soft drinks increased by more than 15 gallons per capita annually.

We've seen a dramatic increase in the consumption of artificially sweetened foods over the past 25 years. Yet the incidence of overweight and obesity has also increased markedly during this period. Despite the superficial logic that consuming fewer calories will lead to weight loss, the evidence is very clear that using artificial sweeteners can, paradoxically, *cause weight gain.*

Research shows that specific artificial sweeteners (such as aspartame and saccharin) are linked to cancer, but all artificial sweeteners are known to cause increased cravings and weight gain, and may subsequently contribute to insulin resistance. According to a study by researchers at the University of Texas San Antonio, middle-aged adults who drink diet soft drinks drastically increase their risk of gaining weight later on. The study monitored the weights and soda-drinking habits of more than 600 normal-weight subjects ages 25 to 64. When researchers followed up with the participants after 8 years, they discovered those who consumed one diet soda a day were *65 percent more likely to be overweight than those who drank none.* Drinking two or more low- or no-calorie soft drinks daily raised the odds of becoming obese or overweight even higher. The real shocker? Participants who drank *diet soda had a greater chance of becoming overweight than those who drank regular soda!*

Artificial sweeteners appear to be a double-edged dieting sword. They don't allow for the leptin release that normally happens when we eat the sugars that signal to the brain that our hunger is satisfied. Moreover, even though artificial sweeteners don't cause your blood sugar to rise, your body still responds as though there is sugar in your bloodstream by secreting insulin. Between the low leptin and high insulin, your appetite and cravings go haywire. Knowing that high insulin is a stepping-stone to type 2 diabetes and obesity, we cannot overlook the connection to the number of diabetic, prediabetic, and overweight people who use these types of products.

AWFUL ASPARTAME

When aspartame is broken down in the body, methanol is produced. Methanol, a neurotoxic alcohol, is hundreds of times more potent than the alcohol in alcoholic beverages. As a result of this chemical change in form, aspartame has been shown to cause neurological diseases and symptoms, including headaches, muscle spasms, dizziness, twitching, memory loss, migraines, and even seizures.

HOT HORMONE FACT

Artificial sweeteners may also disrupt our natural ability to mentally count calories based on the sweetness of the foods we eat, according to research conducted at Purdue University. This disruption may explain why more and more of us seem to lack the natural ability to regulate our appetite and food intake.

Increased consumption of artificial sweeteners and of high-calorie beverages is not the sole cause of obesity, but it may be a contributing factor. It could become more of a factor as more people turn to artificial sweeteners as a means of weight control and, at the same time, others consume more high-calorie beverages to satisfy their cravings.
—SUSAN SWITHERS, associate professor of psychological sciences, Purdue University

Researchers have established that the taste and feel of food in our mouth influences our learned ability to match our caloric intake with our caloric need. For instance, we learn very early on that both sweet tastes and dense, thick foods signal high calorie content. Our natural ability to control how much we eat may be weakened when this natural link is impaired by consuming products that contain artificial sweeteners. These foods and drinks prompt us to eat more because they often have a thinner consistency and texture than regular, sugar-sweetened foods. You may have noticed this textural difference in the past when drinking diet versus regular soda or eating yogurt sweetened with artificial sweeteners.

Beware of One Too Many

Many of us like to enjoy a refreshing cocktail or glass of wine once in a while, but we need to approach these drinks with caution. Alcohol is a known appetite stimulant and frequently causes us to overeat because it also lowers our inhibitions. Just a few drinks, especially those mixed with sugary fruit drinks or soda, can cause a serious insulin spike, resulting in hypoglycemia (low blood sugar). Yes, even healthy people can experience low blood sugar with alcohol consumption.

Even a little bit of alcohol (i.e., more than the recommended four glasses of wine per week for women, seven for men) lowers leptin and raises cortisol. This double whammy leads to disturbed sleep, night waking, and those signature cravings for greasy hangover foods the next day. Over time, chronic alcohol abuse can reduce the body's responsiveness to insulin and cause sensitivity to sugar in both healthy individuals and alcoholics with liver cirrhosis. In fact, a high percentage of patients with alcoholic liver disease are glucose intolerant or diabetic.

In men, alcohol is harmful to the testicles and, as a result, can suppress testosterone production. In a study of normally healthy men who drank alcohol for 4 weeks, testosterone levels declined after only 5 days and continued to fall throughout the study period. In premenopausal women, chronic heavy drinking can contribute to a multitude of menstrual and fertility concerns because alcohol interferes with the hormonal regulation of the reproductive system. Alcohol can increase the conversion of testosterone into estradiol and can contribute to symptoms of estrogen dominance, which boosts breast cancer risk.

Failing to Get Our Fiber

Dr. Robert Lustig, a pediatric endocrinologist at UCSF Children's Hospital, presented a comprehensive review of obesity research published in the August 2006 edition of the journal *Nature Clinical Practice Endocrinology and Metabolism*. In the study, he determined a key reason for the epidemic of pediatric obesity—now the most commonly diagnosed childhood ailment—is that high-calorie, low-fiber Western diets promote hormonal imbalances that encourage children (and adults!) to overeat.

Our current Western food environment has become highly "insulino-genic," as demonstrated by its increased energy density, high-fat content, high glycaemic index, increased fructose composition, decreased fiber, and decreased dairy content. In particular, fructose (too much) and fiber (not enough) appear to be cornerstones of the obesity epidemic through their effects on insulin.

—ROBERT LUSTIG, MD

Changes in food processing over the past 30 years, particularly the removal of fiber and addition of sugar to a wide variety of foods, have created an environment in which our foods are essentially addictive. As Dr. Lustig notes, both excess sugar and insufficient fiber promote insulin production and suppression of leptin activity in the brain.

When and How We Eat

Certainly *what* we eat has an enormous impact on our hormonal health and weight status. But did you know that *when* and *how* we eat also make a huge difference? Eating at the wrong times, in the wrong combinations, and in the wrong amounts can also impede weight loss and play havoc with your hormones. Some of the most common hormone-altering habits I see in my clinical practice include super-sizing; eating late at night; skipping breakfast; restricting calories; eating due to stress; and failing to balance protein, carbohydrates, and fats at meals.

Super-Sizing

Food portions are growing and so are our waistlines. Candy bars are larger. Fast-food restaurants serve bigger meals for just a few cents extra. Even regular restaurants typically serve a lot more food than anyone needs in one meal. Need I say more? Too much food in one sitting (i.e., too many calories) raises blood sugar, sparks an insulin spike, increases inflammation, causes weight gain, and elevates your stress hormones.

Eating Late at Night and Skipping Breakfast

The timing of your meals has very specific effects on your hormones. For instance, eating too close to bedtime raises your body temperature, increases blood sugar and insulin, prevents the release of melatonin, and cuts down on growth hormone release. All these factors interfere with the quality of your sleep and the natural fat-burning benefits of a good night's rest. Furthermore, sleep deprivation leads to more cravings and a greater likelihood of overeating the next day.

Your mom was also right when she told you breakfast was the most important meal of the day. When you skip breakfast, you lose its stimulating benefits on your metabolic rate. You also become more likely to eat unbalanced meals, more calories, and larger amounts of saturated fat throughout the day. Plenty of research shows that those of us who skip breakfast are actually heavier. Missing out on a healthy morning meal also increases stress hormones.

Excessive Caloric Restriction

I've already discussed how excessive caloric restriction messes with your hormones and simply does not work as a dieting strategy. Out-of-control calorie cutting elevates your stress hormones cortisol, NPY, and ghrelin, and decreases leptin. All of these hormonal changes work to perk up your appetite. Insufficient food intake also drops your thyroid hormone and metabolic rate—and depletes your sex hormones, especially testosterone.

Stress-Related Eating

Even when we know what and how much we are supposed to be eating, emotional factors and stress greatly influence our food choices and how much food we consume. High cortisol and NPY brought on by stress cause us to overeat, particularly unhealthy sweet or salty snacks. Giving in to these urges leads to higher insulin levels, more cravings, and weight gain, especially around the abdomen.

Eating can be a very pleasurable experience closely tied to feelings and emotions. Many of us use foods for comfort or to cope with stressful, upsetting situations, especially when we have not developed more effective coping strategies. We also eat when we're bored, feel like celebrating, want to boost our spirits, or want to avoid dealing with anxiety, fear, anger, and resentment. In the very short term, foods can make us feel good. But over the long haul, stress-related eating can leave us with more feelings of guilt and regret, not to mention excess pounds.

Failing to Balance Carbohydrates, Fats, and Protein

This is a biggie! When you eat carbs, the digestive system breaks them down into sugar. Your pancreas then releases a rush of insulin to move the sugar from your bloodstream into your cells. Carbohydrates also trigger the production of serotonin, which creates a "serotonin high" to go with the sugar high for a brief period, until the serotonin is depleted and our blood sugar comes crashing down. That crash makes us crave more carbs, and the destructive cycle continues. These cyclical insulin highs and lows perpetuate further hormonal imbalances, including leptin, sex hormone, and cortisol imbalances.

Eating too many carbs in isolation, like grabbing a muffin for breakfast, is something like letting your car race down the road at lightning speed. By consuming protein and fat together with carbohydrates, we can effectively put the brakes on the sugar entering our bloodstream. Sugar then cruises into our bloodstream in a slow and controlled manner, providing us with consistent energy for a longer period of time and preventing the insulin spike that happens when we eat carbs alone. This glycemically balanced technique, combined with eating often and eating enough, is the guiding principle behind the Hormone Diet nutrition plan to come.

Cooking on High Heat

Grilling, broiling, and frying meat and poultry create damaged proteins called AGEs (advanced glycosylation end products) that trigger inflammation. Research at Mount Sinai School of Medicine showed that diabetics who ate a high AGE-inducing diet experienced a 35 percent jump in inflammation. Those on a low AGE-inducing diet experienced a 20 percent improvement.

In addition to poaching and stewing your meat and poultry, you can also reduce your AGE consumption by choosing fish more often. Broiled fish has about one-fourth the AGEs of broiled steak or chicken.

Poor nutrition habits are a major cause of hormonal imbalance. The Hormone Diet plan is designed to lead you far away from offending foods and egregious eating habits. Get set to clear your cupboards—and your body—of nasty nutrition for good.

CHAPTER 11

THE HORMONE DIET NUTRITION PLAN: THE GLYCI-MED APPROACH

The hormonal benefits you will enjoy from the Glyci-Med eating style are:

- Better fat burning potential through increased glucagon when you eat the right amounts of protein.
- Enhanced melatonin for better sleep (especially when you consume protein, walnuts, or cherry juice and avoid excess carbohydrates at dinner).
- Maximized growth hormone levels when you consume protein, avoid excess sugar before exercising, and have a meal containing protein and carbohydrates within 45 minutes of finishing your workouts.
- Better testosterone status for muscle building when you consume the right amount of protein, carbs, and fats.
- Elimination of harmful excess estrogen when you consume sufficient fiber and enjoy phytoestrogenic foods such as soy, pomegranate, and flaxseeds.
- Prevention of excess estrogen when you avoid high fat intake and too much alcohol.
- Improved serotonin when you avoid excessive carbohydrate restriction and consume enough protein.
- Better appetite control by increasing the appetite-suppressing hormones leptin and CCK when you eat fats and protein at each meal. Consuming enough fiber will have the same benefits on your appetite because, in addition to raising leptin and CCK, it also leads to less insulin release.
- Eating enough and frequently will also prevent the appetite-stimulating hormones ghrelin and NPY from being released.

- Maximized metabolism due to increased thyroid hormone when you eat enough, and frequently enough, and when you obtain the nutrients needed to make thyroid hormone from your diet.
- Increased acetylcholine for muscle function and memory when you include lecithin and eggs among your food selections.
- Reduced insulin and inflammation when you balance your meals and avoid excess sugar, harmful fats, alcohol, and processed foods.
- Better control of cortisol when you avoid skipping meals, consuming excess protein, and severe caloric restriction.

I want you to feel your best. I also want you to enjoy lasting health. In my view, the best ways to accomplish both goals are to avoid foods your body doesn't tolerate well and to leverage the metabolic and hormonal benefits of Glyci-Med eating. When you make these principles part of your life, you can expect to achieve the sought-after results that have eluded you on so many other diets.

The Hormone Diet plan allows you to take control of your health as you gain insight into the close, often overlooked connections between the foods you eat and how you look and feel. Through your process of detoxing and reintroducing foods, you've surely come to realize that one person's pleasure may be another's poison.

Food is the essential fuel that enables your body to do all the wondrous things it can do. But beyond just providing us with energy, the specific foods we eat directly influence our physiology by communicating with our hormones. Your food choices dictate how you feel and function from one moment to the next. Simply paying attention to how you feel after eating a particular food can provide excellent clues to its hormonal effects. Feeling satisfied, focused, and full of energy after eating tells you that the foods you chose had a positive effect on your hormones. If, on the other hand, your meal leaves you tired, foggy, bloated, and craving sweet treats, then you can bet you've just eaten a hormone-hampering meal. The empowering thing about undertaking my plan is that you can enjoy beneficial changes within days or even hours of eating for hormonal balance.

The Glyci-Med Dietary Approach: Balanced Nutrition for Your Metabolism and Your Hormones

The nutritional solution to creating hormonal balance involves blending the food selections characteristic of a Mediterranean diet with the principles of glycemically balanced eating—an eating style I call the Glyci-Med approach. But before we jump into the sample meal plan, here's an outline of the rules. Understanding these rules and the reasons behind them, rather than just following the menu plan, will give you the power to make healthy choices and stay balanced, no matter where you are or what you're up to. These are the rules that you should follow 7 days a week (you are allowed 1 to 2 cheat meals ☺):

1. **Eat the right foods.**
2. **Eat at the right times.**
3. **Avoid the hormone-hindering foods.**

Do this 80 to 100 percent of the time. That's it!

Sticking to these simple rules will help you stabilize your blood sugar balance and boost the hormones that burn fat and control your appetite. It will also prevent the hormonal chaos that can lead to weight gain and overeating.

Now let's go over each rule.

Rule #1: Eat the Right Foods

- Buy fresh, locally grown produce and go for organic or wild sources of food whenever you can. This rule is especially important for meats, eggs, fish, and dairy products, which tend to contain high amounts of hormones and toxins. When you buy produce, I strongly advise you to choose *organic* strawberries, apples, soybeans (and all soy products), apricots, bananas, red and green peppers, tomatoes, lemons, limes, kiwifruit, peaches, grapes, berries (raspberries, blueberries), spinach, lettuce, carrots, green beans, and broccoli. As these fruits and veggies are typically the most heavily sprayed with pesticides, choosing organic will help cut out a lot of hormone-hampering toxins. A fruit and veggie wash is helpful if you are unable to purchase organic foods, and even frozen organic veggies can be a good choice in a pinch.

- Consume Hot Hormone Foods daily. Hot Hormone Foods help you achieve hormonal balance, feel satisfied, fight disease, and lose fat. They include olive oil, broccoli, flaxseeds, green tea, chia, and avocado. To fully take advantage of all the benefits each food has to offer, follow my suggested serving guidelines listed on www.thehormonediet.com. In general, though, you should

Chia is a gluten-free ancient grain that can be added to just about any food. On a per-gram basis, chia is touted to be:

- The highest source of omega-3s in nature—65 percent of its total fat is from omega-3 fatty acids
- The most concentrated source of fiber in nature—35 percent (90 percent insoluble and 10 percent soluble)
- Abundant in the minerals magnesium, potassium, folic acid, iron, and calcium
- A complete source of all essential amino acids
- A great choice for a carbohydrate-conscious eater. The carbs in chia are mostly insoluble fiber, beneficial for digestion

Just $3^1/_2$ ounces of chia offers an amazing 20 grams of omega-3s, the equivalent of $1^3/_4$ pounds of Atlantic salmon. (Source: www.sourcesalba.com) And then there are the hormonal benefits. Chia stabilizes blood sugar, manages the effects of diabetes, improves insulin sensitivity, and aids symptoms related to metabolic syndrome, including imbalances in cholesterol, blood pressure, and high blood sugar. Chia is highly anti-inflammatory. This wondrous little grain also contains high amounts of tryptophan, the amino acid precursor of serotonin and melatonin. It actually has very little taste—another fantastic feature that makes it so easy to blend with other foods.

enjoy all of these hormone-enhancing foods as often as you can.

- I don't advocate counting calories because the source of your calories is the more important factor for hormonal balance, but you should try to avoid overeating in one sitting, since they can cause stress on your body. Pay attention to my recommended serving sizes (measured by your hand/fist or by the number of grams of protein, carbs, and fat). If you feel you need specific numbers as a guideline, the average woman should eat a maximum of 500 calories in one meal, while 150 to 200 calories in snacks is a reasonable amount to try to stick to. The average man may have 500 to 600 calories per meal and 200 to 300 calories per snack.

- Drink as much water as possible between mealtimes throughout the day—at least eight glasses. For the exact number of ounces you should drink, multiply your body weight in pounds by 0.55. Then divide this number by 8 to convert it to cups (a cup has 8 ounces). I weigh 100 pounds, so my calculation would be: 100 x 0.55 = 55 ounces. Fifty-five divided by 8 = about 7 cups of water per day. If you don't enjoy drinking water, try livening up the taste by slicing fresh fruit or cucumbers into it. If you like to store cold water in your fridge, I recommend keeping it in a glass pitcher and drinking your water from a glass tumbler or bottle, rather than plastic. But most important, drink your water, as it keeps your liver focusing on flushing fat and your appetite in check!

- For better appetite control, try having soup or salad before your meal. It fills you up quickly and helps you to eat less for the rest of the meal—and the next meal, too.

- To stabilize blood sugar and insulin and increase metabolism, the Glyci-Med style promotes choosing one serving of lean protein, low-glycemic carbohydrates and healthy fats at each meal. The benefits, best sources, and how much to consume are detailed right after Rule #3.

Rule #2: Eat at the Right Times

Eating at the appropriate times throughout the day will help to maximize fat burning and keep hunger at bay.

- Aim to eat every 3 to 4 hours. Most people eat three meals and one snack, while others may prefer four smaller meals; you're free to find the combination that works best for you. Timing your meals in this way will improve your fat loss by preventing excess insulin, allowing leptin to work its magic on appetite control and metabolism, and by balancing the stress hormone cortisol. You should also enjoy your meals at the same time every day.

- Eat within 1 hour of rising and never within the 3-hour period before bedtime. If you must eat before bed, opt for a light meal or snack that's high in protein and low in carbohydrates and fat, such as a protein shake made with berries and water, salad with grilled chicken, or a shrimp and veggie stir-fry.

- For better appetite control throughout the day, try combining your starchy carbs at lunch, dinner, or after your workouts rather than at breakfast. Stick to eggs or whey protein smoothies for breakfast and you'll eat less throughout the day.

- Always eat within 45 minutes of finishing your workout. This meal or snack is the only one of the day that should not contain much fat and should be higher in carbohydrates. For example, have a smoothie made with juice, fruit, and protein powder, but no flaxseeds or oil.

- Never do your weight training on an empty stomach. You will need energy from your foods to perform optimally. You may, however, complete your cardio before eating if your session will be less than 30 minutes.

- Do not eat while you are doing anything else (i.e., watching TV, working, surfing on the computer, etc.). Focus on chewing your food and relaxing while you eat.
- Eat the protein on your plate first to help speed the signal to your brain that you are full.
- If you have alcohol or wine, do so *after* your meal to enhance the hormones involved in appetite control and digestion.

Rule #3: Avoid These Hormone-Hindering Foods

The following list includes some hormone-hindering foods you should reduce or totally eliminate from your diet. Note that you can have white processed foods, white potatoes, sugar or sweets, and a few other items listed below on special occasions or on your cheat day, even though you need to avoid them 80 percent of the time. (My guess is that you'll feel so bad after eating them that you won't choose to do so very often!) The majority of the rest of the foods are *always* a no-no, even on your cheat day.

- Although it is ultimately up to you, I recommend that 80 to 100 percent of the time you avoid any food you reacted to during your food reintroduction at the end of your detox diet.
- Processed meats and luncheon meats, which are high in chemicals linked to cancer—avoid 100 percent of the time. Instead, look for natural options from your local butcher or deli.
- White flour, white rice, enriched flour, refined flour, white sugar, white potatoes—avoid 80 percent of the time.
- Harmful fats—trans fatty acids (hydrogenated oils, partially hydrogenated oils, shortening, margarines) and unhealthy inflammatory fats such as cottonseed oil, vegetable oil, palm oil—avoid 100 percent of the time.

- Peanuts—avoid 80 percent of the time, unless they're organic and aflatoxin free (aflatoxin is linked to cancer).
- Saturated fats in full-fat dairy products and red meats—avoid 80 percent of the time. Also limit your intake of safflower and sunflower oil, which may become inflammatory if consumed in excess.
- Fructose-sweetened foods or foods containing high-fructose corn syrup, because it cranks up your appetite—avoid 100 percent of the time.
- Foods containing aspartame and artificial sweeteners, which cause you to overeat and experience cravings—avoid 100 percent of the time.
- Large fish known to be high in mercury, including swordfish, tuna, shark, sole—avoid 80 percent of the time. (For more information and to download your free seafood guide, visit www.seachoice.org.)
- Farmed salmon, because it is plagued with toxins—avoid 100 percent of the time.
- Foods containing harmful artificial coloring, preservatives, sulfites, and nitrites—avoid 100 percent of the time.
- Raisins and dates, because they are so high in sugar—avoid 80 percent of the time. These fruits are okay, however, when consumed with protein (like in your smoothies, for example).
- Nonorganic chicken, turkey, pork, or beef—avoid as often as you can.
- Nonorganic coffee—avoid 80 percent of the time. If you do consume coffee daily, stick to 1 cup a day, preferably before your workout, and definitely enjoy it before lunchtime to avoid interfering with your sleep. Decaf coffee should also be avoided unless it is organic, Swiss water decaffeinated.

In the midst of the current obesity epidemic, scientists are striving to understand both our struggle to gain control of our appetites and our tendency to overeat. They certainly have their work cut out for them! The chart below outlines just a few of the countless complex factors that influence our need to feed. You'll be pleased to learn that the three steps in this book cover all the factors and habits that are known to help get a handle on your appetite.

Factors That Spark the Desire to Eat	Factors That Encourage Us to Put Down the Fork
Sight and smell of food	Out of sight, out of mind!
Overweight or obesity	Maintaining a lean body
Variety of foods and mixture of tastes—buffets and standing in front of the fridge grazing are our downfall!	Avoiding buffets or grazing in front of the cupboard or fridge; limiting flavors and varieties of foods in one sitting can help keep appetite in check
Cold body temperature	Warm body temperature
Lack of sunlight or bright light exposure	A healthy dose of sunshine or bright light
Internal body clock—we tend to get hungry at similar times each day; appetite increases in the winter	Eating regularly throughout the day and *always* having breakfast
Dehydration	Staying well-hydrated
Jet lag, sleep deprivation, and shift work	Sufficient, good-quality sleep
High intake of carbohydrates and lack of fiber and fats	Consuming a mix of protein, carbohydrates, and healthy fats at each meal and snack
Brain chemistry imbalance (low serotonin and dopamine); a compromised digestive system	Balanced brain chemistry (sufficient serotonin and dopamine); a healthy digestive system
High-fructose corn syrup and artificial sweeteners	Consuming enough fiber and avoiding processed carbohydrates, artificial sweeteners, fructose, and HFCS

Quit Feeling Guilty about Food!

Feeling guilty is counterproductive. The enjoyment of your food and your life is beneficial to your hormone balance! If you feel guilty every time you have a "bad" food, you are only amplifying the negative

It takes time for hormonal messages to reach the feeding centers of your brain. So the idea of whetting your appetite with a few hors d'oeuvres before a meal may have a solid scientific basis. According to a study in the October 2006 issue of the journal *Cell Metabolism*, researchers found that the very first bites of food sparked brain activity in the hunger centers of rats trained to stick to a strict feeding regimen. The findings also revealed that the brain center responsible for telling us when we are full or satisfied appears to turn on as soon as food hits the stomach, rather than when our threshold of intake has been exceeded. So enjoying a healthy appetizer beforehand and eating slowly throughout the meal are two basic habits that can help you avoid consuming too much in one sitting. If you tend to eat quickly, use chopsticks instead of utensils, count the number of times you chew, or practice putting down the fork between bites.

effects of the poor food choice on your body. Instead, enjoy the moment and acknowledge it as a reminder that your *future intention is to choose primarily healthy foods.*

Your Best Choices for the Building Blocks of the Glyci-Med Dietary Approach

When we speak about macronutrients, we usually discuss the three biggies: protein, carbohydrates, and fats. But if we define a macronutrient as something that's needed in higher amounts in the diet, then I believe *fiber* and *water* should also be added to the list. When we eat (or drink) these nutrients in the right amounts and at the right times, we can crank up our metabolism and create the perfect hormonal balance for fat loss. So, let's get into the juicy details of each of these nutrients—the building blocks of the Glyci-Med approach.

1. Wonderful Water

Health experts suggest that water indirectly aids fat loss by keeping the kidneys functioning at their best. Optimal kidney function leaves the liver free to do its job as one of our primary fat-burning engines. If the kidneys are stressed, the liver has to take up the slack, distracting the liver from its fat-burning role. But water can help us lose weight in another way, too, by controlling our appetites.

We obtain water not only from drinks, but also from foods. In a 1999 study published in the *American Journal of Clinical Nutrition,* researchers from Pennsylvania State University showed that eating foods with a high water content satisfies our appetites more than drinking a glass of water on its own or with solid food.

High-water foods include soups, certain fruits, vegetables, and low-fat dairy products. These low-glycemic foods also tend to be low in calories, which means we can eat significant amounts and use them to control hunger. They also balance our hormones because high-water, high-fiber, low-calorie, low-glycemic foods limit insulin release and also stretch our stomachs. The appetite-suppressing hormone CCK is released from that stretched stomach, which sends the message to our brain that we're full. These "big" water foods sure cause a lot of stretch.

Just as our hormones dictate when and what we want to eat, they also control our thirst. If we are dehydrated, the stress hormone NPY increases and tells us to drink. Beware, however: Dehydration can also cause us to reach for a snack instead of a thirst-quenching beverage. So get plenty of water! It's a very easy way to control your appetite and maximize fat burning. But remember, sugary drinks don't count toward your daily water intake and must be avoided.

2. Fantastic Fiber

We obtain fiber from plant foods, which are essentially carbohydrates. So it's no wonder many people experience constipation on a low-carb diet. You need dietary fiber mainly to keep your digestive system healthy, but getting plenty of it offers many other health benefits. Stable blood sugar, lower cholesterol, cancer protection, weight loss, and improved hormonal balance are just a few examples. In countries with diets traditionally high in fiber, diseases such as obesity, bowel cancer, diabetes, and coronary heart disease are much less common. Unfortunately, the average North American adult consumes only 14 to 15 grams of fiber a day, when 30 to 40 grams a day should be our goal.

3. Cool Carbohydrates

Vegetables, fruits, beans, grains, cookies, pastries, bread, pasta, rice, juice, soda pop, and candies are all sources of carbohydrates. Despite their bad rap in recent years, carbs are a crucial part of our diet because they maintain our moods and provide us with the energy necessary for most bodily functions, including muscle actions and brain activity.

Carbohydrates eventually end up as sugar in the bloodstream. As I'm sure you know, not all carbs are created equal. So-called "good carbs," also called complex carbs, are converted to sugar in much smaller amounts and at a much slower rate than "bad carbs," or simple carbs. As a result, good carbs spark less insulin release, whereas bad carbs initiate more by causing a fast and furious rush of sugar into the bloodstream. You can differentiate good carbs from bad by looking at a food's **glycemic index (GI),** the measurement of how quickly a food ends up as sugar in your bloodstream after consumption.

High-glycemic foods such as white pasta, white rice, potato chips, pastries, cookies, candies, muffins, sodas, bagels, and white potatoes are broken down rapidly. These foods are simple carbs that are also normally low in fiber. As a result, they cause a huge influx of sugar into your bloodstream, followed by loads of insulin release.

Low-glycemic carbohydrates such as berries, green vegetables, and legumes are slowly broken down, allowing sugar to trickle gradually into your bloodstream, thereby limiting insulin release. Most of these foods are also high in fiber, which slows the entry of sugar into the bloodstream. So remember: *Low = Slow = Go for it!*

The **glycemic load (GL)** is a newer measure that builds on the principles of the glycemic index. GL provides an idea of the total glycemic response to a food or meal and also takes into consideration the amount of carbohydrate per serving. On this scale, a low-glycemic load is below 10.

To make it easy for you and so that you do not have to consult glycemic index or load charts, I have provided a list of the best low-glycemic carbohydrate choices, along with their fiber content, on page 254.

Happy Hormone Facts about Carbs

- Consuming the perfect amount of carbs at the proper times and in the right forms helps promote hormonal balance and prevent excess insulin, low leptin, and leptin resistance. This leads to higher metabolism, excellent energy, appetite control, and freedom from cravings.
- Too many, too few, or the wrong types of carbs (high GI) at the wrong times leave you with a hormonal imbalance linked to high insulin, inflammation, aging, weight gain, cravings, erratic fluctuations in energy, foggy thinking, and many other undesirable consequences.
- No matter what all those popular diet books say, cutting carbs completely is not a good weight-loss strategy. Here's what happens when we eliminate carbs:
  - We cause physical stress, which in turn elevates cortisol that can lead to loss of muscle tissue and more abdominal fat gain.
  - Testosterone plummets, leaving our libido flat and our muscles suffering even more.

- Serotonin sags, and we experience cravings, overeating, bingeing, depression, and sleep disruption. No wonder a low-carb diet is associated with irritability, fatigue, and poor performance!
- We adopt an unsustainable way of eating. Remember, your body naturally puts up a fight when you restrict carbs— ghrelin and NPY team up to stimulate your appetite while your sinking thyroid hormone puts the brakes on your metabolism.

So We've Gotta Have Carbs—But When?

You know that infamous 3 p.m. slump? The one that makes you want to reach for coffee and a candy bar? Well, guess what? A balanced breakfast will eliminate it. We know that consuming too many carbs at breakfast increases cravings and caloric intake later in the day. Too many carbs throughout the day will also cause insulin spikes that later leave us yawning, sluggish, and searching for something more. It's best to consume a breakfast that's high in protein for hormonal balance and fat loss.

At the same time, the right type and amount of carbs at dinner can increase serotonin and improve your sleep. Beware, however, of too much sugar (or too many carbs) before bed or after exercise because this prevents growth hormone release, sabotaging the muscle-building and fat-burning benefits we enjoy from these activities.

Carbohydrates: Which Sources Are Best and How Much Should You Have?

The text and tables beginning on page 254 outline the top low-glycemic starch, fruit, veggie, bean, and nut options, as well as your daily suggested number of servings for each. You need to select at least one carbohydrate at each meal. Each table includes serving sizes and fiber content. On most days, your intake of dietary fiber will be very close to your 30- to 40-gram target. You may add a fiber supplement to your diet if you find that you are falling short based on your daily selections from all the categories below.

Rather than using the charts I've provided with your recommended selections and serving sizes, you can also determine you carbohydrate intake by reading labels. Women should consume 25 to 35 grams of carbohydrates per meal; men should aim for 35 to 45 grams. Snack servings should be a maximum of half this amount.

YOUR BEST GLYCI-MED GLYCEMIC LOW-CARB CHOICES
STARCHY CARBS
Most women should choose 1 starch daily; men should choose 2.

Very active people generally need more carbohydrates each day than less active people do. If you are an extremely active person (i.e., someone who exercises intensively with weights and/or does cardio 5 to 6 days a week), you may need 2 (women) or even 3 (men) starches daily. If you begin to experience fatigue or if you can't perform as well during your workouts, you likely need an extra serving. Drop the additional serving, however, if you start to gain weight or experience cravings.

Pasta, Rice, Grains	Suggested Serving Size	Grams of Fiber per Serving
Pearl barley	½ cup	3.0
Brown rice	½ cup	2.0
Buckwheat (kasha)	½ cup	8.5
Ezekiel pasta (Foods for Life)	½ cup	4.4
Kamut pasta	½ cup	6.3
Whole-wheat pasta	½ cup	2.7
Quinoa	½ cup	5.0
Chia*	2 tablespoons	4.5
Wheat bran*	½ cup	12.3
Wheat germ*	3 tablespoons	3.9
Starchy Veggies	Suggested Serving Size	Grams of Fiber per Serving
Sweet potato	½ cup	4.0
Acorn squash	½ cup	4.6
Butternut squash	½ cup	2.8

* Not significant sources of carbohydrates, but excellent sources of fiber.

Breads	Suggested Serving Size	Grams of Fiber per Serving
Ezekiel bread (Food for Life)	1 slice	3.0
Ezekiel tortilla (Food for Life)	1 tortilla	5.0
Kamut	1 slice	4.0
Pumpernickel	1 slice	2.7
Rye	1 slice	1.8
Stone Mills Glycemically Tested Bread	2 slices	4
Whole wheat	1 slice	1.5
Cereals	Suggested Serving Size	Grams of Fiber per Serving
All-Bran	⅓ cup	8.6
Fiber One	½ cup	11.9
40% Bran Flakes	⅔ cup	4.3
Kashi GOLEAN	½ cup	5.0
Oat bran, cooked	½ cup	4.0
Oat flakes	1 cup	3.1
Oatmeal	⅓ cup	2.7
Crackers	Suggested Serving Size	Grams of Fiber per Serving
Ryvita Crispbread (light rye, dark rye, sesame rye, or rye and oat bran)	3 slices	5.0
Ryvita Crispbread (multigrain, sunflower seeds and oat, pumpkin seeds and oat)	2 slices	4.0
Ryvita Snackbread (high fiber)	6 slices	5.0
Wasa Sourdough	4 slices	8.0
Wasa Fiber Rye	4 slices	8.0

FRUITS

Women should choose 2 fruits daily; men should choose 3.

Fruits	Suggested Serving Size	Grams of Fiber per Serving
Apple	1 small	2.8
Applesauce, unsweetened	½ cup	2.0
Apricots, dried	7 halves	2.0
Apricots, fresh	4	3.5
Banana	½ small	1.1

Fruit (continued)	Suggested Serving Size	Grams of Fiber per Serving
Blueberries	1 cup	4.0
Cherries	1 cup	2.3
Goji berries	1 tablespoon	4.0
Grapefruit	½ medium	1.6
Kiwifruit	1 large	3.3
Orange	1 small	2.9
Peach	1 medium	2.0
Pear	½ large	2.9
Pomegranate	½ cup	1.0
Plum	2 medium	2.4
Açaí berries	2 tablespoons	3.0
Prunes	3 medium	1.7
Raspberries	1 cup	3.3
Strawberries	1¼ cups	2.8
Watermelon	1¼ cups cubes	0.6

VEGGIES

Both women and men should choose a minimum of 6 to 10 veggies daily, though you may enjoy unlimited amounts of each.

Vegetables	Serving Size (you may have unlimited amounts)	Grams of Fiber per Serving
Cooked Veggies		
Asparagus	½ cup	2.8
Beets, root only	½ cup	1.8
Broccoli	½ cup	2.4
Brussels sprouts	½ cup	3.8
Carrots	½ cup	2.0
Cauliflower	½ cup	1.0
Green beans	½ cup	2.0
Kale	½ cup	2.5
Okra	½ cup	4.1
Peas	½ cup	4.3
Spinach	½ cup	1.6
Tomato sauce	½ cup	1.7
Turnip	½ cup	4.8

Vegetables (continued)	Serving Size (you may have unlimited amounts)	Grams of Fiber per Serving
Raw Veggies		
Cabbage	1 cup	1.5
Carrots	1 large	2.3
Celery	1 cup	1.7
Cucumber	1 cup	0.5
Lettuce, Romaine	2 cups	1.9
Mushrooms, fresh	1 cup pieces	0.8
Onion, fresh	½ cup chopped	1.7
Green pepper	1 cup chopped	1.7
Tomato	1 medium	1.0

BEANS

Both women and men should choose 1 serving daily.

Beans	Suggested Serving Size	Grams of Fiber per Serving
Black beans	½ cup	6.1
Black-eyed peas	½ cup	4.7
Chickpeas, dried or in hummus	½ cup	4.3
Kidney beans, light red	½ cup	7.9
Lentils	½ cup	5.2
Lima beans	½ cup	4.3
Navy beans	½ cup	6.5
Pinto beans	½ cup	6.1

NUTS

Both women and men should choose 1 serving daily.

Nuts or Seeds	Suggested Serving Size	Grams of Fiber per Serving
Almonds	12 whole	1.6
Cashews	9 whole	0.5
Pecans	10 halves	1.35
Walnuts	7 halves	0.9
Almond butter, smooth or crunchy	1 tablespoon	1.0
Flaxseeds	1 tablespoon	3.3
Pumpkin seeds	1 tablespoon	1.1
Sesame seeds	1 tablespoon	0.5
Sunflower seeds	1 tablespoon	0.5

Fiber information primarily sourced from Harvard University Health, Nutrition Services (May 2004), available at: www.uhs.harvard.edu/assets/File/OurServices/Service_Nutrition_Fiber.pdf (accessed June 24, 2008), which was adapted from J.W. Anderson's *Plant Fiber in Foods,* 2nd ed. (Lexington, KY): HCF Nutrition Research Foundation, 1990).

Reading Nutrition Labels and Making Great Carb Choices

Understanding nutrition labels and the glycemic index will help you be carb-smart when you shop, cook, and eat. Just follow these guidelines.

I. READ NUTRITION LABELS CAREFULLY

- **Read the ingredients.** If the product contains any hormone-hindering ingredients, put it back on the shelf. Do the same thing if the product has sugar listed at the beginning of the ingredients.
- **Check the serving size allocated for the nutrition info.** A serving size of five potato chips doesn't make much sense based on the amount that most of us would really eat in a sitting. Sometimes foods look as though they are a good choice for you, but only because the serving size used to report the nutrition values is completely unrealistic.

- **Check the amount of carbohydrates.** Read the amount listed on the label and measure it against the total amount of carbohydrate you should consume per meal and snack. (Remember, the average woman needs 25 to 35 grams, whereas most men require 35 to 45 grams per meal.) If the product is higher than these amounts, look for something else.

- **Check the amount of protein.** Remember this simple guideline: *If the product contains equal amounts of protein and carbohydrates or more protein than carbs per serving, it is a good choice for you.* For example: Vanilla soy milk has 11 g of carbs and 6 g of protein; plain soy milk has 3 g of carbs and 6 g of protein. In this case, the plain milk is a much better bet. Next, compare it with the amount of protein you should consume per meal and snack (the average woman needs 25 to 30 grams per meal, and men need 35 to 40 grams). This will help you determine your serving size.

> **MAKE YOUR TRIP TO STARBUCKS HORMONE FRIENDLY**
>
> For a quick and easy meal option on the go, order a Vivanno—but first cut the carbs by making these simple requests:
>
> - Orange Mango Blend—order it with half the banana, and half juice, half water.
> - Banana Chocolate Blend—order it with half the banana and low-fat milk or plain soy milk instead of 2% milk.
>
> *HOT HORMONE TIP*

- **Check the fat content.** Compare it with the total amount of fat you should consume in a meal or snack (10 to 12 g per meal for women and 12 to 15 g for men). Check the saturated fat content in particular, and aim for little to none.

- **Check the fiber content.** Products that contain less than 2 g of fiber per serving are not great choices. If you have a number of brands to choose from, select the product that's highest in fiber.

- **Check the sodium content.** Products with less than 140 mg of salt are considered to be low-sodium choices. Remember that you should consume only 2,300 mg of sodium per day (about 1 teaspoon of salt). When comparing products, pick the one that's lowest in sodium.

- **Check the calorie content.** Measure the calorie count against the total number of calories you should be having— remember that 400 to 500 calories per meal is a good guideline for women, 500 to 600 calories per meal for men.

2. GET FAMILIAR WITH THE GLYCEMIC INDEX (GI) AND GLYCEMIC LOAD (GL) OF YOUR FAVORITE PRODUCTS

You don't have to remember the exact GI or GL number for each food; you only need to know whether it is high or low on the charts. I just outlined the best glycemic choices along with their fiber content for you in the charts provided in this chapter. Web sites are listed for your reference in the resource section of the book.

4. Protein Power

In much the same way that carbohydrates are broken down into sugar, proteins are broken down into smaller subunits called amino acids. Amino acids are the essential building blocks of hormones, neurotransmitters, enzymes that assist in digestion, and antibodies that fight infection. Protein is also vital for tissue healing and repair. If you are not recovering well after your workouts, for example, you may need more protein in your diet.

Avoiding excess protein is just as important as getting enough. Too much protein can cause stress on your kidneys, exacerbate osteoporosis, and hamper your digestive system. Diana Schwarzbein, a medical doctor and the author of *The Schwarzbein Principle,* suggests that taking in too much protein in one sitting or eating protein without carbohydrates elevates cortisol and fatigues our adrenals.

Happy Hormone Facts about Protein
- Protein is a necessary building block for many hormones, including serotonin, melatonin, growth hormone, thyroid

hormone, and dopamine. If we fail to get enough in our diet, we can experience mood disorders, memory loss, increased appetite and cravings, decreased metabolism, sleep disruption, muscle loss, and weight gain.

- Protein also packs a hormonal punch because it stimulates the activity of many of our fat-burning and appetite-controlling hormones when we consume it in the right amounts.
- Protein encourages the release of leptin and glucagon, which work opposite to insulin to encourage fat loss.
- Protein also stimulates the release of peptide YY from the gut, suppressing your appetite.
- When consumed before and after workouts, protein increases growth hormone release to stimulate muscle growth, tissue repair, and fat burning.

Protein: Which Sources Are Best and How Much Should You Have?

Although great carb choices are low in sugar, your best protein bets are those that are low in fat. Protein sources high in saturated fats, such as red meats and full-fat dairy products, increase inflammation in your body. And remember, more inflammation only serves to accelerate weight gain, hormonal imbalance, and insulin resistance. You may also notice, as many of my patients do, that reducing or avoiding these inflammatory foods can alleviate joint pain and stiffness within only a few weeks.

Protein requirements vary depending on gender, lean muscle mass, and activity levels. As a very simple guideline you will select a serving of protein about the size and thickness of your palm at every meal, along with a source of carbohydrates and fat. Do this three times a day at mealtimes, and consume about half that much protein in snacks. If

> **HOW MUCH IS TOO MUCH PROTEIN?**
> When the low-carb craze hit its peak, many critics claimed that these diets were too high in protein. Consuming too much protein can definitely cause stress on the body, particularly the kidneys. In most cases, a diet made up of about 30 percent is just right.

HOT HORMONE FACT

you're reading a label, women should aim for 25 to 30 grams of protein per meal and 15 grams per snack. Men should consume 40 to 45 grams of protein per meal and 20 grams per snack.

YOUR BEST GLYCI-MED PROTEIN CHOICES

Both men and women should choose a total 3 servings for meals and $^1/_2$ serving for your snacks daily.

Source	Suggested Serving Size	Special Notes
Fish	Size and width of your palm	Choose organic farmed fish or wild fish as often as possible. Limit your intake of tuna, swordfish, mahi mahi, king mackerel, and other larger fish that often have high mercury content. Avoid nonorganic farmed fish as much as possible, as these typically contain more toxins.
Chicken and turkey	Size and width of your palm	Choose organic whenever possible. Remember ground chicken and turkey are a lower-fat alternative to beef in burgers and chili.
Omega-3 eggs and liquid egg whites	Women: 4 to 5 egg whites or 2 whole eggs. Men: 5 to 7 egg whites or 3 whole eggs.	I recommend always using 1 whole egg and adding in more liquid egg whites rather than throwing out your yolks. (The protein from the whites is better absorbed in the presence of yolk, plus it tastes better!)
Low-fat cottage and ricotta cheese	1 cup = 28 grams of protein (so women should consume 1 cup; men 1½ cups)	Great mixed with yogurt to increase the protein content or eaten alone with fruit.
Fermented soy products	Size and width of your palm; stick to a maximum of 1 serving of soy products per day	If you choose soy-based meat substitutes, pick ones that are low in fat and also free of additives and genetically modified (GM) soy. Tofu, tempeh, soy nuts, and edamame can also be used as sources of protein. I prefer tempeh over tofu because it is a fermented source of soy protein and, therefore, more absorbable.

Source	Suggested Serving Size	Special Notes
Organic pressed cottage cheese (Organic Meadows)	½ cup = 24 grams of protein (so women should have ½ cup; men may have ¾–1 cup)	Excellent for adding texture and protein to soups and chilies.
Scallops	5–7 medium-size or about 15 small scallops provide more than 15 grams of protein	Scallops are almost pure protein.
Shrimp	4 ounces = 23 grams of protein	If you choose shrimp, be aware that it does contain significant amounts of cholesterol (though the effect of this on our cholesterol level is debatable).
Lean cuts of red meat	Size and width of your palm	Again, organic is best. These are high in saturated fat, so keep your intake to only once or twice per month.
Whey protein isolate	25–30 grams for women; 40–45 grams for men	Whey protein isolate is the most bioavailable source of protein. It supports healthy immune system function and is the most useful type of protein to encourage the loss of body fat while maintaining muscle mass. It is also a source of the antioxidant glutathione. A whey protein isolate is easier to absorb than a concentrate and tends to cause less digestive upset for individuals sensitive to dairy. Always choose protein powder supplements that are free of added sugar and artificial sweeteners. Those sweetened with xylitol or stevia are best.
Soy protein powder	Same as whey	Choose fermented soy because it is more easily absorbed. Jarrow makes a very good fermented soy powder that is organic, free of sweeteners and sugar, and does not contain genetically modified (GM) soy.
Rice or bean protein powders	Same as whey	These are good options for vegans and can also be used as an alternative to soy if you are concerned about too much soy in your diet.

5. Fabulous Fats

Consuming excess calories from fat will always contribute to weight gain, but we absolutely need fat and cholesterol in our diet. Fats are essential for maintaining a healthy nervous system, stable mood, and strong heart. They also help keep our skin moist, prevent dry eyes, keep our hair shiny, and help us absorb the fat-soluble vitamins A, D, E, and K. Every single cell membrane in your body is made up of fats. So fats are definitely not all bad, and neither is cholesterol.

Fats for Weight Loss?

Fats also help us feel full and satisfied because of their effects on our appetite-controlling friends, leptin and CCK. They prevent cravings and actually help us to lose weight when we consume them in the right forms and amounts.

Perhaps the most persuasive evidence proving that we need to consume fat to lose fat comes from a team of scientists at the Washington University School of Medicine. Their research showed that *old fat* stored around the belly, thighs, or butt *cannot* be burned off effectively unless we have *new fat* coming in from our diet or our liver. The findings, published in the May 2005 edition of *Cell Metabolism,* revealed that knocking out the fat-producing enzyme from the liver of mice (i.e., making mice unable to produce fats necessary to maintain normal sugar, fat, and cholesterol metabolism) caused the mice to develop fatty liver and show signs of disease even when they were fed a *zero-fat* diet! The mice livers were apparently unable to initiate the fat-burning process and also showed signs of increased inflammation.

> **HOT HORMONE TIP**
>
> **IMFLAMMATORY PROTEIN**
> The inflammatory high-fat proteins you should avoid:
> • Full-fat cheeses
> • Full-fat meat products such as steaks, ribs, and pork
> • Processed meats
> • Deep-fried meats (chicken wings, etc.)
> If you must eat these things, enjoy them on your cheat day and remember to go for a walk after your meal!

Happy Hormone Facts about Fats

- Like protein, fats and cholesterol are necessary building blocks for certain hormones, including progesterone, testosterone, cortisol, and estrogen.
- Cholesterol is an essential constituent of healthy cell membranes, a precursor to bile salts needed for digestion, and a component of vitamin D.
- Eating fats also stimulates the production of other hormones, including appetite-controlling leptin and CCK. Both these hormones play huge roles in telling us when to stop eating.

The Right Fats Help You Stay Slim!

Saturated fats, such as those in red meats and full-fat dairy products, increase the appetite by reducing the appetite-suppressing hormones leptin and CCK. Yes, you should limit your intake of these types of fats, but eliminating fat altogether is not the answer either. Instead, choose healthy options such as avocado, olives, olive oil, walnuts, and almonds. These healthful, calorie-rich, nutrient-dense foods will actually keep your appetite in check and your cravings under control.

GET YOUR DAILY DOSE OF OLIVE OIL

A diet rich in olive oil not only prevents belly fat accumulation, but also the insulin resistance and drop in adiponectin typically seen in people who eat a high-carbohydrate diet. According to a study in the *Journal of the American College of Nutrition* (October 2007), this was especially the case when olive oil was consumed at breakfast. I recommend my patients take a supplement called **Glyci-Med Forte** that's rich in olive and avocado oil at breakfast for these reasons. You can learn more about this supplement through my Web site. But here's the really amazing tidbit. Research published in the *British Journal of Nutrition* (December 2003) showed that olive oil, besides helping us lose weight, balance our hormones, reduce inflammation, and keep insulin under control, also breaks down fat cells we already have!

HOT HORMONE TIP

Fats: The Good, the Bad, and the Ugly

Fats are sometimes hard to get a handle on because there are many types and remembering which fats are "good" and which are "bad" can be a challenge. Here's a brief overview.

- Good fats *reduce* inflammation, ease pain, and promote heart health. These include the monounsaturated fats (which always remain liquid at room temperature); olive oil; canola oil; and the fats found in walnuts, Salba, and avocados.
- Bad fats *increase* pain; exacerbate inflammation; cause heart disease, diabetes, and Alzheimer's disease; and increase the risk of cancer. These include marbled meats; deep-fried foods; foods containing sunflower and safflower oils, which can become inflammatory when consumed in excess (baked chips, crackers, etc.); full-fat cheeses; hydrogenated oils; vegetable oil; saturated fats in animal products (meat and dairy); cottonseed oil; shortening and margarines (yes, I believe *butter is better* even though it's a saturated fat—though *olive oil is best*).

Fats: Which Sources Are Best and How Much Should You Have?

In keeping true to the principles of the Glyci-Med style, *olive oil must be consumed daily,* so be sure to select it as one of your servings of fat. When reading labels, keep in mind that women should have 10 to 12 grams of fat per meal; men should have 12 to 15 grams. Men and women should have about 5 grams in a snack.

YOUR BEST GLYCI-MED FAT CHOICES

Both women and men should consume 3 servings daily.

Healthy Fats	Serving Size
Olives	3–5 (women)
	5–7 (men)
Extra-virgin olive oil	1 tablespoon (women)
	1½ tablespoons (men)

Healthy Fats (continued)	Serving Size
Organic canola oil	1 tablespoon (women) 1½ tablespoons (men)
Avocados	⅛–¼ of an avocado, depending on overall size of fruit
Macadamia nuts	3 or 4
Butter	1 teaspoon maximum
Omega-3 eggs	2 yolks (women) 3 yolks (men)
Guacamole	1 tablespoon (women) 1½ tablespoons (men)

The Sample Menu Plan

The following is an example of a 7-day menu plan for the Hormone Diet nutrition program, which encompasses all of the rules of the Glyci-Med approach. When creating your own plan, you may also continue using the daily meal plans outlined in your detox step. The main difference between the two sample meal plans is that the detox meals are free of gluten, dairy, and red meats. You should not choose meals containing these foods during this step (or moving forward) if you noticed reactions to the foods during your reintroduction process.

Eating well does not have to be complicated; it just takes some planning. And I guarantee you will never go hungry!

THE GLYCI-MED PLATE

According to your Glyci-Med dietary guidelines, about two-thirds of your plate at mealtimes should be occupied by carbohydrates: one-third salad and one-third veggies. The remaining third should be your protein. Your fats may fall on top of your carbohydrate selections (as salad dressing, for instance) or be consumed within your protein selections. Add spices to your meals as often as you can. Once a day, include your serving of starchy carbohydrate. I recommend including the starch with your evening meal (to improve your sleep and to maintain consistent energy throughout the day) or after your workout, but some of you may prefer having your starch at lunch.

HOT HORMONE TIP

Day 1
Breakfast: Awesome Omelette (page 412)
Lunch: Lovely Lentil Soup (page 420) and tomatoes with Balsamic Vinegar and Olive Oil Dressing (page 415)
Snack: The Simply Bar (See the Resource Section, page 449)
Dinner: Veggie Chili (page 426)

Day 2
Breakfast: Antiaging Smoothie (page 409)
Lunch: Super Salmon Salad with 1 slice 100 percent rye bread (page 430)
Snack: Hummus and Veggies (page 437)
Dinner: Baby Spinach with Grilled Ginger Scallops (page 431)

Day 3
Breakfast: Pure Energy Smoothie (page 407)
Lunch: California Avocado and Chicken Salad (page 418)
Snack: Black Bean Dip and veggies (page 436)
Dinner: Beef Fajita with Side Salad (page 433)

Day 4
Breakfast: Anti-Inflammatory Smoothie (page 412)
Lunch: Sweet Potato, Squash, and Ginger Soup (page 419) and tossed mixed greens side salad (page 423)
Snack: Simple Apple Snack (page 439)
Dinner: Anti-Inflammatory Curry (page 427)

Day 5
Breakfast: Dopamine Delight Smoothie (page 410)
Lunch: Zippy Three-Bean Salad (page 421) with tossed mixed greens side salad (page 423)
Snack: Almond Butter Protein Bar (page 438)
Dinner: Sweet Garlic Chicken Stir-Fry (page 428)

Day 6

Breakfast: Super Satisfying Shake (page 410)
Lunch: Antioxidant Chicken Salad (page 417)
Snack: Berry-Apple Ricotta Cheese (page 439)
Dinner: Mediterranean Tilapia (page 425) with baked asparagus and tossed mixed greens side salad (page 423)

Day 7

Breakfast: Serotonin-Surge Smoothie (page 411)
Lunch: Warm Black Bean and Turkey Salad (page 422)
Snack: Simple Apple Snack (page 439)
Dinner: Zesty Chicken Salad (page 424)

Now you have a good idea of what, when, and how much to eat every day, as well as a complete menu of healthy, satisfying meals and snacks to choose from. We are ready to move on to the second part of Step 2—replenishing your body, topping up your energy, and balancing your hormones with supplements.

CHAPTER 12

REPLENISH WITH SOMETHING EXTRA: BASIC SUPPLEMENTS TO SUPPORT HORMONAL BALANCE AND FAT LOSS

These are the hormonal benefits you can expect to enjoy from the Hormone Diet's basic supplement plan:

- Increased metabolism by replacing the nutrients needed to make thyroid hormone
- Reduced insulin and inflammation
- Improved mood, motivation, and craving control via support of the production of serotonin and dopamine
- Better growth hormone and melatonin for nighttime repair and enhanced fat-burning benefits from sleep
- Increased vitamin D for enhancing mood, insulin activity, and immunity

Now that you've learned everything you need to know to make the Glyci-Med eating style a part of your life, we need to take your nutrition plan to the next level with supplements to support hormonal balance and fat loss. At this point, you may be wondering why you can't simply get all the nutrients you need through your diet. So let's address this question right away.

Why Should You Take Supplements?

Over the past 50 years, our food has grown more and more vitamin deficient. Once upon a time, soils were replete with nutrients, which were transferred into the plants they fed. But as farming techniques have changed dramatically over the last half century, so has the nutrient content of crops. Many of the foods on our supermarket shelves have been transported, frozen, cooked, or processed in ways that strip away much-needed vitamins and minerals. Add in our insatiable desire for foods made with white flour, trans fats, and sugar, and it's no surprise that few of us are getting the nutrition we need from our daily meals.

Then there are the lifestyle factors. Living with air pollution, drinking coffee, taking medications, consuming alcohol, and even exercising—all of these increase our vitamin and mineral requirements. Add the various forms of stress to the mixture, and our need for nutrients is higher still. Some sources say our vitamin C is completely sapped after 20 minutes under stress. A deficiency of any nutrient can cause fatigue, poor concentration, malaise, anxiety, increased susceptibility to infections, and, if left untreated, can eventually lead to a more serious medical condition.

Unless you are ready to leave the city and start growing all your own organic food, the best way to ensure that you're meeting your many vitamin and mineral requirements is through supplementation. Now, taking a raft of supplements every day may not make you feel like turning cartwheels in the street, but simply taking vitamins C and E daily can reduce your risk of Alzheimer's disease by 58 percent. Is it not worth a little bit of effort now to be sharp and active at 85?

The documented health benefits of multivitamins continue to accumulate. In fact, most major health organizations now recommend the use of a multivitamin daily. Certain nutrients such as vitamin D, folic acid, vitamin B_6 and vitamin B_{12} have gained particular attention for their cancer-preventing and health-promoting benefits. Highly promising findings about the effects of vitamin D for cancer protection have prompted the American Cancer Society, American College of Rheumatology, National Council on Skin Cancer Prevention, and the World Health Organization (WHO) to recommend daily use of vitamin D supplements or a multivitamin high in vitamin D.

The Hormone Diet Supplement Plan

I believe supplements are an absolutely vital component of any wellness and fat-loss plan. Seeing patients who have lost a lot of weight without taking the right nutrients to support the cleanup of toxins released from fat cells always gives me cause for concern. Recently, one patient's cellular health showed significant signs of deterioration, even though she had made favorable changes in her body composition by gaining 4 pounds of lean muscle mass and losing 8 pounds of fat within a 3-month period. I'm certain her cells were suffering because her body wasn't able to eliminate the resulting toxins effectively. I immediately prescribed antioxidants and liver detoxification support. I also suggested she do 10 sessions in the infrared sauna to sweat out all that harmful waste! Thankfully, within 4 weeks her readings returned to optimal levels.

All this being said, you don't necessarily have to take a pile of daily supplements to reap abundant health rewards. I consider just five supplements to be essential to the Hormone Diet plan, though I believe there are three categories of supplements needed to *completely* restore hormonal balance and vibrant good health. They are:

1. **Basic supplements or foundation products.** These are the basic products required for the Hormone Diet plan covered in *this* chapter, including an omega-3 fish oil, a multivitamin (complete with 800 to 1,000 IU of vitamin D$_3$), basic antioxidants, a calcium-magnesium combination, and a whey protein supplement.

2. **Products to correct specific hormonal imbalances.** If you have identified any hormonal imbalances or signs of inflammation through your Hormonal Health Profile or blood work, you need to treat these in order to reach your optimal weight and achieve lasting wellness. Your options to correct specific signs of an imbalance are presented in the *next* chapter. The supplements you need in this category will change as your signs

and symptoms improve. You may no longer need them at all once your optimal balance is restored.

3. **Additional supplements to optimize health and wellness.** These include supplements to increase metabolism, energy, immunity, antiaging benefits, and antioxidant protection. Examples of these types of products are glutamine, creatine, co-enzyme Q10, CLA, alpha-lipoic acid, N-acetylcysteine, lutein, DMAE, acetyl-l-carnitine, turmeric, resveratrol, green foods, and more.

The Basic Supplements for Hormonal Balance

Taking high-quality products is important. Unfortunately, many products on the market fail to contain nutrients at the doses we require, while others have ingredients that can be harmful. To learn about my complete and easy-to-use Clear Essentials—Morning and Evening Packs, or to look for one of the brands I have listed for you here, visit www.thehormonediet.com. When you are ready to shop, there are four essential supplements you should be looking for.

1. A High-Quality Multivitamin

Remember, a deficiency of just one nutrient is enough to slow your metabolic rate and increase your risk of disease, especially if your body is not properly supported during detox and weight loss. A daily multivitamin supports your energy, metabolism, and body "cleanup" during fat loss. Your multivitamin should also provide 800 to 1,000 IU of vitamin D_3.

RECOMMENDED BRANDS

- Clear Essentials—Morning and Evening Packs
- MultiThera 3 (ProThera) or Nutrient 950 (Pure Encapsulations)
- New Chapter Multivitamin
- Other reputable brands include Douglas Labs, Natural Factors, Source Naturals, New Roots, and Allergy Research Group

CHOOSING YOUR MULTIVITAMIN

When taking vitamins, you need to consider a number of factors about yourself and your lifestyle. Your age and gender should ultimately dictate your requirements. Your secondary concern should be dosing frequency, as overdosing on multivitamins can create more problems than it solves. Too much iron, for example, can increase your risk of heart disease. Because men tend to accumulate iron as they age, their multivitamins should be iron-free. Menopausal women, who are also normally less susceptible to iron deficiencies, should choose an iron-free multi that's also high in calcium for bone health. Conversely, women in their reproductive years should take a multivitamin containing iron and high amounts of folic acid (600–1,000 mcg).

I recommend taking your multivitamin twice daily with meals. This consistent routine is easier to maintain and also provides your body with a steady supply of nutrients. The recommended dosage of the nutrients that should be present in your multi are on www.thehormonediet.com.

2. Omega-3 Fish Oil High in DHA

Since each and every cell membrane in our body is made of fat, our dietary fatty acid intake determines the healthy composition of all our cells. When you eat fatty acids such as those in fish oils—eicosapentaenoic acid (EPA) and docosahexaenoic acid (DHA)—your cell membranes become more fluid and more receptive to insulin. The more insulin receptors you have on the surface of your cells, the lower your insulin levels and the less prone to weight gain we become. Healthy

HOT HORMONE TIP

EXERCISE + OMEGA-3S = PERFECT PAIRING FOR FAT LOSS
When Professor Peter Howe and his colleagues at the University of South Australia studied the effects of diet and exercise on the body, they found that fish oil supplements and exercise made a powerful fat-loss combination. During the study, overweight to obese adults with metabolic syndrome and a greater risk of heart disease took omega-3 fish oil daily in combination with moderate aerobic exercise three times a week for 12 weeks. Body fat stores, particularly ab fat, were significantly reduced in the fish-oil-plus-exercise group, but not in those who used fish oil or exercise alone. Fish oils make great sense for fat loss, especially when you are exercising.

cell membranes allow you to enjoy greater wellness benefits and weight loss as you prime your body for better insulin balance.

Saturated fats such as those found in animal products have the opposite effects on your cells. You definitely need to choose your fats wisely for wellness! You can, however, prevent the harmful effects of saturated fats by including a supplement of DHA in your diet. When rats fed saturated fats were also provided with DHA fish oils, symptoms of insulin resistance were vastly improved or prevented entirely.

There are many benefits of omega-3 supplements. One of my favorites is that all forms moisten our skin from the inside out, though a fish oil that is higher in DHA is optimal for fat-burning effects.

Dosage: Take 2 to 4 grams per day with meals.

RECOMMENDED BRANDS
- proDHA capsules or ProEFA (Nordic Naturals)
- Super DHA capsules or liquid MedOmega Fish Oil (Carlson)
- EPA/DHA Extra Strength Capsules (Metagenics)
- Clear Omega (Clear Medicine)

5 WAYS FISH OILS HELP WITH FAT LOSS

1. They stimulate secretion of leptin, one of the hormones that decreases your appetite and promotes fat burning.
2. They help us burn fat by activating our PPARs.
3. They encourage storage of carbs as glycogen (in your liver and muscles) rather than as fat.
4. They are natural anti-inflammatory agents. Remember, inflammation causes weight gain and can prevent fat loss by interfering with our PPARs.
5. They possess documented insulin-sensitizing effects.

3. Whey Protein Isolate Supplement

Whey is fantastic for fat loss, building muscle, and boosting our fat-burning hormones. It is also rich in the antioxidant glutathione, aids immunity, and supports the removal of harmful heavy metals. Available in powder form, whey protein isolate is simple to mix into smoothies and is easily absorbed by the body. Choose a product free of artificial sweeteners and sugar.

RECOMMENDED BRANDS
- Dream Protein
- Proteins+ (Genuine Health)
- American Whey Protein (Jarrow or AOR)

4. Calcium-Magnesium Supplement in a Citrate Base with Vitamin D₃

I recommend the citrate form of calcium because it is most absorbable. I also prefer a product that offers a 1:1 ratio of calcium to magnesium. Many formulations have twice the amount of calcium. Taking your calcium-magnesium combination before bed is a great idea, since it's a natural muscle relaxant and can assist with your sleep. Also, calcium is best incorporated into your bones while you sleep.

Most men and women require 1,000 to 1,200 mg of calcium and a minimum of 600 to 800 mg of magnesium daily. Keep this figure in mind when adding up your calcium and magnesium intake from both your multi and your cal-mag supplements.

ADDITIONAL SUGGESTIONS FOR THOSE WHO ARE 40+
1. COENZYME Q10: I recommend 60 to 100 mg every day for *anyone over 40 years of age* and for those who are taking cholesterol-lowering medications. Coenzyme Q10 is a potent antioxidant that is naturally highest in the heart muscle but

that decreases as we age. CoQ10 supplements can increase your energy and brain power and aid your heart health. They are also fantastic for your skin. CoQ10 also has documented benefits for maintaining the health of muscle cells, which typically deteriorate as we age.

2. SAW PALMETTO AND LYCOPENE: Lycopene is a powerful antioxidant that is abundant in tomatoes and pink grapefruit. Saw palmetto is an herb that has been widely studied for its benefits for prostate health. This combination is very valuable for men age 40 and older when used daily for protection of the prostate gland.

ADDITIONAL OPTIONAL SUPPLEMENTS

1. MIXED VITAMIN E: Mixed vitamin E contains all eight types of vitamin E, especially gamma-tocopherol. Most vitamin E products out there contain only the alpha-tocopherol form of vitamin E, so be sure to look for a mix. Gamma-E is insulin sensitizing (and therefore a good adjunct to support fat loss) and has documented benefits for protection from breast cancer.

> **PROTECT YOUR MUSCLES AND GIVE 'EM A BOOST!**
> Mitochondria are the energy centers within your cells. When they are compromised by aging, stress, or disease, muscle cells can deteriorate and die. Supplementing with coenzyme Q10 not only protects those precious mitochondria from damage, but can also give them a welcome boost of energy.
>
> HOT HORMONE TIP

2. LUTEIN: This antioxidant protects our eyes and can help reduce the risk of cataracts. Today the incidence of cataracts and the surgery required to fix them is skyrocketing. Take 6 mg every day with a meal.

3. CREATINE AND GLUTAMINE: You will learn more in the exercise chapter about these supplements, which are excellent for promoting muscle growth and boosting energy.

4. A GREEN-FOOD SUPPLEMENT: According to a study presented in

the *American Journal of Preventative Medicine* (2007), only about 35 percent of adults met the USDA minimum guidelines for daily consumption of vegetables (three or more servings) from 1988 to 1994. Just 27 percent met the daily guideline for fruit (two or more servings). Even though a national fruit and vegetable campaign was launched in 1991, the results from 1999 to 2002 were not much more encouraging. Overall, a mere 11 percent of adults meet the USDA guidelines for both fruits and vegetables. Apparently we need to develop some new approaches to promote healthy eating!

Simply eating fruits and vegetables aids in the prevention of just about every disease associated with aging, yet most of us fail to include these essential foods in our daily diet. A green-food supplement, or a multivitamin similar to the one I recommend for use with my patients (Clear Essentials, which is mixed with a green-food supplement), can definitely help fill the gaps. These products offer an easy and effective way to increase your intake of greens and have documented benefits for energy, immunity, and bone health.

Your Summary of Instructions for Supplements for Hormonal Balance

Beginning a supplement program can be daunting. Spend your time and money wisely by following my suggestions closely. Don't waste your cash or your energy taking the wrong products in the wrong amounts and wrong combinations.

Achieving better health and aging gracefully require preparation. By staying active, getting hormonally balanced, and filling in nutrition gaps with proper supplementation, you'll be better prepared for what lies ahead in your life. You can even expect to enjoy an energy boost—one of the most common benefits reported by patients of all ages once they begin taking supplements. Happy shopping!

Your Bare Essentials Supplementation Plan

BASIC SUPPLEMENT PLAN	
When to Take It	**Supplement**
With breakfast	Multivitamin
	2–4 grams omega-3 fish oil high in DHA (it's best to begin with a higher dosage)
	Whey protein smoothie
With dinner	Multivitamin
	2 Cal/mag/vitamin D3 combination capsules (or take at bedtime)

Your Deluxe Supplementation Plan

Your deluxe version may include the products in the chart above along with any products listed in the next chapter that you wish to add to address your individual signs of imbalance. Use the Hormonal Health Profile or the blood test results explained in Appendix A to pinpoint any imbalances you may have.

ADVANCED SUPPLEMENT PLAN	
When to Take It	**Supplement**
On rising (no food)	Probiotic supplement
	* Green-food supplement
With breakfast	* Multivitamin, 1 mixed vitamin E (high in gamma-tocopherol), a 60–100 mg capsule of coenzyme Q10, and 1 tablet lutein
	2–4 g omega-3 fish oil high in DHA
	Whey protein smoothie
With dinner	† Multivitamin, 2 cal/mag/vitamin D3 combination capsules, 1 antioxidant combination containing A, C, E, selenium, and zinc

* Alternatively, you may choose the Clear Essentials—Morning Pack, which provides all of these nutrients as well as your green-food supplement.
† Alternatively, you may choose the Clear Essentials—Evening Pack, which provides these nutrients.

CHAPTER 13

GETTING BACK IN BALANCE: ADVANCED SUPPLEMENTS AND BIOIDENTICAL HORMONE REPLACEMENT

If you succeeded in completing the Hormonal Health Profile in Chapter 2 without any high scores, congratulations! Your hormones appear to be in good shape and you do not need to include this section of Step 2 in your program at this time. You can move on to Step 3. However, if you wish to add supplements to *enhance* certain hormones or to *address specific signs of imbalance* that were revealed by your profile or blood work—read on.

If you choose to add supplements from this chapter, note that *they are the one aspect of the Hormone Diet you will need to alter from time to time to meet your changing needs.* You will experience plenty of changes in your body—for a number of reasons, such as aging, stress, and so forth. Depending on the number of hormonal imbalances you currently have, you may need to continue modifying your supplement regimen for a number of weeks or months.

This plan is certain to offer you amazing results because of the precise way it identifies and effectively overcomes the major fat-packing factors that prevent weight loss. It enables you to determine why you haven't been able to beat those last stubborn pounds and then leads you to a place where your healthy work in the gym and the kitchen will be most highly rewarded—with the help of your Hormonal Health Profile results, the Treatment Pyramid, and the contents of this chapter.

Create Your Own Treatment Pyramid

Transfer your scores from the Treatment Pyramid in Chapter 2 (page 53) to the appropriate numbered space below.

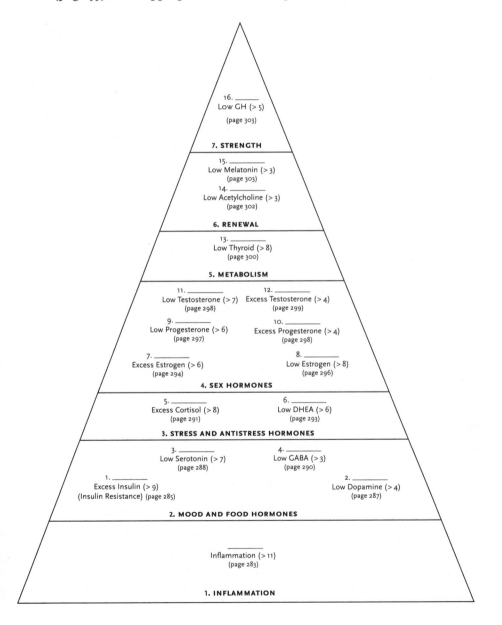

16. _____
Low GH (> 5)
(page 303)

7. STRENGTH

15. _____
Low Melatonin (> 3)
(page 303)
14. _____
Low Acetylcholine (> 3)
(page 302)

6. RENEWAL

13. _____
Low Thyroid (> 8)
(page 300)

5. METABOLISM

11. _____   12. _____
Low Testosterone (> 7)   Excess Testosterone (> 4)
(page 298)   (page 299)

9. _____   10. _____
Low Progesterone (> 6)   Excess Progesterone (> 4)
(page 297)   (page 298)

7. _____   8. _____
Excess Estrogen (> 6)   Low Estrogen (> 8)
(page 294)   (page 296)

4. SEX HORMONES

5. _____   6. _____
Excess Cortisol (> 8)   Low DHEA (> 6)
(page 291)   (page 293)

3. STRESS AND ANTISTRESS HORMONES

3. _____   4. _____
Low Serotonin (> 7)   Low GABA (> 3)
(page 288)   (page 290)

1. _____   2. _____
Excess Insulin (> 9)   Low Dopamine (> 4)
(Insulin Resistance) (page 285)   (page 287)

2. MOOD AND FOOD HORMONES

_____
Inflammation (> 11)
(page 283)

1. INFLAMMATION

Use Your Hormonal Health Profile Results to Create Your Road Map to Hormonal Balance

If your profile revealed *only one* high score, go ahead and address it now with one of the options listed below for the associated hormonal imbalance.

If you have *more than one* high score, start with whichever one appears lowest on the Treatment Pyramid. You will work your way up to the highest imbalance over time. This method is important because correcting a lower-level imbalance may be enough to correct or improve other imbalances noted in the levels above. For example, look at your score in Level 1. If it is high, start to address it now with one of the recommendations listed below. If you do not have a high score in Level 1, move up to Level 2 or keep going up until you reach the next level with one or more high scores. Each level of the Treatment Pyramid builds upon the next, which means that besides starting from the bottom, *you should also address imbalances within the same level at the same time.*

As an aside, taking *all* the supplements I have listed for each hormonal imbalance is *neither needed nor recommended.* Carefully read the information about each product and choose the supplement you feel best suits your needs. You can also visit www.thehormonediet.com for product sources and brand recommendations.

How Long Should You Use a Certain Supplement?

Stick with treatment suggestions for each specific imbalance until you feel your symptoms have improved. The length of time you will need to treat each imbalance will depend on the severity and duration of the imbalance and, of course, your body's response to the treatment steps.

Then, when you feel you're ready, return to your pyramid and address the next high score. But first go back and review the associated group of questions in the profile to identify whether this hormone is still a concern for you. If it is, carry on with the specific treatment suggestions for that hormonal imbalance noted in this chapter.

Don't be surprised if, when you do go back to the profile, symptoms you once had have cleared up. Remember, as you work your way up the pyramid, each level of hormones helps to restore the next.

Keep going through all the levels of the pyramid in this way until you have addressed all your imbalances. After this point, I recommend revisiting the Hormonal Health Profile at least once or twice a year to ensure that you're maintaining balance.

Level 1 Treatment
Inflammation
SUPPLEMENT OPTIONS

1. TURMERIC: Turmeric has anti-inflammatory, antioxidant, anti-aging, immunity-enhancing, and hormone-balancing effects. It works naturally to cut inflammation, pain, and swelling. Turmeric also supports liver function and detoxification. Take 500 to 1,500 mg per day on an empty stomach. Alternatively, take a product that contains turmeric along with a mixture of herbs to cut inflammation, such as Zyflamend (New Chapter) or Inflavonoid (Metagenics).

2. RESVERATROL: A number of studies show this natural red-wine extract assists with weight loss. Have you heard of the "French paradox"—the fact that the French seem to eat and drink what they want but still remain slim? It appears this may be due to the resveratrol from all the red wine they tend to consume. Now we have access to this in a bottle—but not a wine bottle! Data published in the journal *Nature* (November 2006) showed that resveratrol protected mice from the harmful effects of a high-calorie diet, including heart disease, weight gain, and diabetes. Resveratrol appears to act on adiponectin and also possesses natural anti-inflammatory properties. You might recall that adiponectin is produced by our fat cells, but actually helps us lose fat by improving our insulin sensitivity. Resveratrol also provides us with plenty of antioxidant

protection. Take 100 to 200 mg per day on an empty stomach. Resveratrol Extra from Pure Encapsulations is an excellent choice. *Turmeric and resveratrol are both fantastic because they crank up our fat-burning PPARs, too.*

3. WOBENZYM: Wobenzym is the most researched systemic anti-inflammatory enzyme formulation in the world. It is used by Olympic athletes, doctors, and millions of Europeans to help normalize all types of inflammation, speed injury recovery, promote healthy aging, aid surgery recovery, relieve arthritis and tendonitis, and improve circulation. Wobenzym contains bromelain and other enzymes in enteric-coated tablets that pass through your digestive tract and allow the enzymes to enter your bloodstream. The enzymes are distributed throughout your body along with nutrients and oxygen to benefit all your tissues and organs by breaking down inflammatory proteins. Wobenzym rids the blood of these harmful proteins that can damage joints, blood vessels, and other tissues. Take three to eight tablets two or three times a day on an empty stomach. *This is my favorite choice for pain relief.*

4. NATTOKINASE: This enzyme is a by-product of the fermentation of soy. It works like a charm for cutting inflammation and aiding circulation. *I use it specifically for reducing elevated hs-CRP, a blood marker of inflammation.* Take 38 to 50 mg twice a day on an empty stomach for 3 months, then retest hs-CRP.

5. GREEN TEA: Recent research has found that the catechin antioxidants in green tea help to increase fat burning as well as reduce the risk of cancer, high cholesterol, and diabetes. Besides its natural anti-inflammatory effects, green tea may also lower blood sugar by inhibiting enzymes that allow starch and fat absorption in the intestine. Green tea contains theanine, which has a calming yet energizing effect on the body. Typical dosage is 3 or 4 cups of tea per day or a 300- to 400-mg capsule of green tea extract one to three times daily on

an empty stomach. *Green tea is one of my favorite choices for supporting weight loss and cutting inflammation.*

FOODS OR HABITS TO DECREASE INFLAMMATION
- The three steps!

Level 2 Treatment: Mood and Food Hormones
Hormonal Imbalance 1: Excess Insulin

SUPPLEMENT OPTIONS

1. CONJUGATED LINOLEIC ACID (CLA): CLA is naturally present in dairy products and beef. It has anticancer and antidiabetic properties and may be useful in reducing arterial disease as well as osteoporosis. A paper entitled "Dietary Fat Intake, Supplements, and Weight Loss," published in the *Canadian Journal of Applied Physiology* (December 2000), reported that CLA is one of only a few supplements proven to reduce body fat and assist in increasing lean muscle mass without a change in caloric intake. These powerful effects are due to its insulin-sensitizing properties. CLA also shows anti-inflammatory benefits and seems to reduce fat storage in the fat cells while also increasing fat-burning activity in the muscles (it turns on our PPARs). The minimum dosage is 1,500 mg twice daily with food for at least 3 months. Look for CLA from Pure Encapsulations or for any product containing the conjulite form of CLA, which I feel is highly effective. *CLA is one of my favorite choices for the treatment of insulin resistance and inflammation. It's also my top choice for preserving precious muscle during weight loss.*

2. HOLY BASIL: This important herbal medicine has been found to reduce cortisol and help the body adapt to stress. It also improves blood sugar balance and the activity of insulin in the body. Take two gel caps per day. *Holy basil from New Chapter is my favorite choice for aiding insulin resistance when stress is also a factor.*

3. CINNAMON: Besides adding a nice flavor to cooking and baking, cinnamon has wonderful insulin-balancing effects. A study published in *Diabetes Care* (December 2003) showed that cinnamon may cause muscle and liver cells to respond more readily to insulin. Take 1 to 2 g per day, with or without food.

4. ALPHA-LIPOIC ACID: This supplement improves our cellular response to insulin. It has favorable effects on blood sugar balance, abdominal fat, aging, and all of the complications of metabolic syndrome. Take 200 mg one to three times daily, with or without food. *This is my favorite choice for prevention of long-term complication of high insulin.*

5. MINERALS:

   a) Chromium. As a key mineral involved in regulating the body's response to insulin, chromium deficiency may result in insulin resistance. Chromium polynicotinate, a highly absorbable form of chromium, may help with weight loss because of its positive effect on insulin response. Dosage is typically 200 to 400 mcg per day. Prediabetics or patients with type 2 diabetes often benefit from 800 to 2,000 mcg per day, taken with food.

   b) Magnesium. Most insulin-resistant patients have a magnesium deficiency. Magnesium improves our cellular response to insulin, stabilizes blood sugar, prevents cravings, and reduces anxiety. Take 200 to 400 mg per day, with or without food. *Magnesium is one of my favorite supplements to include when high blood pressure or sleep disruption is a concern.*

   c) Biotin. This mineral is involved in the action of insulin. Take 1 to 3 mg per day.

   d) Zinc. Essential for blood sugar balance and insulin action. Take 25 to 50 mg per day with food.

6. PGX: Kudos to Dr. Michael Lyons, coauthor of *Hunger Free Forever,* and researchers from the University of Toronto, who have developed this water-soluble fiber blend. When con-

sumed before meals, PGX aids weight loss and effectively reduces cholesterol, insulin, and blood sugar levels. It comes in powder or pill form. Begin with 2.5 g once a day before a meal (with water) and gradually increase to 2.5 to 5 g two to three times daily. Use this approach to reduce possible side efects of increasing your fiber intake like gas, bloating, or diarrhea.

FOODS OR SPECIFIC HABITS TO DECREASE INSULIN

- The three steps!

Hormonal Imbalance 2: Low Dopamine

SUPPLEMENT OPTIONS

1. L-TYROSINE: The amino acid L-tyrosine is a building block of dopamine, so supplements can definitely help perk up production of this important mood-influencing hormone. Take 500 to 1,000 mg on rising on an empty stomach. Another dose may be added later in the day, but because L-tyrosine is a stimulating supplement, it should not be taken after 3 p.m. nor by anyone with high blood pressure. This product should be taken for at least 4 to 6 weeks to reach full effectiveness. *L-tyrosine is the best choice if low thyroid hormone or underactive thyroid is also suspected.*

2. D- OR DL-PHENYLALANINE: Like L-tyrosine, phenylalanine is a building block of dopamine. A study published in one German psychiatry journal showed that phenylalanine was as effective as certain antidepressant drugs, though both the D and DL forms have been found to be beneficial for depression. Take 500 to 1,000 mg per day on an empty stomach before 3 p.m. Like L-tyrosine, phenylalanine must be taken for at least 4 to 6 weeks for full effectiveness. *And DL-phenylalanine may be the better choice if you also have body aches and pains.*

3. RHODIOLA: Rhodiola can enhance learning capacity and memory and may also be useful for treating fatigue, stress, or

depression. Research suggests rhodiola may enhance mood regulation and fight depression by stimulating the activity of serotonin and dopamine. Take 200 to 400 mg per day in the morning on an empty stomach for a minimum of 1 month.

4. CHASTEBERRY EXTRACT (VITEX): Chasteberry has been shown to increase both dopamine and progesterone, making it an excellent choice for *women who experience symptoms of depression in conjunction with PMS or irregular menstrual cycles.* Take 200 mg of a 10:1 extract each morning before breakfast for 1 to 6 months.

FOODS OR SPECIFIC HABITS TO INCREASE DOPAMINE

- All proteins (meat, milk products, fish, beans, nuts, soy products). Turkey is high in phenylalanine. In fact, phenylalanine is found in most protein foods, so eat them when you want to feel sharper. Coffee may also stimulate dopamine release.
- Exercise
- Sex
- Massage
- Sources of L-tyrosine to increase the production of dopamine are almonds, avocados, bananas, dairy products, lima beans, pumpkin seeds, and sesame seeds.

Hormonal Imbalance 3: Low Serotonin
SUPPLEMENT OPTIONS

1. 5-HTP: A derivative of tryptophan and one step closer to becoming serotonin, 5-hydroxytryptophan (5-HTP) has been found to be more effective than tryptophan for treating sleeplessness, depression, anxiety, and fibromyalgia. Take 50 to 400 mg per day, divided between two doses throughout the day or all at once before bed. This product should be taken for at least 4 to 6 weeks to reach full effectiveness. *I think this is your best choice, often combined with St. John's Wort.*

2. ZENBEV: Specially formulated from powdered pumpkin seeds,

Zenbev can be taken during the day or in the evening to provide a powerful source of tryptophan, a precursor for serotonin and melatonin. Consume as directed on the label.

3. VITAMIN B6: Vitamin B_6 supports the production and function of serotonin in the brain. Take 50 to 100 mg before bed.

4. RHODIOLA: Rhodiola may enhance learning capacity, memory, and mood regulation. It may also help fight depression by stimulating the activity of serotonin and dopamine. Take 200 to 400 mg each day, preferably in the morning.

5. ST. JOHN'S WORT: This herb has been proven effective at easing mild to moderate depression. It appears to work as a natural SSRI (selective serotonin reuptake inhibitor) by preventing the breakdown of serotonin in the brain. It takes at least 4 to 6 weeks to reach full effectiveness. Recommended dosage is 900 mg per day, on an empty stomach. MediHerb and Metagenics make a St. John's wort that is particularly effective.

6. INOSITOL: Naturally present in many foods, inositol improves the activity of serotonin in the brain. As a supplement, it is an excellent choice for alleviating anxiety and depression and supporting nervous system health. I use it in powdered form (Cenitol by Metagenics) and add it to my daily smoothie. Take 4 to 12 g per day. When mixed with magnesium, inositol is very effective at calming the nervous system. *I recommend including this product in all treatment plans for low serotonin, as well as vitamin D_3.*

7. Vitamin D_3 (2,000 to 4,000 IU) and EPA/DHA (4 to 6 g) taken daily with meals will help serotonin to work more effectively in the brain.

FOODS OR SPECIFIC HABITS TO INCREASE SEROTONIN

- Eating carbohydrates will boost your serotonin. Choose slow-release, complex carbs, including whole grain breads, rice, or pasta to keep you sustained, energized, and balanced. Simple carbs such as white bread and pastries will only give you a momentary boost followed by a crash. Plus they pack on the fat!

- The best food sources of serotonin-boosting tryptophan are turkey, brown rice, cottage cheese, meat, peanuts, and sesame seeds. The grain chia contains tryptophan, too.
- Sun exposure
- Staying warm
- Meditating or focusing your mind on one thing. Avoid multi-tasking!
- Exercise
- Massage

Hormonal Imbalance 4: Low GABA

SUPPLEMENT OPTIONS

1. GABA is an inhibitory neurotransmitter—a brain chemical that has a calming effect. If you are anxious, have trouble sleeping, and experience muscle tension or pain, this supplement is a good choice for you. Take 500 to 2,000 mg an hour or two before bed. Alternatively, take GABA 10 to 20 minutes before your evening meal. The standard dosage of 200 mg three times daily can be increased to a maximum of 500 mg four times daily if needed. This latter dosage should not be exceeded. *This is my favorite choice for low GABA.*

2. PASSIONFLOWER: This calming herb appears to improve the activity of GABA. An excellent choice for anxiety and sleep disruption—even in children. Take 300 to 500 mg at bedtime.

3. TAURINE: This amino acid plays a major role in the brain as an inhibitory neurotransmitter. Similar in structure and function to GABA, taurine provides a similar antianxiety effect that helps calm or stabilize an excited brain. Taurine is also effective for treating migraines, insomnia, agitation, restlessness, irritability, alcoholism, obsessions, depression, and even hypomania/mania (the "high" phase of bipolar

disorder or manic depression). Take 500 to 1,000 mg a day. Taking your last dose before bed is often most helpful. Taurine should be taken without food.

4. MAGNESIUM: Magnesium has wonderful relaxing effects on tense muscles, racing mind, and overactive nervous system. Take 200 to 400 mg per day.

FOODS OR SPECIFIC HABITS TO INCREASE GABA

- Fish (especially mackerel) and wheat bran may increase GABA
- Relaxation
- Sleep
- Yoga
- Massage

Level 3 Treatment: Stress and Antistress Hormones
Hormonal Imbalance 5: Excess Cortisol

SUPPLEMENT OPTIONS:

1. VITAMIN C: Vitamin C is naturally highest in our stress glands (adrenal glands), so it's no wonder stress can deplete our vitamin C stores. Vitamin C is a potent antioxidant, essential for healthy immune system function and collagen formation in the skin, tendons, and ligaments. Take 2,000 to 6,000 mg spread throughout the day for stress protection and immune support. Make sure that your vitamin C contains bioflavonoids, which enhance the activity of vitamin C in the body.

2. B VITAMINS: Endurance athletes and stressed or fatigued individuals should take extra B vitamins, especially vitamin B_5, which helps the body adapt to stress and supports adrenal gland function. When taken at bedtime, vitamin B_6 is useful in correcting abnormally high cortisol release throughout the night. B vitamins are water soluble and are easily depleted with perspiration and stress. Take 200 to 500 mg of vitamin B_5 and/or 50 to 100 mg of B_6 per day. These are often available in combination.

3. RELORA: This supplement is a mixture of the herbal extracts *Magnolia officinalis* and *Phellodendron amurense*. It is medically proven to reduce stress and anxiety. It significantly reduces cortisol and raises DHEA, sometimes within as little as 2 weeks of use. Relora can be used to prevent health conditions associ-ated with stress, including poor immunity, high blood pressure, insomnia or sleep disruption, hot flashes, loss of vitality, and weight gain, especially in relation to metabolic syndrome. Take two capsules, 250 mg each, at bedtime and one on rising for at least a month. It is best taken on an empty stomach. I find the most effective formulas include a mixture of B vitamins and folic acid, like Relora Plex from Douglas Labs. *Relora is my favorite choice for reducing cortisol; raising DHEA; and relieving stress, low libido, abdominal weight gain, fatigue, and disrupted sleep.*

4. ASHWAGANDHA: Ayurvedic practitioners use this herb to enhance mental and physical performance, improve learning ability, and decrease stress and fatigue. Ashwagandha is a general tonic that can be used in stressful situations, especially insomnia, restlessness, or when you are feeling overworked. The typical dosage is 500 to 1,000 mg twice a day for a minimum of 1 to 6 months. Capsules should be standardized to 1.5 percent withanolides per dose. *Ashwagandha is my favorite choice for reducing cortisol; increasing thyroid hormones; and treating stress combined with a sluggish metabolism, anxiety, poor concentration, and tension.*

5. HOLY BASIL: This herbal medicine has been found to reduce cortisol and help the body adapt to stress. It also improves blood sugar balance and the activity of insulin in the body. Take two gel caps per day for at least a month. *Holy basil is my favorite choice for reducing cortisol when insulin resistance or hypoglycemia symptoms are also present.*

6. HYDROLYZED MILK PROTEIN: No matter whether the stress you are under is physical, emotional, psychological, or environ-

mental, milk protein hydrolysate is documented to prevent the associated rise in cortisol by calming the stress response pathway. Dosage is 75 to 300 mg per day. I love this supplement, and patients consistently report that it "takes the edge off." I use NuSera, a chewable, butterscotch-flavored product, because chewing the product allows it to take effect quickly. *This product can be used in all cases of high cortisol and is often very effective when conbined with other products.*

7. PHOSPHATIDYLSERINE (PS): This supplement is ideal for alleviating nighttime worrying. It curbs the inappropriate release of stress hormones and protects the brain from the negative effects of cortisol, such as memory loss and poor concentration. PS may also reduce the negative effects of cortisol on muscle tissues during exercise. Take 100 to 300 mg before bed.

8. RHODIOLA: This herbal supplement can enhance learning capacity and memory and may also be useful for treating fatigue, stress, or depression. Research suggests rhodiola may enhance mood regulation and fight depression by stimulating the activity of serotonin and dopamine. Take 200 to 400 mg per day in the morning, on an empty stomach, for at least 6 weeks. *Rhodiola is my favorite choice for reducing cortisol and increasing serotonin and dopamine—stress with anxiety, depression, cravings, fatigue, and poor concentration (even ADHD symptoms, too).*

FOODS OR SPECIFIC HABITS TO DECREASE CORTISOL
- The three steps!

Hormonal Imbalance 6: Low DHEA

SUPPLEMENT OPTIONS

1. RELORA: It significantly reduces cortisol and raises DHEA in only 2 weeks of use. Relora can be used to prevent the health conditions associated with stress, including poor immunity, high blood pressure, insomnia or sleep disruption, loss of vitality, and weight gain, especially in relation to metabolic

syndrome. Take two capsules, 250 mg each, at bedtime and one on rising. It is best taken on an empty stomach. I find the most effective formulas, like Relora Plex from Douglas Laboratories, contain a mixture of B vitamins and folic acid as well.

2. DHEA: DHEA should be taken under the medical supervision of a licensed health-care provider. I prefer low dosages of 5 to 25 mg twice daily with meals.

3. 7-KETO DHEA: Unlike straight DHEA, 7-keto DHEA does not convert to estrogen or testosterone, making it a good choice for younger people who, in most cases, would not benefit from increased amounts of these hormones. Also, 7-Keto has documented metabolism-enhancing effects, promotes fat loss, protects us from the harmful effects of excess cortisol, and appears to prevent the decrease in metabolism known to occur when we're dieting. Take 25 to 100 mg twice a day. One hundred mg twice a day has been proven effective for weight loss in clinical trials, according to a report in *Current Therapeutic Research* (2000).

FOODS OR SPECIFIC HABITS TO INCREASE DHEA

- Meditation
- Exercise; weight training
- Sex
- Sleep
- The three steps!

Level 4 Treatment: Sex Hormones
Hormonal Imbalance 7: Excess Estrogen
SUPPLEMENT OPTIONS

1. THE CLEAR DETOX PRODUCTS: There are very few products that support hormonal detoxification, so I formulated my own. Clear Detox—Hormonal Health and Clear Detox—Digestive Health contain all of the nutrients needed to support the breakdown and elimination of excess estrogen, including those listed next. *This is my favorite choice for treating excess estrogen.*

2. INDOLE-3-CARBINOL (I3C): Formulated from extracts of broccoli and other cruciferous vegetables, I3C is known to increase the breakdown and excretion of harmful estrogen metabolites. It may be useful in the treatment and prevention of breast and prostate cancer. Take 200 mg twice a day for 1 to 3 months.

3. CALCIUM D-GLUCARATE: This calcium salt is heavily involved in detoxification and the removal of estrogen from the body. Some evidence suggests it protects against cancers of the colon, breast, and prostate. Take 500 mg twice a day for 1 to 3 months.

4. TURMERIC, ROSEMARY EXTRACT, GREEN TEA, AND MILK THISTLE: Together these herbs support the elimination of estrogen by enhancing the liver detoxification pathways. Look for a product containing a mixture of all these ingredients, such as my detox formula.

FOODS OR SPECIFIC HABITS TO DECREASE HARMFUL ESTROGEN

- Consume weak phytoestrogenic foods such as pomegranate, flaxseeds, pears, apples, berries, organic non-GM fermented soy, wheat germ, oats, and barley.
- Eat yogurt and high-fiber foods to aid the breakdown and elimination of estrogen.
- Choose organic dairy and meat products to reduce your exposure to hormone additives.
- Add plenty of detoxifying foods to your diet, including broccoli, cauliflower, Brussels sprouts, kale, cabbage, beets, carrots, apples, ginger, onions, and celery.
- Avoid alcohol.
- Avoid exposure to xenoestrogens from plastics, cosmetics, and the birth control pill.
- Avoid unfermented soy products.
- Use infrared sauna treatments.
- Exercise.
- Lose fat with your three steps!

Hormonal Imbalance 8: Low Estrogen

SUPPLEMENT OPTIONS

1. BI-EST BIOIDENTICAL CREAM: This topical cream is a mix of 80 percent estriol and 20 percent estradiol. See your MD, ND, or compounding pharmacy. The dosage will depend on your specific condition. I recommend applying the cream to areas of thin skin (wrist, elbow crease, behind the knees, neck, etc.) rather than over fatty tissue (inner thigh, abdomen, back of the arms).

2. PHYTOESTROGENIC HERBS: Black cohosh, *Angelica,* red clover extract, sage, or licorice can be used to support healthy estrogen balance.

   a) Black cohosh can be used to treat hot flashes, night sweats, vaginal dryness, urinary urgency, and other symptoms that can occur during menopause. Take 40 mg twice daily on an empty stomach.

   b) *Angelica* has been used for ages to treat many symptoms of menopause (hot flashes, etc.), lack of menstrual cycle (amenorrhea), and PMS. It is anti-inflammatory and may help to relieve menstrual cramps due to its antispasmodic properties. Take 400 mg on an empty stomach one to three times a day.

   c) Red clover contains high quantities of plant-based estrogens (called isoflavones) that may improve menopausal symptoms, reduce the risk of bone loss, and lower the risk of heart disease by improving blood pressure and increasing HDL cholesterol. Research on the effectiveness of red clover for the treatment of menopause has yielded conflicting evidence—some reports show it is beneficial, whereas others claim it is no more helpful than a placebo. You can try taking 80 mg of red clover per day to see if it does the trick for you. Look for Promensil, which appears to be the most extensively researched product.

d) Sage is an excellent choice to support healthy estrogen balance, especially if sweating and hot flashes are your predominant menopause symptoms. Take 400 mg on an empty stomach once a day.

e) Licorice has phytoestrogenic properties and is an especially great choice if you're feeling burnt out or stressed out. Take 300 to 900 mg per day before 3 p.m. Because licorice is stimulating, it shouldn't be taken later in the day or if you have high blood pressure.

FOODS OR SPECIFIC HABITS TO IMPROVE THE SYMPTOMS
OF LOW ESTROGEN

- Phytoestrogenic foods such as soy products, flaxseeds, fennel, pomegranate, fennel, etc.

Hormonal Imbalance 9: Low Progesterone

SUPPLEMENT OPTIONS

1. BIOIDENTICAL PROGESTERONE CREAM: I prefer a 3 to 6 percent natural progesterone cream. See your MD, ND, or compounding pharmacy. If you're using this product for PMS, apply it on days 14 to 28 of your cycle, when progesterone is naturally highest. For the treatment of menopause symptoms, it may be used for 25 days followed by 5 days off, or it may be applied on a schedule that more closely matches a woman's natural menstrual cycle. *This is my favorite choice for treating low progesterone.*

2. CHASTEBERRY EXTRACT (VITEX): Chasteberry increases progesterone by stimulating the production of luteinizing hormone. Take 200 mg per day, on an empty stomach, for 1 to 6 months.

3. EVENING PRIMROSE OIL (EPO): While flaxseed oil appears to be estrogen enhancing, EPO is touted as a progesterone-enhancing compound. Take 1,000 to 2,000 mg per day with food.

Hormonal Imbalance 10: Excess Progesterone

SUPPLEMENT OPTIONS

1. Option 2, 3, and 4 (the Clear Detox products) listed for excess estrogen (page 294) can be helpful for excess progesterone.
2. Progesterone may also rise when the stress response is chronically overstimulated. Supplements of hydrolyzed milk protein, which decreases stimulation of the stress response pathway, may indirectly help to reduce excess progesterone.
3. Avoid evening primrose oil, since it appears to increase progesterone.

Hormonal Imbalance 11: Low Testosterone

SUPPLEMENT OPTIONS

1. BIOIDENTICAL TESTOSTERONE CREAM: See your MD, ND, or compounding pharmacy.
2. INDOL-3-CARBINOL (I3C): Supplements of this extract from cruciferous vegetables may help to preserve testosterone by preventing the conversion of testosterone to estrogen. Take 200 mg twice daily.
3. *TRIBULUS TERRESTRIS:* Also known as puncture vine, *Tribulus* may boost testosterone by increasing the secretion of luteinizing hormone (LH) from the pituitary gland. Other studies suggest it boosts testosterone by increasing DHEA. Take 500 to 1,000 mg per day on an empty stomach. *This is my favorite choice because Tribulus also increases DHEA.*
4. TONGKAT ALI (*EURYCOMA LONGIFOLIA,* JACK, OR LONGJACK): Dubbed the "Asian Viagara," longjack has been found to raise testosterone and aid weight loss in men and women. Take 150 to 200 mg per day. Ensure it's a standardized 50:1 extract.
5. L-ARGININE: L-arginine can improve testosterone. Take 3,000 mg per day on an empty stomach, preferably at bedtime. *I include L-arginine and zinc in all treament plans for low testosterone in women and in men.*

6. ZINC: This mineral is needed to maintain testosterone levels in the blood. A deficiency of zinc causes a decrease in the activity of LH, the hormone that stimulates the production of testosterone. Zinc also appears to inhibit the conversion of testosterone to estrogen via the aromatase enzyme. Take 25 to 50 mg per day with food.

7. OATS *(AVENA SATIVA)*: As an herbal medicine, oats are touted to increase bioavailable testosterone in the blood by freeing it from sex hormone binding globulin (SHBG). Take 100 to 250 mg twice a day on an empty stomach.

FOODS OR SPECIFIC HABITS TO INCREASE TESTOSTERONE

- Sleep
- Exercise
- Sex
- Exposure to morning sunlight
- Protein
- Sufficient fat and avoidance of excess carbohydrate restriction
- Cuddling (women)
- Competitive sports (men)
- Success in competitive activities or ventures

Hormonal Imbalance 12: Excess Testosterone

SUPPLEMENT OPTIONS

1. SAW PALMETTO: This herb appears to inhibit the enzyme that supports the conversion of testosterone to dihydrotestosterone (DHT). It may also reduce the risk of prostate enlargement and hair loss commonly associated with DHT. Saw palmetto may improve a woman's breast size if shrinkage has occurred due to excess testosterone exposure. Take 160 mg twice a day on an empty stomach. Supplementing plant sterols also protect the prostate via similar means.

2. OPTIONS FOR HORMONES 1 AND 5: Because high testosterone in

women is usually a result of excess insulin or cortisol, choose supplements that improve insulin sensitivity (Hormonal Imbalance 1) and lower cortisol (Hormonal Imbalance 5) to restore testosterone balance.

3. OPTIONS FOR LIVER DETOX: Support of liver detoxification is also beneficial to aid the breakdown and elimination of testosterone. Therefore, milk thistle, calcium-d-glucarate, and turmeric can be helpful for this imbalance. Clear Detox—Hormonal Health contains all of the nutrients to support the breakdown and elimination of excess testosterone.

Level 5 Treatment: Metabolism
Hormonal Imbalance 13: Low Thyroid Hormone
SUPPLEMENT OPTIONS

1. ASHWAGANDHA: This supplement may increase both thyroxine (T4) and its more potent counterpart, T3. Both ashwagandha and guggulipids appear to boost thyroid function without influencing the release of the pituitary hormone TSH (thyroid-stimulating hormone), indicating that these herbs work directly on the thyroid gland and other body tissues. Good news, since thyroid problems most often occur within the thyroid gland itself, or in the conversion of T4 into T3 in tissues outside the thyroid gland. Take 875 to 1,000 mg twice a day. *Ashwagandha is my favorite choice for supporting the thyroid when stress is also a concern.*

2. FORSKOLIN: Extracted from an herb called *Coleus forskohlii,* forskolin may increase the release of thyroid hormone by stimulating cAMP, a substance that is comparable in strength to TSH, which prompts the thyroid to produce more thyroid hormone. Take 250 mg two or three times per day. *Forskolin is one of the top supplement choices when both weight loss and thyroid support are the goals.*

3. GUGGULIPIDS (*Commiphora mukul*): Guggulipids enhance the

conversion of T4 to the more potent form, T3. Dosage is 500 mg three times a day. *Guggulipids may also lower elevated cholesterol and aid weight loss, so choose this one if you're concerned about high cholesterol or weight loss as well as sluggish thyroid function.*

4. L-TYROSINE: The amino acid L-tyrosine is necessary for the production of thyroid hormone in the body. The recommended dose is 1,000 mg on rising, before breakfast. Do not take this supplement if you have high blood pressure. *L-tyrosine is one of my favorite choices for low thyroid, especially when cravings, low motivation, low libido, or fatigue are concerns.*

5. NATURAL THYROID HORMONE: See your MD or ND for a prescription for natural thyroid. This supplement contains a natural mixture of T3 and T4 thyroid hormone. Using a mix of both will reduce the risk of low T3 in those who fail to properly convert thyroid medication (synthetic T4) to T3. Natural thyroid can be considered as an alternative to synthetic thyroid hormone (Synthroid) or as an adjunct treatment if symptoms of hypothyroidism are still present when using prescription thyroid.

FOODS OR SPECIFIC HABITS TO INCREASE THYROID HORMONE

- Exercise—but do not overexercise!
- Get enough sleep. Sleep deprivation decreases thyroid hormone and your metabolic rate.
- Eat regularly and avoid excessive caloric restriction.
- Consume foods that contain the nutrients necessary for the production of thyroid hormone.
  L-TYROSINE: almonds, avocados, bananas, dairy products, pumpkin seeds, and sesame seeds.
  IODINE: fish (cod, sea bass, and haddock), shellfish, and sea vegetables such as seaweed and kelp. Kelp is the richest source of iodine.
  SELENIUM: brewer's yeast, wheat germ, whole grains (barley, whole wheat, oats, and brown rice), seeds, nuts (especially

Brazil nuts), shellfish, and some vegetables (garlic, onions, mushrooms, broccoli, tomatoes, and radishes).

Level 6 Treatment: Renewal
Hormonal Imbalance 14: Low Acetylcholine
SUPPLEMENT OPTIONS

1. ACETYL-l-CARNITINE: Acetyl-l-carnitine is a potent antioxidant for the brain. It is an anti-inflammatory that provides a source of the acetyl group needed to make acetylcholine, as well as l-carnitine, which assists with fat burning. Take 500 to 1,000 mg per day, preferably in the morning before breakfast. *Acetyl-l-carnitine is my favorite choice for boosting acetylcholine, aiding weight loss, and slowing aging of the brain.*

2. PHOSPHATIDYLCHOLINE (PC): PC provides choline, which is needed to make acetylcholine. Take 1,200 to 2,400 mg per day with food. *PC is my favorite choice for use during pregnancy. It supports development of the baby's brain and nervous system, and I swear the babies in my practice are smarter for it!*

3. DMAE (dimethylaminoethanol): DMAE is an anti-inflammatory and antioxidant that increases the production of acetylcholine. It is useful for both cognitive function and for improving muscle contractions. Take 100 to 300 mg per day with food. As an aside, DMAE may also be used topically to improve skin tone and firmness.

4. l-ALPHA-GLYCEROPHOSPHOCHOLINE (ALPHA-GPC): Glycerophosphocholine plays an important role in the synthesis of acetylcholine. It maintains neurological health and may also help to enhance growth hormone. The standard dose is one or two 500 mg capsules per day on an empty stomach.

FOODS OR SPECIFIC HABITS TO INCREASE ACETYLCHOLINE
- Exercise.
- Consume healthy fats and sources of choline such as

lecithin, egg yolks, wheat germ, soybeans, organ meats (liver, kidney, etc.), and whole wheat products.

Hormonal Imbalance 15: Low Melatonin

SUPPLEMENT OPTIONS

1. MELATONIN: Take 0.5 to 3 mg per day sublingually (under the tongue) at bedtime to aid sleep.
2. CHERRY JUICE EXTRACT: This juice appears to provide a rich source of melatonin and may help us sleep better. Cherry juice is also anti-inflammatory and may help to reduce high uric acid, which is commonly associated with gout.

FOODS OR SPECIFIC HABITS TO INCREASE MELATONIN

- Sleep in total darkness.
- Expose yourself to bright light immediately on rising and during the day; keep the lights dim after dinner.
- Consume protein, particularly sources that contain the tryptophan needed to make melatonin, such as cherry juice, pumpkin seeds, Salba, and walnuts.
- Follow the Hormone Diet habits for healthy sleep.

Level 7 Treatment: Strength
Hormonal Imbalance 16: Low Growth Hormone

SUPPLEMENT OPTIONS

1. OPTIONS FOR HORMONE 14 (ACETYLCHOLINE): Supplements that boost acetylcholine will also enhance growth hormone because acetylcholine is known to stimulate the production of growth hormone (GH).
2. SPECIFIC AMINO ACIDS: The amino acid precursors to growth hormone are L-arginine, lysine, ornithinine, and glutamine. Supplements of these amino acids taken together before bed or after exercise may be useful to support growth hormone production. Aim for the following dosages:

- L-arginine: 2,000 to 3,000 mg per day
- L-glutamine: 2,000 mg per day
- L-ornithine: 2,000 to 6,000 mg per day
- L-lysine: 1,200 mg per day
- L-glycine: 1,000 mg per day
- L-tyrosine: 1,000 mg per day

These amino acids are most effective when combined with vitamin B_3, vitamin B_6, vitamin C, calcium, zinc, and potassium.

FOODS OR SPECIFIC HABITS TO INCREASE GROWTH HORMONE
- Sleep
- Exercise
- Consume sufficient protein
- Manage stress with the three steps!

Remember the Body-Fat Map from Chapter 5? Well, use this chart to find your fat spot(s) and then to pick your solution(s)!

FIND YOUR FAT SPOT(S)

Fat-Storage Site	Hormonal Imbalance: Men	Hormonal Imbalance: Women	Reference "Spot" for Your Solutions
Belly or abdomen (apple shape)	Excess estrogen	Excess estrogen	Hormonal imbalance 7 (p. 294)
		Low estrogen (postmenopausal)	Hormonal imbalance 8 (p. 296)
		Excess testosterone (premenopausal)	Hormonal imbalance 12 (p. 299)
	Low testosterone		Hormonal imbalance 11 (p. 298)
	Excess cortisol	Excess cortisol	Hormonal imbalance 5 (p. 291)
	Excess insulin	Excess insulin	Hormonal imbalance 1 (p. 285)
	Low growth hormone	Low growth hormone	Hormonal imbalance 16 (p 303)

Fat-Storage Site	Hormonal Imbalance: Men	Hormonal Imbalance: Women	Reference "Spot" for Your Solutions
Back of the arm (triceps)	Excess insulin	Excess insulin	Hormonal imbalance 1 (p. 285)
	Low DHEA	Low DHEA	Hormonal imbalance 6 (p. 293)
		Excess testosterone (more fat in arms in general)	Hormonal imbalance 12 (p. 299)
Hips/buttocks/ hamstrings (pear shape)	Excess estrogen	Excess estrogen	Hormonal imbalance 7 (p. 294)
		Low progesterone	Hormonal imbalance 9 (p. 297)
"Love handles" (above the hips)	Insulin and blood sugar imbalance	Insulin and blood sugar imbalance	Hormonal imbalance 1 (p. 285)
Chest (over the pectoral muscles)	Excess estrogen (often coupled with excess insulin and low testos- terone)	Excess estrogen	Hormonal imbalance 7 (p. 294)
			Hormonal imbalance 1 (p. 285)
			Hormonal imbalance 11 (p. 298)
Back ("bra fat")	Excess insulin	Excess insulin	Hormonal imbalance 1 (p. 285)
		Excess testosterone	Hormonal imbalance 12 (p. 299)
Thighs	Low growth hormone	Low growth hormone	Hormonal imbalance 16 (p. 303)

Remember, you do not need to—and should not—take all of the supplements suggested for each hormonal imbalance. Review the properties of the products in order to *match your specific signs* of imbalance and determine which one(s) will do the trick for you. Also, recall that you may need to change your selections over time as your body responds to the treatments. Fixing one imbalance may be all you need to bring all the others in line. Also, be sure to address each imbalance in the order presented here, and you may not even need to address more than one.

Once your hormones are brought back into healthy balance, you'll be ready to move on to the third and final step in your program. Your body will be ready to respond *wonderfully* to exercise!

STEP 3

RESTORE STRENGTH, VIGOR, AND RADIANCE

YOUR FINAL 2 WEEKS

Movement is a medicine for creating change in a person's physical, emotional, and mental states.

CAROL WELCH

CHAPTER 14

SEX AND SWEAT: WHY WE NEED BOTH FOR HORMONAL BALANCE

Love is the answer, but while you are waiting for the answer,
sex raises some pretty good questions.
WOODY ALLEN

Here's what you will learn in this chapter:
- Many of us are not enjoying the sex we should
- How sex revs up your fat-burning hormones
- How sex can satisfy cravings and control your appetite
- The benefits of exercise on your hormones for fat burning and metabolism
- The common workout mistakes that slow fat loss and hamper the hormone-enhancing benefits of exercise

Now that you have primed your hormones in Steps 1 and 2, you are set to enjoy the explosive benefits that great sex and exercise have on your hormones, metabolism, and weight loss. If you are not in the habit of getting physical on a regular basis, I hope this chapter will persuade you to change. When I say "getting physical," I mean enjoying two very basic hormone-enhancing, fat-burning, stress-busting activities: sex and exercise. Both involve working up a sweat. Both have wonderful hormone-boosting effects when we engage in them regularly. And, believe it or not, when we do one, we often have more desire to do the other.

Any amount of pleasurable sex is beneficial for you, as is any amount of exercise, when done properly. So, I guess in this sense, every workout counts and every make-out session counts—but doing both a few times weekly is even better! Unfortunately, the majority of us don't exercise, and just as many of us don't enjoy sex as often as we should.

We can come up with a whole host of reasons why we don't exercise: we're too busy, too tired, don't have enough time, not in the mood, don't like it, don't feel well enough, don't know how to do it, don't think we're good at it, can't last long enough, wouldn't know how to start, don't like to do it alone, don't like doing it in public. And I suppose all of these excuses could apply to sex, too.

In my practice, I have at times *begged* patients to begin working out. In some cases I have actually told them not to come back to see me but to spend their money on personal training, instead. One patient in particular was terrific about taking her supplements and was spending plenty of good money doing so. I told her she would probably need *half* the products if she would exercise.

I truly believe there is no better way to change your life than to start exercising. If there's one thing I pray you'll do after reading my book, it's to make exercise a part of your life, if it isn't already. If it already is, perhaps you'll learn something from the second part of this chapter that will allow you to enjoy better results from your efforts. But let's start with sex first. It's always a good attention grabber!

Bringing Sexy Back!

Sex is something we can get by without, whether we are in a relationship or not, but we shouldn't have to. Sex can be a complicated issue because it involves emotions, relationships, past sexual experiences, and physical and spiritual components. It also depends heavily on your current hormonal state, although some experts say your prior sexual functions and relationships are more important variables in determining how much sex you have or how enjoyable it is for you in the here and now.

When a patient comes to see me, I ask two basic questions: How's your energy? and How's your sex drive? When a patient tells me either of these aspects of his or her life has changed, I know immediately that there's a bigger health problem at play. Sadly, I've found that a surprising number of people ignore these changes for years, simply accepting them as normal or feeling too embarrassed to deal with them.

If this scenario sounds familiar to you, I hope to inspire you to think differently and to take steps to get your "mojo" back. You may be one of the millions of adults who experience sexual dysfunction, the incidence of which appears to be at an all-time high. According to an extensive study published in the *Journal of the American Medical Association,* the obesity epidemic is certainly not our only concern at this point. The results revealed that about 43 percent of women and 30 percent of men experience symptoms of sexual dysfunction, including lack of desire, arousal issues, inability to orgasm or ejaculate, premature ejaculation, painful intercourse, lack of enjoyment, erectile dysfunction, and performance anxiety.

If you think sex has fallen away just because you're getting older, are not in a relationship, or haven't done it in a long time, think again. Pleasurable sex is something every adult should enjoy for a lifetime—with or without a partner. And remember, sex doesn't mean intercourse alone. Masturbation (on your own or with a partner) and other forms of sexual play that get your hormones revving are definitely recommended. If you're currently having great sex, keep at it because it's good for you. Have sex all your life, and your body, brain, muscles, and fat cells will thank you for it. Do it over and over—that's right, don't stop.

Are Your Hormones Hampering Your Sex Life, or Is It the Other Way Around?

The answer is both. Sexual dysfunction is a global concern, as shown by the Global Study of Sexual Attitudes and Behaviors (GSSAB). After 13,882 women and 13,618 men from more than 29 countries were surveyed, the researchers concluded: "Sexual difficulties are relatively common among mature adults throughout the world. Sexual problems tend to be more associated with physical health and aging among men than women."

Sexual Issues for Men

An estimated 1 in 5 men currently experience erectile dysfunction (ED). Although psychological reasons play strongly in cases in men 35 years of age and younger, physiological factors are the main cause for men 50 and up. But ED at any age can provide a much bigger picture of a man's health than just what's happening below the belt. We now know, for example, that the state of a man's penis is a very good indication of cardiovascular wellness. Problems in this area are linked to arterial disease, heart attacks, stroke, and diabetes.

Ever since that now-famous little blue pill topped $1.5 billion in sales in 2001, becoming a pharmaceutical smash hit practically overnight, drug companies have been working feverishly to produce second-generation medications to deal with ED. Think about that figure—$1.5 billion! And realize at the same time that about 30 to 50 percent of patients can't even take Viagra because of contraindications such as heart disease. Since this family of drugs hit the market in the late 1990s, the number of American men with health complaints has increased by 50 percent. Evidently sex is an important issue and a great source of motivation for seeking medical intervention. Viagra is certainly working wonders for many people, although in my view it represents a "quickie" solution when a "long-term love affair" with lasting lifestyle change is certainly what's needed. That's right, I mean the three steps.

That Viagra sales, obesity, and stress rates are at all-time highs is no coincidence: The hormonal distress associated with abdominal obesity is a major contributing factor to impotence and erectile dysfunction. All healthy men experience a gradual decrease in testosterone, about 1.5 percent each year after age 30. (This percentage appears to be increasing, however—possibly due to toxin exposure.) Although the link between men's testosterone levels and their desire for sex is not entirely clear, the connection between lower free testosterone and weakened orgasmic function and/or erectile function is definite, according to a 2002 study from the *British Journal of Urology*.

The hormonal changes men naturally experience as they age tend to happen more gradually than the ones women undergo with menopause, although they can still result in symptoms of reduced energy, poor sex drive, declining muscle mass, increased abdominal fat, or irritability. These symptoms may seem uncomplicated, but they are increasingly common in my clinical practice among men in their 30s and 40s and are definite signals of high risk in the field of preventive medicine. Remember, low testosterone in men is linked to heart disease and even death.

Sexual Issues for Women

Drug companies are also scrambling to tap into the sexual dysfunction market for women. Sadly, this market is also huge and, unlike the case with men, the distribution of difficulties is fairly even among women 18 to 59 years of age. About 20 percent of women experience problems with arousal and, as a result, experience poor lubrication. Drug companies are now looking at ways to understand the female brain and develop a means of stimulating the arousal centers. But more pharmaceuticals are not always the answer. The three steps of the Hormone Diet have the potential to create the perfect hormonal balance for both a healthy libido and successful fat loss, especially because of their wonderful ability to calm the cortisol that can crush a healthy sex drive, even under the best of conditions.

Stress is certainly quick to kill that lovin' feeling, but menopause is often no help, either. The natural dip in estrogen, testosterone, and progesterone that are part and parcel of this stage of life can lead to problems in almost all areas of sexual function, including interest, responsiveness, and enjoyment. These same hormones also affect mood, sleep, where we store fat, and how well we lose it. Considering the incredible impact these hormones have on your life, restoring their balance—either with bioidentical hormone replacement therapy or herbal medicines—is extremely important.

Good Sex Is So Good for You

Sexual function is a lot like lean muscle—if we don't use it, we lose it and the health and hormonal benefits that come with it. Guys, if your sex life is in the doldrums lately, you likely have less testosterone as well. The fix is pretty straightforward. Research shows that if we can get you back to enjoying more frequent sex, your testosterone can, ahem, rise again. A group of Italian researchers looked at men with erectile issues and measured their testosterone status before and after treatment (though not with testosterone replacement). Those whose ED treatment was successful had higher testosterone compared with those whose treatments failed to yield improvements. If you needed a strong argument for having sex tonight, now you have one.

Ladies, the same principles apply to you. Women who enjoy more love in the bedroom have increased estrogen and testosterone. When present in the proper balance, these hormones add fire to sexual desire, give us more sex appeal, improve mood and memory, and can even prevent abdominal fat gain. A little precoital cuddling, however, is also very important. Scientists at Simon Fraser University measured the levels of testosterone in women before and after sex, cuddling, and exercise. Although the women's testosterone levels were higher both before and after sexual intercourse, cuddling gave the biggest testosterone boost of all.

Sex Busts Stress

Do I really need to go into detail on the benefits of sex for stress relief? Most of us know that a healthy sex life can help knock the pants off stress. A great orgasm also encourages the release of oxytocin, which makes us feel calmer and more relaxed and can even lower our blood pressure. Orgasms also spark an antiaging surge of DHEA. So having at least two orgasms a week can slow the aging process and indirectly support fat loss, while also offering some protection from the adverse effects of cortisol.

Wait, there's more. Depending on the duration and "energy level" of the session, sex can help you burn calories and improve the fitness of your heart. Sex (including masturbation) improves your sleep and reduces the risk of depression, both of which are essential in preventing fat gain and improving hormonal imbalance. It also causes the release of endorphins, which can help ease pain and boost immunity. Some research even suggests having sex three times a week can slow aging and prevent wrinkling around the eyes. Sounds better than any eye cream I've ever tried.

Sex Can Curb Your Appetite

Sex is a basic human need, just like food and shelter. You won't be surprised to learn, then, that our desire to "get some" is controlled by the hypothalamus, which also regulates appetite, body temperature, and circadian rhythms. I once heard Sam Graci, author of *The Path to Phenomenal Health*, speculate that Mother Nature may start selecting against us when our sex engines cool, simply because of the basic laws of evolution or survival of the fittest. This ideal resonated with me and has certainly motivated me to stay active—and I don't mean in the gym.

Your libido (that's scientific lingo for sex drive) is determined by a set of complex physiological processes that involve delicate interactions between your brain, body, and hormones. For instance, an appetite-suppressing compound in the brain controls sexual arousal as well by stimulating the release of oxytocin. Also involved in sexual responsiveness and orgasm, the hormone oxytocin counteracts stress and depression by combating the harmful effects of cortisol.

Frequent hugs between spouses or partners are associated with lower blood pressure and higher oxytocin levels in premenopausal women. Having regular massages can also help to stimulate oxytocin.

The dose of dopamine we get from sex, which increases steadily to the point of orgasm and then declines, also helps curb our need to feed. Apparently, the dopamine pathways in the brain involved in stimulating desire for both sex and food are shut down by the hormones released immediately after we have an orgasm. Can you imagine better news for appetite and craving control?

So if you remember nothing else after reading this book, I am certain this little snippet of advice will stay with you: *Have more sex.* If you satisfy your sexual appetite, you can satisfy your growling stomach and your need to nibble on candy, too.

There's No Pressure, Though

Perhaps you are like many women and men with a lowered sex drive who find the idea of "jumping" into an active sex life hard to imagine. This can change, however, *if* you want it to. Following the recommendations of the Hormone Diet will help to improve your hormone balance and overall well-being, which will help a languishing libido. But you can also fuel sexual desire further with visualizations or small acts of intimacy. For instance, try thinking of positive words on waking—even if you don't feel positive—like love, joy, peace, strength, happiness, beauty, etc. Next, tailor this simple exercise to help your lowered sex drive by adding words you find sexy—like hot, sensual, sultry, or touchable. You can also slowly bring intimacy back into your life with activities to help you feel close and connected again, such as back rubs, foot rubs, or date nights.

> **SEX KEEPS YOUR HORMONES YOUNG**
>
> Scientists have looked at 100-year-old men and women who have maintained sexual intimacy, love, and function well into their advanced years. Turns out these centenarians living in Okinawa, Japan, and Bama, China, have higher levels of testosterone, DHEA, and estrogen than typical 70-year-olds in the United States!

HOT HORMONE FACT

The Challenges of Sex and Aging

As we age, we tend to have less sex. A good deal of research suggests this decline is caused by hormonal changes that naturally occur with age. But at the same time we know that less sex alters our hormones. It's a real catch-22.

Experiencing both a decrease in the desire for sex and changes in sexual responsiveness is common for both men and women. As we age, women may notice vaginal dryness or discomfort, decreased lubrication, and even pain with intercourse, whereas men may experience more difficulty achieving an erection or erections that are not as firm as they once were. Orgasms may also become less intense for both sexes. All these symptoms are due to the inevitable hormonal shifts that come about as we age. They will occur more rapidly if we stop having sex, because then we lose all the wonderful hormone-enhancing effects sex has to offer.

Natural Help for Sexual Concerns (Besides the Three Steps)

If your sex life is stuck in neutral, you don't have to live with it and you don't necessarily need to turn to pharmaceuticals, either. Here are a few simple tips you can try to get your love life back in gear.

Concern	Helpful Tips for Women	Helpful Tips for Men
Low Libido	For men and women individually, consider the following:	
	Try my supplement recommendations in Chapter 13 for low testosterone, low DHEA, low dopamine, or excess cortisol. If your concern is associated with menopause, look at the suggestions for low progesterone and low estrogen, as well.	Try my supplement recommendations in Chapter 13 for low testosterone, low DHEA, low dopamine, or excess cortisol. You may also wish to consider the options for excess estrogen if you have excess abdominal fat or other signs of estrogen dominance.
	Several supplements can be used to enhance the hormones involved in a healthy sex drive for men and women. Two herbs in particular, maca and ashwagandha, have shown promise for increasing libido in both sexes.	

Concern	Helpful Tips for Women	Helpful Tips for Men
	Investigate other ways to stimulate your sexual interests, including sex toys, books, DVDs, a sex class (tantric sex, etc.), and so forth. I recommend the book *Mating in Captivity* by Esther Perel.	
Vaginal Dryness	Local use of an estriol cream can be very helpful. See your local compounding pharmacy or your MD/ND for a prescription.	
Erectile Dysfunction		Certain herbs and supplements may enhance penile bloodflow: • Ginkgo • L-arginine • Ginseng • Horny goat weed • Magnesium

Get Sweaty: Exercise!

I'm passionate about exercise. Yet despite the well-documented and actively promoted benefits of regular workouts, statistics show that not everyone shares my enthusiasm. Recent research shows that the number-one cause of death in the United States is poor diet and lack of exercise. Believe it or not, these factors kill more North Americans each year than smoking! In other words, failing to exercise is just as harmful as smoking, if not more so.

Recall the hormonal catch-22 we can get into without sex—a hormonal imbalance can cause *and be caused by* a lack of love-making. Well, a hormonal imbalance is unlikely to prevent us from working out (except perhaps depression), but a lack of physical activity sure can bring about a hormonal imbalance. Moreover, too much sex is not an issue for most healthy people, but overexercising or working out incorrectly can cause us more harm than good.

The Benefits of Exercise for Fat Loss

The effects of exercise on your hormones and your weight will vary depending on the type of activities you choose (e.g., cardio, weight training, or yoga) and the intensity and duration of your sessions. But no matter what type of exercise we do, working out is just plain good for us. Here's why:

- CALORIE BURNING: We burn calories while we exercise and, if we do strength training, we burn calories well after the session is completed.

- MUSCLE BUILDING: Exercise can help us build metabolically active muscle. For every pound of muscle you gain, you'll burn an extra 30 to 50 calories, even when you're doing absolutely nothing!

- STIMULATION OF MUSCLE-BUILDING HORMONES: A 2002 study published in the *Journals of Gerontology Series A: Biological Sciences and Medical Sciences* looked at hormonal changes occurring in menopausal women who completed endurance training (40 minutes of cycling at 75 percent maximal exertion) and resistance training (3 sets of 10 reps of 8 exercises) compared with the control group that didn't exercise. Endurance and resistance training both significantly increased estrogen, testosterone, and growth hormone. Only the resistance training, however, increased DHEA. Testosterone will rise higher when you play a competitive sport and even higher still if you win.

- STIMULATION OF OUR FAT-LOSS FRIENDS: Exercise stimulates the hormones that are our fat-loss friends, including thyroid hormone, noradrenaline, testosterone, growth hormone, serotonin, leptin, and dopamine.

- REDUCTION OF OUR FAT-LOSS FOES: It also reduces the hormones that interfere with fat loss, including excess stress hormones that can wear the body down, and excess estrogen, which can increase breast cancer risk. Researchers selected a group of postmenopausal women from Seattle who did not exercise. Half of the women were instructed to begin a moderate-intensity walking program (45 minutes, five times per week); the others were told to do only stretching exercises. The women who walked decreased their harmful estrogen within 3 months.

- MOOD ENHANCEMENT: Exercise stimulates your mood and mental function; decreases anxiety and depression; and reduces pain by increasing dopamine and endorphins, our natural pain killers. According to a 2005 study from the *European Journal of Sports Science*, just 15 minutes of cardiovascular exercise two or three times a week can boost serotonin enough to prevent anxiety and treat depression.
- FAT BURNING AND INSULIN BALANCING: Exercise cranks up our PPARs, the regulators of fat metabolism and insulin sensitivity in our muscle cells.
- APPETITE CONTROL AND REDUCTION OF INFLAMMATION: Exercise has positive effects on fat-cell hormones such as leptin and adiponectin, which control inflammation and influence our appetite.

10 Workout Mistakes That Sabotage Fat Loss

You'll enjoy all the hormonal benefits of exercise I've just shared *providing you perform the right type, frequency, intensity, and duration of exercise.* Here are a few of the top workout mistakes and misconceptions that can *interfere* with our fat-burning results so you can be sure to avoid them going forward.

Workout Mistake #1: Completing Your Cardio Before Your Weight Training

I used to think cardio worked best as a warm-up before doing weights. I now know that saving my strength and completing my weight workout first is a much better plan. You can work out harder and lift more when you avoid fatiguing yourself with cardio first. Plus, you will continue to burn fat should you decide to follow your weight session with some cardio. Just hop on the bike or walk for 3 to 5 minutes, as a warm-up, to loosen up a bit before your weights.

Although I've personally used the weights-then-cardio approach for years, I certainly didn't come up with the idea. A study from the University of Tokyo found that people who did a total-body strength workout before cycling burned 10 percent more fat than participants who only cycled. The author of the study, Dr. Kazushige Goto, also found that less fat was burned and less growth hormone was released by the group that completed cardio first, followed by weights.

At the same time, adding cardio to the end of a particularly taxing weight-training session can cause a spike in your cortisol because the entire workout ends up being too long and stressful. For these reasons, I recommend you do your weights and cardio sessions at separate times. If you do wish to do them together, keep your cardio short. But dividing your workout may actually give you better fat-burning potential; the same study from the University of Tokyo showed that splitting cardio into two sessions maximized the post-workout fat burn. I'm sure the same theory would apply to dividing cardio and weight training into two separate sessions.

If you're still not convinced, I think you'll feel differently once you begin the Hormone Diet exercise plan. Then you'll see that resistance-training workouts can be intense enough that you won't have much zip left for cardio immediately after. Your heart certainly gets pumping when you do your strength training exercises effectively, with little rest in between sets. Resistance training can yield the most amazing changes in your body composition *when you do it properly.* If you want to stand in front of the mirror and love your look, resistance training is the way to achieve your goal. And finally, another great benefit of this approach to exercise is that it keeps your workouts short and sweet.

Workout Mistake #2: Pumping Iron for Hours at a Time

Unless you are an athlete training for a specific sport or event, workout sessions that last longer than 45 minutes are not necessary and may even be harmful. Although exercise is a wonderful long-term stress reliever, working out does put physical stress on your body in the short term. So when your workout is too long, your cortisol goes up, up, up. Cortisol is destructive to muscle tissue, especially when it's present without the muscle-protective hormones growth hormone and testosterone. Keeping your workouts shorter, though still intense, will help prevent excessive cortisol release, which usually starts to happen after about 40 minutes or so of continuous exercise. Compacting your workout in this way will give you the best gains in the shortest amount of time. It also means less wear and tear and quicker recovery.

Workout Mistake #3: Getting Socially Active between Sets

If you are the gym's social butterfly, you need to turn over a new leaf. You don't have time for chatting any more. Most of the workouts outlined for you in Chapter 15 are no longer than 30 minutes, which leaves no time for chitchat during your session. Power through your routine and socialize only after you are done. Studies show this no-nonsense, heads-down approach is the best way to maximize muscle gains and elicit the hormonal response you're looking for.

In a study published in *Medicine and Science in Sports and Exercise Journal* (2005), Kazushige Goto and his team at the University of Tokyo found that a group of test subjects who worked out continuously, with no rest between exercises, had greater increases in growth hormone, noradrenaline, and adrenaline during their workouts and netted greater muscle gains after 12 weeks than those who were instructed to rest between exercises. These findings can help you understand why I recommend completing your exercises in a circuit two or three times before having a rest. I truly don't want to torture you; I simply want you to get the best rewards from your efforts. Give each workout your all and you won't believe how quickly your body will respond.

Workout Mistake #4: Thinking Cardio Is the Best Way to Lose Weight

I know I'll probably ruffle more than a few feathers with this one, but neither running nor continuously training in the "fat-burning zone" is the golden ticket to your best body composition. Shorter workouts with intervals are far more effective than running or using a cardio machine for 40-plus minutes every other day. An interval is a short period of exercise performed at a higher intensity for a specific length of time. Each interval is separated from the next by a short period of rest or lighter activity. To truly take advantage of the benefits of interval training, you must be willing to shake the mindset that endless (and boring!) cardio training is the key to weight loss.

For example, 25 minutes of running can be more effective than 40. How? You burn more fat during and after your workout if you run for 10 minutes at a steady pace, then alternate 1 minute fast and 1 minute slow for the next 10 minutes, and then run at a slower pace for the last 5 minutes to cool down. Even though you're exercising for a shorter period, you'll still net greater fat loss using this method.

A number of studies lend very strong support to the value of interval training. One piece of research by Tremblay and colleagues, published in the journal *Metabolism*, showed greater muscle gains and fat loss in one group of subjects who exercised using intervals at a higher intensity for 15 weeks than a second group who exercised at a steady pace for 20 weeks. Although more *calories* were burned by the steady group, the interval-training group lost much more subcutaneous fat. Moreover, researchers at the University of New South Wales in Sydney, Australia, found 20 minutes of interval training to be more effective in sparking our fat-burning hormones than 40 minutes at a steady pace. How great is this? *More* fat burning with *less* time spent exercising. Clearly, intervals are the secret to shorter workouts with more fat-loss success!

Workout Mistake #5: Having Sports Drinks Before or After Workouts

When you're working out for 30 to 40 minutes, you don't need sugar to get you through your session. The only thing you should be guzzling is water. Consuming so-called sports drinks (i.e., a sugar blast in a plastic bottle) before or after your workout will do nothing but interfere with fat loss and hormonal balance. Too much sugar before or after exercise can also blunt growth hormone release. (An aside: Fatty foods after a workout have also been found to have the same dampening effect on growth hormone.) Sports, energy, and other drinks containing high-fructose corn syrup have no place in your diet at any time.

Workout Mistake #6: Lifting Weights on an Empty Stomach

Your muscles need fuel to reach full force of contraction and strength during exercise. Always consume a blend of protein and carbohydrates before and after your resistance-training sessions. This combination is proven to stimulate more growth hormone release and to encourage more muscle gains.

About an hour before your workout, have a snack that includes the macronutrients you need, such as a slice of Ezekiel bread with almond butter; a bowl of oatmeal with soy milk and blueberries; a Simply Bar (see Appendix C and the Resources section); or a protein shake with flaxseed oil, soy milk, and whey protein. Follow your workout with an Elevate Me! Bar (see Appendix C) or a protein shake made with fruit juice, soy or skim milk, bananas, and whey protein. Do *not* add the fat (flaxseed oil or flaxseeds) to your smoothie after your workouts because it can hamper growth hormone release. Always consume your shake within 45 minutes of finishing your exercise session for the greatest muscle-repair benefits. Remember, this is the one period of the day that you can get away with eating more carbs.

When you do your cardio, on the other hand, you can do it on an empty stomach (although you don't have to), provided you stick to a session that's 30 minutes max. You should still have your smoothie within 45 minutes of finishing your cardio, and it shouldn't contain much fat.

Workout Mistake #7: Believing the More Exercise, the Better for Maximum Fat Loss

I started lifting weights and going to the gym regularly after my first year of college. Ten years later I met a personal trainer who finally told me to stop working out for an hour at a time. In fact, he used to *yell* at me if I ran or exercised on the days I was supposed to rest. For months I couldn't wrap my head around the idea of exercising less. But guess what happened? When I finally followed his advice, *I got in the best shape of my life.*

Overtraining or overuse of cardio is an incredibly common mistake among people who love to work out or are enthusiastic about weight loss. This misguided approach, however, only serves to raise your cortisol and interfere with your ability to build metabolically active muscle. You should train with weights a maximum of four times a week (the Hormone Diet program recommends three) and do your cardio no more than two or three times a week. On the days you are not supposed to work out, don't! When we are trying to maximize the hormonal benefits of exercise, sometimes less truly is more. Stick to your routine, take the time off you need for rest and recuperation, and *trust me,* you will notice greater gains.

You wouldn't believe the results I've seen in my patients who have heeded my advice and gotten away from lengthy stints on the treadmill. Instead, they turned to interval training, yoga, and weights, and now they look amazing! Their body-fat percentages have dropped and they are more toned than ever.

Workout Mistake #8: Thinking Lifting Weights Causes Women to Bulk Up

Ladies, if you've always avoided the weight room for fear of ending up looking like a member of the Russian men's power-lifting team, you need to think again. Most, if not all, women will not bulk up from lifting weights. We women naturally possess only 5 to 10 percent of the testosterone that men do. *Testosterone* is what causes men to build muscle, whereas women are far more reliant on *growth hormone* to build muscle.

Remember, the more muscle you have, the more fat you'll burn, even when you're sleeping. So building more lean muscle mass will absolutely help your fat-loss progress. Using weight training will allow you to build strong, lean muscles without looking too pumped up or masculine, guaranteed.

In fact, exercise for weight loss *must* include resistance training. A comprehensive review of hundreds of studies completed by Miller and colleagues and published in the *International Journal of Obesity* proved this to be the case when *little benefit was found* in subjects who used moderate *cardiovascular exercise and dieting over diet alone.* Meanwhile, it's well documented that people who use a combination of resistance training *and* cardio lose fat while losing *little or no* metabolically active muscle.

Does this mean cardiovascular exercise is a waste? No, cardio boosts your mood, keeps your heart and lungs fit, and helps to maintain body weight, especially after a calorie-reduced diet. But, it's definitely not the answer to lasting fat loss.

Workout Mistake #9: Thinking Heavy Weights Are Just for Guys

Wrong! Ladies, don't be afraid to lift heavier weights. Just make sure you use proper form so you don't run the risk of injuring yourself.

I'm small but can lift a lot of weight and have been doing so since 1999—right about the time I met that trainer who persuaded me to stop overexercising.

Heavier weights tone muscle and boost growth hormone much more than the lighter weights most women tend to use. A 2006 study led by William J. Kraemer, a professor of kinesiology, physiology, and neurobiology at the University of Connecticut at Storrs, found greater gains of growth hormone in women who did fewer repetitions with heavier weights than in those who did higher reps with moderate weight. The study, published in the *American Journal of Physiology—Endocrinology and Metabolism,* showed that women who underwent 6 months of moderate- or high-intensity training and aerobic exercise had higher amounts of growth hormone.

This common workout mistake was the driving force behind the recent setup of the strength training studio at my clinic, staffed by a team of top trainers. Now my patients enjoy the benefits of an integrated approach involving care from an ND, MD, and exercise expert as we guide them through the Hormone Diet program. I want all my patients to learn how to exercise—properly!

Workout Mistake #10: Believing That Yoga Is Just for Girls

Years of weight lifting and running, especially without proper stretching, can shorten tendons and cause stiffness, misalignment, and joint and back pain. With its full spectrum of poses, yoga can bring the body back into its natural alignment, level out imbalances, and strengthen physical weaknesses. If you're an athlete, yoga can improve your performance by increasing your flexibility, relaxation, breathing, and balance. Anyone can improve his or her posture, energy, and endurance with regular yoga practice.

If you think yoga is too easy or too gentle a workout, how wrong you are! We have a yoga studio at Clear Medicine, and when my husband the hockey jock tried it, he couldn't believe how hard yoga was.

This type of workout can be very challenging and can make you feel inadequate if you compare yourself with other practitioners who appear more limber. Just remember, yoga is a solo sport; the only person you should be competing with is yourself. As with all sports or skills, you will definitely see improvements with practice. No matter what your ability level, yoga offers fabulous benefits for calming your nervous system, restoring hormonal balance, *and* strengthening your muscles.

Yoga can also be a terrific stress reliever. Numerous studies, including one completed in 2003 by the Center of Integrative Medicine at Thomas Jefferson University Hospital, in collaboration with the Yoga Research Society, have shown that yoga can lower blood cortisol levels in healthy males and females. It's also known to reduce adrenaline and stimulate our calming brain chemical GABA. Research from Boston University School of Medicine and McLean Hospital published in the *Journal of Alternative and Complementary Medicine* (May 2007) suggests that yoga should be explored as a possible treatment for disorders often associated with low GABA levels, such as depression and anxiety.

If you have excess ab fat or sleep disruption, yoga is one stellar choice of a workout for you. It's also excellent if you have fertility concerns. So leave your gender biases at the door and give yoga a try.

There you have it—all the hormonal benefits of sex and getting sweaty. Now we're ready to make you move—on to the exercise prescription we go!

CHAPTER 15

STRENGTH, STAMINA, AND STRETCHING:
THE HORMONE DIET
EXERCISE PRESCRIPTION

These are the hormonal benefits you will enjoy from exercise:

- Less inflammation
- Reduced insulin resulting in fewer cravings, better energy, and easier fat loss
- Diminished harmful effects from an accumulation of excess estrogen
- Increased DHEA, your antiaging and muscle-enhancing hormone
- A boost in testosterone for increased motivation and muscle-building benefits
- A dose of dopamine for your mood, motivation, and appetite control
- Tamed cortisol and a balanced nervous system when you exercise properly
- Increased metabolic rate due to increased thyroid hormone
- Increased growth hormone for better growth and repair of skin, bone, and muscle cells
- More of serotonin's beneficial effects on mood, sleep, and cravings
- Increased leptin sensitivity for fat burning and appetite control

Up to this point in my three steps, any exercise other than walking has been an optional component, because I wanted you to focus entirely on understanding and implementing the essentials of hormonally balanced nutrition, sound sleep, stress recuperation, and your anti-inflammatory detox. But now that you've done all the prep work involved in Step 1 and Step 2, your body is absolutely primed for the fantastic benefits of the Hormone Diet exercise plan. I cannot wait for you to experience the incredible body benefits of this approach!

Although reducing our food intake certainly sparks an initial loss of body weight, only the increase in metabolism that happens with exercise will maintain our efforts. The good news is that exercise allows us to enjoy more freedom with our food choices once we have reached our goal. Exercise truly is the more critical determinant of your lasting success than continually cutting your calories.

A weekly exercise routine you can use to stay fit for the rest of your life is outlined in this chapter. I have been using this workout for years, but the program you're about to enjoy also includes the expertise of three wonderful trainers from Clear Medicine: Reggie Reyes, Jason Gee, and Vanessa Bell. I thank them for their generosity and contributions.

The Hormone Diet Exercise Philosophy

HOT HORMONE TIP

GET FIT QUICK WITH THE HELP OF TWO SUPPLEMENTS: CLA AND CREATINE

Exercise is proven to combat the loss of muscle that unfortunately, but inevitably, happens with aging. But here's some good news. According to new research from the Public Library of Science, supplements of creatine monohydrate (5 g per day) and conjugated linoleic acid or CLA (3 to 6 g per day) can boost the benefits of exercise even further. Naturally produced by your body and present in meat, creatine is known to supply your muscles with energy. CLA, a naturally occurring fatty acid in beef, helps to preserve muscle tissue while encouraging safe fat loss. When used in conjunction with exercise, these two supplements pack a powerful muscle-building and antiaging punch. Look for Clear Recovery on the Hormone Diet store, which provides a highly absorbable form of creatine.

Before you begin, take a look at the principles behind the Hormone Diet exercise plan that will help you maximize hormonal and fat-burning benefits.

1. **Keep it short and sweet.** All workouts are 30 minutes (or a maximum 40 minutes).
2. **Give every workout your all.** High intensity and maximum effort—to the point where you just can't squeeze out one more rep—are *musts* for effective fat-burning and hormonal

benefits. When you're pushing yourself hard in the gym (or wherever you exercise), just remember that your workout is short and it will all be over soon!

3. **Complete your exercises with little rest between each circuit.** Circuit training keeps your heart rate high throughout your workout. When you use this method, you basically get your cardio workout and resistance training all in one shorter session. Circuit training is also the best type of workout for improving insulin response, boosting testosterone, and stimulating growth hormone. You spend less time exercising but you reap even more benefits.

4. **Work multiple muscle groups with each strength training session (but train each muscle group only once or twice a week).** This approach is designed to increase growth hormone and stimulate more muscle groups at once. It also lets you complete more work in less time and ensures that your muscles get the proper recuperation time they need *between* sessions.

5. **Keep cardio sessions short and use intervals**. Remember, intervals are a series of shorter periods of intense exercise separated by periods of brief rest or lighter activity. This method of training offers the most fat-burning potential and the greatest health benefits. Even cardiac patients can use interval training to improve their fitness.

6. **Use yoga for its hormone-enhancing effects**. Besides challenging and stretching your muscles, yoga can lower blood cortisol levels, reduce adrenaline, and stimulate brain-calming GABA.

7. **Consume the right stuff before and after your workouts for hormonal effects.** Always consume a blend of protein and carbohydrates about an hour before and within 45 minutes after your resistance-training sessions. Limit fat in your post-workout meal. This combination is proven to stimulate more growth hormone release and encourage muscle gains. You can

do cardio on an empty stomach, but eat your snack of protein and carbs (again, no fat) within 45 minutes of finishing your session. Drink only water during your workouts—no sports drinks allowed.

Tools of the Trade

Whether you choose to work out in the gym, outside, or at home, there are a few key pieces of equipment you need to get the job done properly. Most gyms provide these items for you; if you work out elsewhere, you may have to purchase them for yourself. Here's all the equipment required to complete your weekly exercise routine.

    a. **A stability ball:** These come in different sizes, so be sure to purchase/use the proper one for your height.

    b. **A set of dumbbells:** 3, 5, 8, 10, 12, and 15 pounds for women; 10, 15, 20, 25, and 30 pounds for men.

    c. **A support bench:** A weight bench or other stable bench is helpful, but not necessary if you have a stability ball.

    d. **A medicine ball:** You can also use a dumbbell.

    e. **Options for indoor cardio:** A stationary bike, treadmill, stair stepper, or elliptical machine for home use. (You can also walk, bike, or run outside when weather permits.)

    f. **Music:** Listening to your favorite tunes while working out is a great motivator.

The Hormone Diet Workout Weekly Schedule

For maximum health and hormonal benefit, I recommend you exercise 6 days a week. You'll complete three types of workouts each week.

    1. Three days a week you'll complete 30 to 40 minutes of strength training.

    2. Once a week you'll do cardio (20 to 30 minutes). A second cardio session is optional. If you simply *must* do more cardio, you can do so at the *end* of your weight-training sessions. Don't

overdo it, and don't add more than 15 minutes to your workout.

3. Once a week, preferably twice (but not on your strength-training days), do yoga for 30 to 90 minutes. This is the one workout that may be longer in duration.

One day a week you will rest and do no exercise, though fun activities like in-line skating or a leisurely swim, bike ride, or walk are fine. ☺

Do your best to follow the weekly exercise routine as laid out for you here. The program is specifically designed to keep you working hard during each session and progressing each week, allowing specific muscle groups to recuperate while others are being pushed to develop. A sample schedule of weekly workouts may look something like this:

Monday	Tuesday	Wednesday	Thursday	Friday	Saturday	Sunday
Rest	Day 1 Strength-Training Routine	Cardio Interval Training* Yoga	Day 2 Strength-Training Routine	Yoga†	Day 3 Strength-Training Routine	Cardio (optional 20 minutes of cardio at a steady pace or interval)*

*If you wish to do cardio and strength training on the same day, sometimes it's better to split them into two different workouts (e.g., cardio in the morning and strength training in the afternoon).

†Avoid yoga on the same day as strength training. A yoga class or a yoga DVD at home are both excellent options. As far as the type of yoga is concerned, we prefer Hatha, Ashtanga, or Vinyasa at Clear Medicine, but I'll leave it up to you to decide which you like best.

Selecting the Right Amount of Weight

Time and time again, I see people at the gym who fail to get results, either because they don't lift enough weight to challenge their muscles or because they're lifting too much and using improper form. Choosing the right weight and using correct form are absolutely *essential* to get the results you want and avoid injury.

When you are just starting out, choose a weight light enough to allow you to complete all the suggested repetitions for each exercise without compromising your form. Remember, if your posture is poor or you are swinging your weights instead of lifting them in a controlled manner just to finish the last few reps, you're not doing yourself any favors! In fact, you can really hurt yourself. As your workouts progress, you'll decrease the number of repetitions and increase your weight to the point that you can barely complete the last few repetitions.

Hiring a personal trainer may seem like a daunting or expensive proposition, but don't be afraid to try it, even for just a few sessions, if you feel you need help getting started and someone to show you proper form. (Some trainers will even charge less if you do your session with a partner.) Besides, we're talking about an investment in your long-term health and well-being. I fully believe it's some of the best money you will ever spend and I encourage *all* my patients to do so.

The Hormone Diet Strength-Training Workout

If you've never exercised or have been inactive for a very long time, you can follow the basic strength-training routine for beginners that I have outlined on my Web site under the Book Extras section. Certain to crank up your fat-burning potential, it involves full-body circuit training 3 days a week. Otherwise, you can jump right into the strength-training component of the plan presented here. Remember, every workout counts. Even once a week is better than none, but don't expect great results until you can increase to a minimum of three times a week.

I encourage you to try switching up your workout *even* if you have been exercising successfully on your own. As most exercise experts will agree, the change will challenge your muscles, force your body to adapt, and further your fitness gains.

The exercises are to be done consecutively in sequence with no rest in between sets. Rest for 1 minute at the end of each circuit before moving on to the next. Each workout should take you about

30 minutes, even when you have worked your way up to 3 sets. (By then your fitness level will have improved and you'll be able to finish the exercises faster.) Warm up by riding the bike, walking, or jogging for 4 to 5 minutes before beginning your strength-training session.

You can keep progressing by increasing the weight lifted (while still maintaining form) and by altering your exercise choices. You may also change the order of the circuits within each workout or the exercises within each circuit as a means to keep your body guessing. For more information on these exercises, and for ideas and exercise options that will help you stay challenged, visit www.thehormonediet.com. I promise you'll never get bored. I've been doing this workout for years and years and still love it.

DAY 1 STRENGTH-TRAINING ROUTINE: CHEST, BACK, AND CORE

Circuit Grouping	Exercise	Repetitions	Weight	No. of Times to Repeat Circuit
1	Crunches over the Ball	20	None	2
	Leg Raise with Pulse up to Ceiling	15	None	
	Plank	Hold for 20 to 60 seconds	None	
Rest 30 seconds to 1 minute while setting up for circuit 2				

Crunches over the Ball

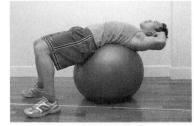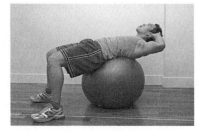

Leg Raise with Pulse up to Ceiling

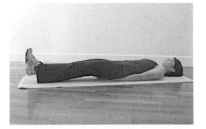

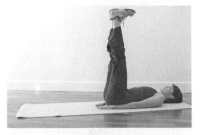

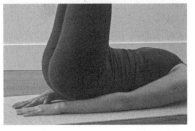

Plank

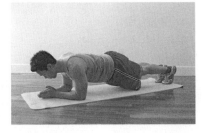

Circuit Grouping	Exercise	Repetitions	Weight	No. of Times to Repeat Circuit
2	Chest Dumbbell Press on Ball	15	Light first set, moderate second set, heavy third set	3
	Straight-Leg Deadlift (with Dumbbells)	15		
Rest 30 seconds to 1 minute while setting up for circuit 3				

Chest Dumbbell Press on Ball

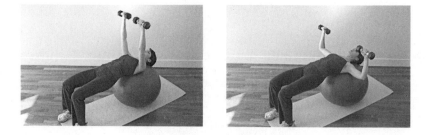

Straight-Leg Deadlift (with Dumbbells)

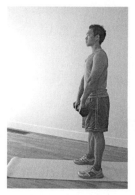
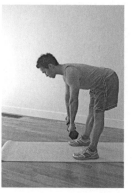

Circuit Grouping	Exercise	Repetitions	Weight	No. of Times to Repeat Circuit
3	Dumbbell Fly	15	Moderate first set, heavy second set (for very advanced, add a third set)	2 (3)
	Bent-Over Dumbbell Row (Double or Single Arm)	15		
Rest 30 seconds to 1 minute while setting up for circuit 4				

Dumbbell Fly

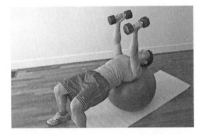 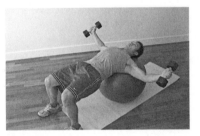

Bent-Over Dumbbell Row (Double Arm)

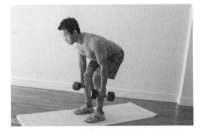 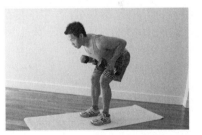

Bent-Over Dumbbell Row (Single Arm)

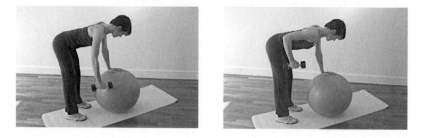

Circuit Grouping	Exercise	Repetitions	Weight	No. of Times to Repeat Circuit
4	Push-Ups	15	None	2 (3)
	Back Extensions on Ball	15	None	

Push-Ups

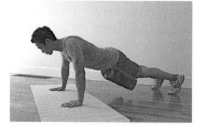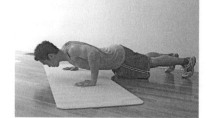

Back Extensions on Ball

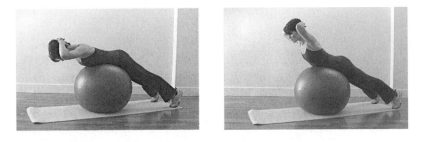

DAY 2 STRENGTH-TRAINING ROUTINE: LEGS AND CORE

Circuit Grouping	Exercise	Repetitions	Weight	No. of Times to Repeat Circuit
1	Standard Crunch	20	None	2
	Back Extensions	20	None	
	Seated Oblique Twists with Medicine Ball	20 per side	4- to 10-pound medicine ball	
Rest 30 seconds to 1 minute while setting up for circuit 2				

Standard Crunch

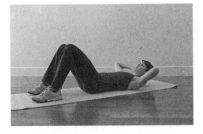
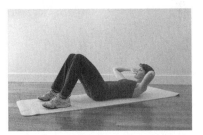

Back Extensions

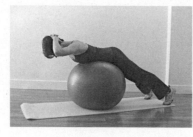 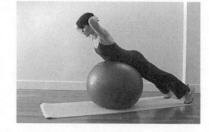

Seated Oblique Twists with Medicine Ball

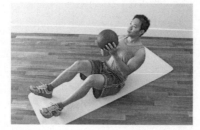 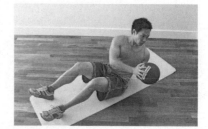

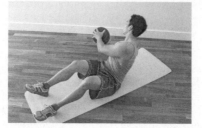

Circuit Grouping	Exercise	Repetitions	Weight	No. of Times to Repeat Circuit
2	Squats	15	Light first set, moderate second set, heavy third set	3
	Leg Raises with Ball between Feet	15	None, just the ball	
Rest 30 seconds to 1 minute while setting up for circuit 3				

Squats

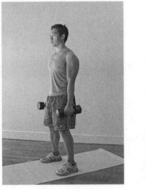 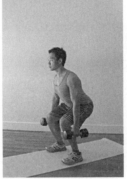

Leg Raises with Ball between Feet

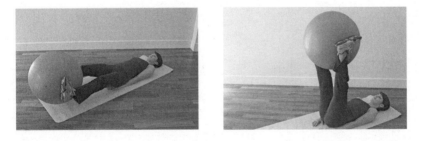

Circuit Grouping	Exercise	Repetitions	Weight	No. of Times to Repeat Circuit
3	Lunges with Biceps Curl	10–15 each leg	Moderate first set, heavy second set (for very advanced, add a third set)	2 (3)
	Hamstrings Curls with Feet on Ball	15–20	None	
Rest 30 seconds to 1 minute while setting up for circuit 4				

Lunges with Biceps Curl

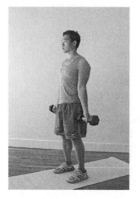 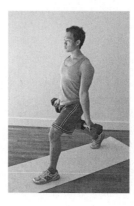 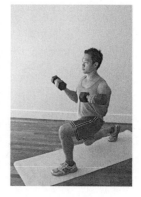

Note: Your arms will fatigue. When necessary, continue to lunge without the biceps curl.

Hamstrings Curls with Feet on Ball

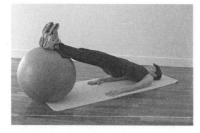 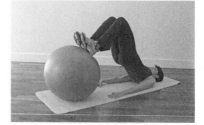

Circuit Grouping	Exercise	Repetitions	Weight	No. of Times to Repeat Circuit
4	Bent-Knee Dumbbell Deadlift with Calf Raise	15	Moderate first set, heavy second set	2 (3)
	Plank	Hold 30 seconds to 1 minute	None	

Bent-Knee Dumbbell Deadlift with Calf Raise

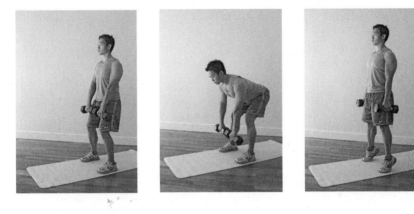

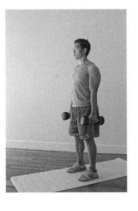

Plank

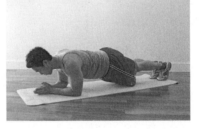

Circuit Grouping	Exercise	Repetitions	Weight	No. of Times to Repeat Circuit
1	Ball Pull-Ins with Push-Up	15	None	2
	Side Jackknife	15 per side		
	Side Plank	Hold 20–60 seconds per side		
Rest 30 seconds to 1 minute while setting up for circuit 2				

Ball Pull-Ins with Push-Up

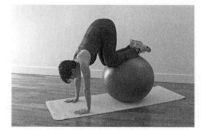 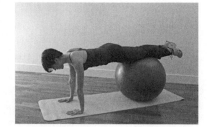

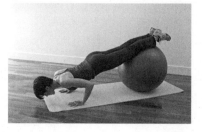

Side Jackknife

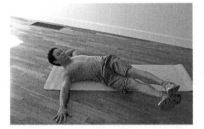 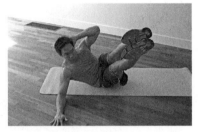

Side Plank

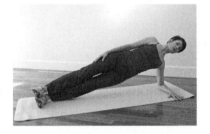

Circuit Grouping	Exercise	Repetitions	Weight	No. of Times to Repeat Circuit
2	Standing Hammer Biceps Curls into Shoulder Press	15	Light first set, moderate second set, heavy third set	3
	Lying Triceps Dumbbell Skull-crushers on Ball (or Bench)	15		
Rest 30 seconds to 1 minute while setting up for circuit 3				

Standing Hammer Biceps Curls into Shoulder Press

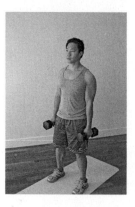 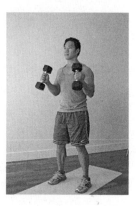

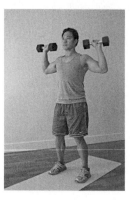 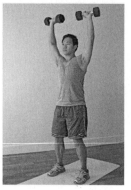

Lying Triceps Dumbbell Skullcrushers on Ball (or Bench)

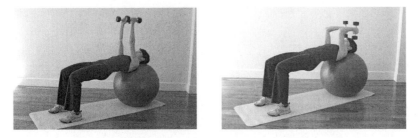

Circuit Grouping	Exercise	Repetitions	Weight	No. of Times to Repeat Circuit
3	Standing Shoulder Lateral and Front Dumbbell Raise	15	Moderate first set, heavy second set (for advanced, add a third set)	2 (3)
	Standing Alternating Biceps Curls	15		
	Lying Triceps Dumbbell Extensions (on Ball)*	15		
Rest 30 seconds to 1 minute while setting up for circuit 4				

*Optional. Repeat the skullcrushers from the previous set, but alternate your arms.

Standing Shoulder Lateral and Front Dumbbell Raise

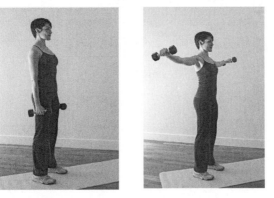

(continued)

Standing Shoulder Lateral and Front Dumbbell Raise

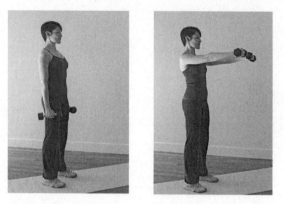

Standing Alternating Biceps Curls

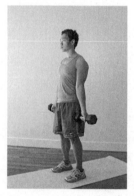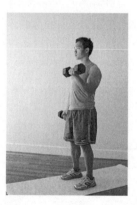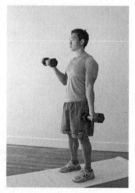

Circuit Grouping	Exercise	Repetitions	Weight	No. of Times to Repeat Circuit
4	Bent-Over Reverse Dumbbell Fly	15	Moderate first set, heavy second set (for advanced, add a third set)	2 (3)
	Triceps Dips	15	None	

Bent-Over Reverse Dumbbell Fly

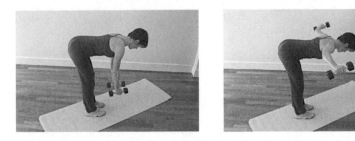

Triceps Dips

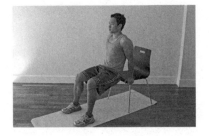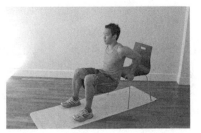

ADD MUSIC TO YOUR WORKOUTS!

Did you know that just 15 minutes of music a day can improve your immunity and reduce pain? It can also decrease your blood pressure, lower your heart rate, and slow your breathing simply because it helps drop your cortisol and boost your endorphins. Incredibly, researchers in Florida have found that 20 minutes a day of music is enough for patients to report a reduction of more than 50 percent in osteoarthritic pain in just 14 days!

If you are currently exercising without music, you had better get some earphones on ASAP. The newest research from Brunel University in England shows that upbeat music can enhance our aerobic endurance, motivation, and drive. Fast-tempo music will inject vigor into your workouts. Slow-tempo, soothing music, on the other hand, can aid relaxation during cooldown and stretching. In essence, music can make you work harder without realizing it. It offers a pleasant distraction from the discomfort of physical exertion and causes your workout to pass by quicker.

But music does more than make your individual workouts more enjoyable. A 2005 study completed at Fairleigh Dickinson University in New Jersey found that routinely listening to music while exercising made people more consistent with their workouts and boosted weight loss results.

Get the most out of music for your workouts and your overall health. Choose tunes you love to listen to and consider the following:

1. Pick upbeat exercise music to help you work harder and maximize your fitness results.
2. Play soothing music while stretching in your car or while you commute to reduce tension, anxiety, or pain. Relax with chill-out music for 15 minutes at the end of your day. I recommend the Sonic Aid series by Dr. Lee Bartel for relaxation and enhancing brain activity.

3. Bring some music with you for an added mood-enhancing, pain-reducing boost when you go out in the morning for your daily dose of sunshine.

4. Crank up your tunes just for fun or when you feel you need a stress release or mood boost. Even better, dance! Dancing elevates endorphins, raises serotonin, and balances out the sympathetic nervous system by lowering cortisol and dopamine. A December 2005 study published in the *International Journal of Neuroscience* proved that 12 weeks of dance sessions raised serotonin and lowered dopamine (often high when we are stressed). Remember that low serotonin also means more cravings and less motivation. So moving to your favorite tunes is an awesome way to have some fun, burn a few calories, and beat cravings for sugar and carbs!

The Hormone Diet Interval Cardio Training

Sticking to a regular exercise routine can be tough. So choosing an activity you enjoy—one you know you'll keep up with consistently—is always your best cardiovascular fitness option. However, if you want the most bang for your cardio buck, then high-intensity interval training on the treadmill (walking or running), elliptical trainer, stationary bike, or indoor/outdoor track is your secret to success.

Short bursts of intense exercise not only improve your cardiovascular fitness but also increase your fat-burning capacity, even during low- or moderate-intensity workouts. What's more, high-intensity training provides a boost of feel-good and appetite-controlling hormones, which can truly be your secret weapons against unwanted weight gain—especially during the cold, dark winter months when many of us are prone to depression and cravings for comfort foods.

Don't rush into interval training if you have heart disease, high blood pressure, or joint problems, or if you are over the age of 60.

If you fit any one of these categories, you should definitely consult your doctor first.

Here are a few examples of interval training to choose from. You'll do cardio at least once a week for 20 to 30 minutes. A second cardio workout is optional.

Four Examples of Interval Training

I. STEADY-PACE INTERVALS OF WALKING, JOGGING, RUNNING, CYCLING, ETC.

- 5-minute warmup at a gentle or moderate pace of the activity of your choice.
- 1 minute at a fast pace or high intensity, followed by 1 minute at a moderate pace. Alternate 5 to 8 times.
- 5-minute cooldown at a gentle or moderate pace.

2. INTERVALS THAT INCREASE IN SPEED OR INTENSITY THROUGHOUT THE WORKOUT

The example I have included here applies to running on a treadmill. A similar approach could be taken, however, by changing the tension or peddling faster on a stationary bike; by increasing the level or moving faster on your elliptical machine; or by walking on an incline on the treadmill while increasing the speed or incline.

5-minute warmup at 5.5 mph
- 1 minute at 7 mph
- 1 minute at 6 mph
- 1 minute at 7.5 mph
- 1 minute at 6 mph
- 1 minute at 8 mph
- 1 minute at 6 mph
- 1 minute at 8.5 mph
- 1 minute at 6 mph

- 1 minute at 9 mph
- 5-minute cooldown

3. INTERVALS THAT VARY BY DURATION

Rather than increasing the speed or intensity, as in the example above, your intervals could range in duration—for example, 30 seconds, 60 seconds, 90 seconds, 60 seconds, 30 seconds—with 1-minute, low-intensity sessions between each interval.

4. ADVANCED OPTION: SPRINTING (ONLY 15 MINUTES Or SO)
- Warm up with a light jog for 5 to 10 minutes.
- Sprint 50 to 100 meters and lightly jog or walk back to your starting point. Repeat 10 times.
- Cool down with a light jog for another 5 to 10 minutes.

You could also use this approach on hills by running (or speed walking) up the hill and lightly jogging down.

A Few Simple Tips to Keep You Active

If you've never exercised before, you must know that getting started is often the hardest part. I am confident that, by now, the first two steps of the Hormone Diet have given you the motivation to make the leap into physical fitness, but here are a few more tips.

- **Schedule your workouts on your calendar.** This habit will help keep you on track and ensure that you make time for exercise.
- **Pick a time that fits with the rest of your daily activities, whether it's first thing in the morning or right after work.** Going home first or working out after dinner, whether you do it at home or at a gym, can make your workout routine much tougher to stick to.

- **Record what you've done during each workout.** Monitoring your progress is a great source of motivation. And reviewing all the hard work you've done feels truly rewarding.
- **Get a friend on board the workout train with you.** It's so much more fun and also gives you a way to fit friend time into your busy schedule. Just make sure you're both working for 30 minutes and save your socializing for afterwards.
- **Hire a personal trainer.** Or enroll in a program like ours at Clear Medicine that integrates your health care with your fitness goals. I believe exercise is medicine. As such, it should be dispensed and explained like any prescription.

Enjoy the changes you see in your body; you'll never look back! And speaking of looks, now that you have your exercise routine in place to take care of all your inner workings, you're ready to optimize your outer appearance—with all-natural, toxin-free skin care.

CHAPTER 16

LOOK LOVELY, LIVE WELL:
THE IMPORTANCE OF NATURAL SKIN CARE

Here are the hormonal benefits you can expect to enjoy from choosing natural skin care:

- Protection from harmful chemicals that can mimic estrogen in your body
- Less inflammation
- Protection from the aging effects of other products

Everyone wants soft, supple skin that feels good and looks healthy. To truly make sure your skin looks its best, you must take care of it from the inside out, which, until now, has been the focus of my discussion. So let's start talking about how you can approach your skin from the outside in. You'll be looking fresh in no time.

Skin care is *big* business. On a daily basis we are bombarded with marketing messages about the latest product guaranteed to make us look years younger. But someone once advised me that I should never put anything on my skin that I wouldn't put in my mouth. Think about it—several medications come in cream or patch form because this allows the drug to absorb quickly and easily into the body. This fact led me to realize that I should pay more attention to the products I apply to my skin! After all, the skin *is* our largest vital organ.

That's right, vital organ. Just like the heart, brain, liver, and more,

LET THE SUNSHINE IN
Sunlight, in reasonable doses,
enables natural immunity, promotes skin growth and healing,
stimulates hormone production
(e.g., our happy hormone, serotonin) and contributes to an
overall sense of well-being. Getting some sunlight for 15 to 20
minutes a day enables the body
to manufacture vitamin D and is
responsible for the synthesis of
the pigment melanin, the skin's
natural sunscreen. Just make
sure you don't go overboard.
Excess sun exposure is a leading
cause of skin cancer and premature aging.

your skin performs several essential biological functions. It blocks viral and bacterial
infections from entering your body. It controls your body temperature through sweating. When exposed to sunshine, it supports
the production of the vitamin D we need
for bone health and insulin balance.
Through its intricate network of sensory
nerves, it also informs us about our surroundings and allows us to feel a myriad of
sensations, including the pleasure of touch.
Your skin is crucial for life and for your
ability to interact with the world.

Skin consists of three main layers: epidermis, dermis, and subcutaneous tissue
(fat). You can almost imagine your skin
like a dessert with several layers.

The "Meringue": Your Epidermis

The epidermis is the top layer of skin. It is made up of different types
of cells that make the protein keratin—melanin, which is the pigment responsible for your skin color and tone, and immune cells
that protect you from infections. As we age, the function of these
immune cells of the epidermis weakens, our wounds take longer to
heal, and our skin doesn't recuperate from damage the way it once
did. Therefore, the benefits of maintaining healthy immune system
function are certainly not limited to experiencing fewer colds and
flus. (Good thing the three steps offer a completely natural immunity boost.)

Most of your epidermis comprises the cells that make keratin.
They begin at the bottom of the epidermis as fresh cells but lose
water and flatten out as they move upward. They end up as dead
cells on your skin's surface. Eventually these dead cells are sloughed

off and replaced by new ones. Somewhat like the meringue topping on a pie, your epidermis is moist on the inside with a delicate but crusty outer surface.

The state of your epidermis determines how fresh your skin appears. *By now, the favorable inner changes you have been making over the past month or so while following your three steps are surely starting to show on the outside, since epidermal cells renew every 4 to 5 weeks.* In fact, most of my patients continue to report substantial improvements in their skin during the first 3 to 6 months after adopting the healthy lifestyle habits prescribed by the Hormone Diet.

The Cream Filling: Your Dermis

Sandwiched between your epidermis and subcutaneous fat is the dermis, the thickest layer of your skin. (Note that some experts view the dermis and subcutaneous fat as one layer.) Nerve fibers, blood vessels, sweat and sebaceous glands, hair follicles, and lymphatic tissue are all found in this layer of your skin.

The dermis is important for your skin's circulation, oil and moisture content, oxygenation, and further protection from invading bacteria or viruses. When your skin fails to produce enough sebum (oil), dryness and wrinkling occurs, whereas overproduction leads to acne and blackheads. You shouldn't be surprised to learn that your sebum and sweat glands respond to your hormones. Testosterone, progesterone, and DHEA are known to increase the production of sebum and are linked to acne breakouts. DHEA, testosterone, and estrogen can also cause or contribute to excess sweating and even body odor.

The dermal layer is also heavily involved in the structural support, elasticity, and resiliency of your skin. If you have wrinkles now, they are rooted within your dermis. A protein called collagen provides skin's structural framework and tone, whereas another called elastin is involved in the suppleness and elasticity of your skin.

Because the dermis is composed of collagen and elastin, your dietary intake of protein and other protein building blocks will affect the health and appearance of your skin. Thinning, wrinkling, and sagging are signs of deficient collagen or elastin production. Estrogen is also an important factor involved in the collagen and elastin production in this layer of your skin.

The Graham Cracker Crust: Subcutaneous Fatty Tissue

This layer of your skin is the one you hope stays in place as you age. Just as the crust is to a tasty pie, subcutaneous fatty tissue is the foundation of firm, fresh-looking skin. Unfortunately, this layer tends to shrink away with aging, which results in sagging and wrinkling. According to an October 2004 report by the American Society of Plastic Surgeons, sun exposure and the loss of fat play far greater roles than gravity in the aging of our faces. Plastic surgeons are now rejuvenating faces by replacing lost facial fat with wrinkle fillers such as collagen and fat cells.

As with the dermis, estrogen also plays an important role in maintaining this layer of your skin. Many women notice thinning and sagging skin as part of menopause. These changes occur because estrogen, which declines during menopause, plays a vital role in maintaining both the elasticity and firmness of your skin.

Your Hormones and Your Skin

Glowing skin; thick, shiny hair; and smooth, flexible nails are all hallmarks of health and hormonal balance. When your hormones are out of whack, visible signs of aging turn up in the look and feel of your hair and skin. Here's a brief summary of just a few of the ways in which hormones affect hair and skin.

Insulin

Foods high in sugar, such as pastries, muffins, white pasta, white rice, and juice, cause spikes in blood sugar and insulin, which can cause inflammation and contribute to wrinkles and aging.

Cortisol

Our long-term stress hormone has documented aging effects on our skin cells. (Anything that beats stress basically beats aging, too.)

Estrogen

As already mentioned, the drop in estrogen production that naturally occurs with age makes our skin thinner and less elastic, which leads to more wrinkling and sagging. As estrogen dips, less collagen and elastin are produced. Estrogen also helps skin stay moist by boosting hyaluronic acid. A 1997 study of 3,875 postmenopausal women concluded that estrogen supplementation helped aging women have younger-looking skin. It also maintained skin's collagen, thickness, elasticity, and ability to retain moisture. According to the Life Extension Foundation, these effects can be enhanced even further with supplements of both estrogen and testosterone.

Testosterone

In both women and men, excess testosterone may result in acne on the face, chest, or back. With age, some women experience an increase in testosterone along with a decrease in estrogen. Meanwhile, men tend to experience the opposite—an increase in estrogen and a decrease in testosterone, which causes the skin to dry out.

DHEA

Dry skin increases with age. Interestingly, DHEA tends to decline with stress, as well as with aging and menopause. DHEA turns on oil production and seems to help combat this problem and improve hydration. It also increases the production of collagen, making skin appear smoother and younger looking. Our skin's natural protective barrier also appears to improve with DHEA.

Melatonin

Both melatonin and serotonin are produced in your skin from the amino acid tryptophan. According to a July 2005 article from the journal *Endocrine,* melatonin is involved in hair growth and protection against melanoma. As an antioxidant hormone, melatonin guards us from UV radiation and appears to play a role in repairing burned skin. New research led by Dr. Russel Reiter, a cell biologist at the University of Texas in San Antonio, also suggests that melatonin supplementation may offer extra protection from skin cancer. Whether it's applied topically or taken internally, melatonin may shield us from environmental and internal stressors.

Progesterone

Ever wonder why pregnant women seem to have that special glow? The secret is the high level of progesterone common in a healthy pregnancy. Progesterone is very beneficial for skin elasticity and circulation.

Growth Hormone

Since growth hormone tends to drop off as we get older, supplements are promoted as a way to "reverse" the effects of aging. Growth hormone is essential for skin-cell repair and the prevention of sagging.

Natural Skin Care

Considering the impact hormones can have on your skin, hormonal imbalances can clearly affect how you look as well as how you feel. We need to choose our skin-care products wisely to ensure they don't disrupt the delicate hormonal balance that keeps us looking our best.

Think about how many different products come in contact with your body every morning before you even leave the bathroom: shampoo, conditioner, body wash or soap, shaving cream, body cream, face wash, moisturizer, toothpaste, deodorant—and the list goes on, especially if you wear makeup or cologne. Before you take your first breath of outdoor air, you've already been exposed to hundreds of chemicals. Imagine how the daily absorption of these chemicals adds up over a lifetime!

This long-term exposure is a definite hormonal health concern. Some of the chemicals found in a variety of cosmetics— including phthalates, acrylamide, formaldehyde, and ethylene oxide—are listed by the US Environmental Protection Agency and the state of California as carcinogens or reproductive toxins. That's serious!

Recall our discussion of phthalates in Chapter 8. This group of industrial chemical plasticizers is used in many cosmetic products from nail polish to deodorants—products that are linked to birth defects, low testosterone in men, and the feminization of baby boys. Unfortunately, phthalates are just one of many examples.

By following the principles of the Hormone Diet, you have made a commitment to ridding your life of hormone-imbalancing habits and toxins. Now that you have optimized your skin's appearance by making so many healthy changes on the inside, natural skin-care products are the absolutely perfect way to round out your three-step plan and get gorgeous from the outside. And guys, this advice is not just for ladies only.

Cleanse and Moisturize

Your cleansing products should be free of sodium lauryl sulfate, a harsh detergent present in shampoos and cleansers. This chemical is highly astringent, which means it strips your skin of natural moisture. It's also used to clean machinery and industrial flooring, if that tells you anything. The skin-care lines Caudalie, John Masters,

Naturopathica, Burt's Bees, and Juice Beauty offer a selection of chemical-free cleansers to choose from.

Contrary to popular belief (prompted by prominent marketing messages), we should avoid using abrasive, scratchy products or brushes to exfoliate our skin. If you really like the feeling you get from such products, make sure the exfoliating ingredient consists of fine particles that won't scratch or damage your skin. Better yet, choose products with natural, fruit-based acids such as lactic acid or alpha hydroxy acid (AHA) to lift off dead skin cells without any abrasive action. Note that you can still overexfoliate, even with these milder fruit acids. Years of abnormally increasing cellular turnover in your skin may accelerate the aging of your skin later on.

If you do choose a mildly grainy exfoliating compound for your body, it should contain natural oils and be free of additives. Alba Organics' Sugar Cane Body Polish is a good choice that's available at most health food stores. The sunflower oil base and added macadamia oil, vitamin E, and honey make it a treat for dry, flaky winter skin. To gently exfoliate and brighten facial skin, try using Environmental Defense Mask from Naturopathica or Juice Beauty's Green Apple Peel twice a week after cleansing.

The moisturizers you use on your body or face should be free of the following: methylparabens, propylparabens, formaldehyde, imidazolidinyl urea, methylisothiazolinone, propylene glycol, paraffin, isopropyl alcohol, sodium lauryl sulfate, and other chemical tongue twisters. I dare you to go into your bathroom right this second and read all the labels you find. No doubt you'll realize almost everything should go directly into the recycling bin. Parabens, in particular, have been identified as estrogenic substances that disrupt normal hormone function and may increase the risk of breast cancer.

Instead, choose products containing pure oils, protective vitamins, and natural scents. Burt's Bees, available in most health food stores and natural pharmacies, makes an excellent line of natural skin-care products for both babies and adults. Two of my personal favorites are Apricot Baby Oil (fabulous on damp skin after bathing) and Milk & Honey Body Lotion. Both of these products smell delicious and include vitamin E and other antioxidants to protect skin cells. I have also discovered Korres, a wonderful natural skin-care line from Greece, whose body lotions and butters are divine. Plus, their lip balm is quite possibly the best I've ever tried.

PERSONAL-CARE PRODUCTS AND THEIR HARMFUL CHEMICALS

Personal-Care Product	Harmful Chemical
Body wash, shampoos, facial cleansers, toothpaste	Sodium lauryl sulfate (a harsh chemical cleanser)
Lipstick	Certain brands may contain lead (which can accumulate and cause lead toxicity)
Most products	Synthetic dyes and fragrances (these increase our risk of allergy and the chemical content of products)
Body wash, shampoo, conditioner, makeup, eye creams, deodorants, body and facial moisturizers	Parabens (methylparabens, propylparabens, etc., are linked to breast cancer)
Nail polish	Formaldehyde (a carcinogen)
Toothpaste	Fluoride (potentially harmful to our thyroid function when present in excess)
Shampoo, lotions, creams	Cocamide DEA (listed in the United States as likely to cause cancer in humans)

Save Face

If preventing aging is your goal, ingredients proven to stimulate collagen production and reduce fine lines, free radical damage, sun damage, and uneven skin tone are a must in your daily skin-care regimen. Look for hyaluronic acid, vitamin C, coenzyme Q10, alpha-lipoic acid, vitamin E, or vitamin A. Applying these nutrients topically has documented antiaging effects. DMAE has also been found to freshen skin and prevent sagging.

The stores are full of skin-care creams that promise wrinkle-free, younger-looking, smooth and toned skin. Realize that little clinical data are available to support these claims. But take heart. Clinical studies have proven a few ingredients to be effective in reducing fine lines and evening out skin tone.

ALPHA-LIPOIC ACID: Lipoic acid is an antioxidant compound involved in healthy blood sugar balance and insulin action. This dual action provides highly protective, antiaging benefits for our skin by reducing the risk of glycation—the abnormal attachment of sugar to our skin cells, causing wrinkling and aging.

Alpha-lipoic acid is both water and fat soluble, making it protective for most tissues in the body. One study reported a 50 percent reduction in fine lines and wrinkles with the topical use of a high-potency lipoic acid cream.

EXTRACTS OF WHITE AND GREEN TEA: A 2003 study from the University Hospitals of Cleveland and Case Western Reserve University found that certain antioxidant compounds in white tea extract are effective in improving skin-cell immunity and offering protection from the damaging effects of the sun. Evidently, a skin cream containing these tea extracts may offer potent antiaging and anticancer benefits.

The Skin Study Center at University Hospitals of Cleveland also found that the antioxidants in green tea can reduce the harmful effects of sunburn. In addition, Dr. Stephen Hsu from the Medical College of Georgia Department of Oral Biology found the polyphenols in green tea help to eliminate free radicals, which can cause cancer by altering cell DNA. As our outer epidermal cells naturally slough off, skin cells from deep within the epidermis make their way to the surface about every 4 weeks. By about day 20, cells are basically hanging out on the upper layer waiting to die. The most abundant polyphenol in green tea, EGCG (also used for its benefits in weight loss), appears to bring dying skin cells back to life when it is applied to the surface of the skin. Besides making us look fresher, these effects of green tea may be very useful for improving skin conditions and for the prevention of scarring. It seems EGCG is the fountain of youth for our skin cells! You might want to look for John Masters's Green Tea & Rose Hydrating Face Serum—I think it's the best, and I received compliments on my skin when first trying it out.

COENZYME Q10: A 1999 study found that topical application of the antioxidant coenzyme Q10 (CoQ10) improved the skin's resistance to the oxidative stress of UV radiation. When applied long term, CoQ10 may reduce the appearance of crow's feet, those nasty lines around the eyes.

DMAE: Dimethylaminoethanol (DMAE) boosts the production of acetylcholine, as well as phosphatidylcholine, a component of cell membranes. DMAE may be the first clinically proven agent to effectively combat facial sagging. Many of Dr. Nicholas Perricone's skin-care products contain DMAE. Visit www.perriconemd.com for more information.

VITAMIN C: Topical use of a product containing stabilized vitamin C can increase the production of collagen in the skin. It can also promote skin-cell growth and aid in cell regeneration, which translates to younger-looking skin and improved firmness. The form of vitamin C used in your skin-care products is important because it has the potential to become unstable and even a potentially harmful source of free radical stress. Ascorbyl palmitate, the fat-soluble form of vitamin C, appears to be the most beneficial and stable type for use in skin-care products. It should be present in significant concentrations to boost collagen production in the skin.

Choose a product that is white or, even better, a colorless serum.

This way you can easily toss your topical vitamin C product if it turns yellow, orange, or brown—a sign it has become oxidized. When this happens, it will do more harm than good.

VITAMIN A: Topical products containing natural forms of vitamin A (retinol, retinyl palmitate, retinoic acid, retinaldehyde) or vitamin A derivatives (called retinoids) have proven to be beneficial for skin damaged by the sun. According to some sources, retinyl palmitate is the best source, since it appears to be less irritating. These products also slow down the signs of aging. *Dermatology Surgery* (June 2004) reported that vitamin A is an effective, well-tolerated treatment for photodamaged facial skin and also reduces fine and large wrinkles, acne, liver spots, and surface roughness.

To avoid overexfoliating the skin, I recommend using a vitamin A cream only once or twice a week. These products should not be applied before sun exposure.

All-natural face care may cost a little more, but getting proven results without harmful toxins is far better than spending a ton on questionable products from your local drugstore or department store. Your local Whole Foods Market, natural spa, or health food store will usually offer the best source of all-natural, age-defying face products, or you can visit the Life Extension Foundation at www.lef.org. You may also visit a compounding pharmacy in your area.

Get Gorgeous

If you use makeup, the products you choose should, like your skin care, be all natural. Dr. Hauschka and Jane Iredale make natural cosmetics from skin-friendly, beautifully colored mineral powders. The products are made in a base of vitamin E and olive oil and actually contain minerals such as zinc, which provides a natural sunscreen.

Don't Forget the "Care" in Your Skin Care

No matter what products you choose, caring for your skin and keeping the effects of aging at bay requires a gentle approach. Consider these suggestions to make the most of your natural skin-care regimen.

- Wash your face with warm, not hot, water, which may damage your skin and accelerate aging.
- Apply your body moisturizer and facial moisturizer immediately after getting out of the shower, when your skin is still damp. In the winter or after shaving, I sometimes follow up my moisturizer with a natural oil to seal in the moisture. The same approach can be used on your face at night after applying your night cream. Evening primrose oil and natural vitamin E can be very soothing and moisturizing without blocking your pores.
- If facial cleanser is part of your routine, use it only at night. In the morning simply wash with water to avoid stripping your skin of its natural moisture.
- I recommend exfoliating twice a week with a product that contains fruit acids or vitamin A. Do not overexfoliate; it can harm your skin and upset your natural cycle of skin-cell regeneration.
- Use a hyaluronic acid serum on your skin after cleansing morning and night to maintain your skin's moisture and boost collagen production. Hyaluronic acid is a smaller building block of collagen that's more readily absorbed into the skin.
- Before applying your moisturizer, use a vitamin C serum once or twice daily to maintain the collagen production in your skin and to prevent free-radical stress.
- Warm your moisturizer before applying by rubbing it between your fingertips. Apply with short strokes or tap it on lightly. Don't stretch, pull, or rub your skin.

Well, it seems the old adage is true: Beauty really does come from within, especially when it comes to your skin. If you want to look (and feel) your best, inside and out, consistently follow these steps: Eat a nutritious diet complete with healthy fats, adequate protein, and low sugar; take your supplements; hydrate; sleep; maintain a healthy digestive system; and manage stress. Without these essential steps, the appearance and even the structure of your skin will suffer, even if you use the very best products available. Here's looking at you!

CHAPTER 17

YOU'RE ALMOST THERE!
A REFRESHER TO KEEP YOU GOING

Do more than exist, live.
Do more than touch, feel.
Do more than look, observe.
Do more than read, absorb.
Do more than hear, listen.
Do more than listen, understand.
Do more than think, ponder.
Do more than talk, say something.

JOHN H. RHOADES

By now I hope you are well on your way to reaching your weight-loss and wellness goals. More important, I hope you are motivated to maintain them. My wish is that this book has provided you with a practical and clear way to improve your health and well-being, not just for a few months, but for a lifetime.

Above all, I hope this plan has taught you to pay attention to early-warning symptoms and to recognize that your health is not defined solely by the number on the bathroom scale. I want you to look good and feel great about every aspect of your life, because you deserve to be happy and well. Take charge of your health and visit your doctor annually for complete blood work. Know your risk factors and continue to track them every year. My mom, who is now living with liver cancer, regrets that she did not take this one simple step.

This chapter gives you a quick, three-section refresher of the Hormone Diet plan. I will leave you with an outline of the perfect hormonally balanced day, a reminder to complete your 6-week check-in, and, lastly, a few final tips to keep you going if your fat loss has stalled.

Refresher #1: Your Hormonally Balanced Day

Reading about hormone-balancing habits is one thing. Making sure they are part of your everyday life is another. Here's an overview of what your hormonally balanced day should look like. Do your best to stick to this regimen 6 days a week. On your cheat day, eat and do whatever you wish—just remember to stay away from the hormone-disrupting foods that are to be avoided 100 percent of the time. Hey, you're even off the hook for shunning sugar on your cheat day, since you only need to avoid it 80 percent of the time!

Note that the specific hormonal benefits of each activity and task are identified in parentheses.

Between 6 and 8 a.m.

Wake up without a loud alarm clock (↓ cortisol). Open your blinds/curtains right away (↑ serotonin, ↓ melatonin, ↑ energy) to set your body clock on "awake."

Take your green-food drink and your probiotics; fit in your workout if you can. Always have breakfast *before* your strength-training workouts. If you aren't working out now, try to head outside for at least 15 minutes of natural sunlight—eat your breakfast outside, walk the dog, etc. (↑ serotonin, ↑ testosterone in men, ↑ fertility/ovulation in women).

Within an hour of waking, eat a breakfast that contains protein, carbohydrates, and fats, preferably a smoothie that includes all three macronutrients (all your meals should illicit this hormonal response: ↑ leptin, ↑ glucagon, ↑ serotonin, ↑ PYY, ↑ CCK, ↓ cortisol, ↓ ghrelin, ↓ neuropeptide Y). Enjoy your cup of organic coffee, if you wish (↑ dopamine, ↑ adrenaline). Take your Clear Essentials—Morning Pack or your multivitamin, vitamin D_3, and omega-3 fish oil (↓ inflammation; ↑ fat burning, energy, and metabolism).

Listen to music, books on tape, motivational material, or whatever you enjoy listening to on the way to work to reduce the stress of driving or commuting. Breathe (↓ cortisol, ↑ serotonin).

9 a.m.

At work, try as much as possible to minimize your exposure to harsh fluorescent lighting; consider earplugs or headphones if you work in a noisy or open office environment (↓ cortisol).

Fill your glass water bottle and grab a cup of green tea a few times throughout the day (↓ cortisol and NPY, ↑ thyroid hormone, ↑ metabolism and appetite control).

Between 11 a.m. and 1 p.m.

Enjoy a lunch that contains protein, good carbs, and healthy fats. Get outside for your dose of sunshine if you didn't get it in the morning, though morning is best (↑ serotonin, ↑ energy, better digestion throughout the day and night).

3 p.m. to After Work

Grab a snack that contains protein, good carbs, and healthy fats. Head for your workout if you haven't done so already (↓ cortisol, ↓ insulin, ↑ growth hormone, ↑ DHEA, ↑ testosterone, ↑ dopamine, and ↑ serotonin). Engage in competitive sports if you want an extra testosterone boost.

Within 45 minutes of finishing your workout, have a snack with protein and carbohydrates or have your dinner (see below). Minimal fat is needed at this time; the meal after your workout is the only one where you can get away with more carbohydrates (↑ growth hormone).

7 p.m.

Have a dinner that includes protein, good carbs, and healthy fats, but limit fat if it is after your workout. Take your Clear Essentials— Evening Pack or your multivitamin and calcium-magnesium.

8 to 10 p.m.

It's time to dim the lights in your house until bedtime (↑ serotonin, ↑ melatonin, ↓ cortisol, better digestion of carbs from your evening meal). If you watch TV or movies, remember that your selections will affect your hormones, so choose accordingly (the right choice should ↑ growth hormone, ↑ progesterone, ↓ cortisol).

If you enjoy alcohol, have it by 9 p.m. Any later and it could interfere with your sleep (because it ↑ insulin, ↑ cortisol, and ↓ melatonin). Consuming one glass right after dinner is best, if you have any at all. Remember, only four glasses per week for women; seven for guys.

Definitely shut down your computer and turn off your TV by 10 p.m., if you haven't done so already (otherwise ↑ dopamine can keep you too stimulated for sleep). Have a hot bath or shower at this time or earlier to improve your sleep, if necessary (↑ melatonin, ↓ cortisol). Showering at night, rather than in the morning, is helpful for your sleep and can sometimes give you more time in the morning.

Enjoy some cuddling, kissing, caressing, or sex (↓ cortisol, ↑ oxytocin, ↑ testosterone, ↑ DHEA, ↑ progesterone). Get to bed 10 to 20 minutes earlier if you want extra time to work your mental magic on your life's plan—visualize or meditate (↑ serotonin, ↑ DHEA, ↓ cortisol, ↓ adrenaline).

11 p.m.

Go to sleep by 11 in total darkness. Remember to create the perfect environment for slumber and follow the sleep rules to maximize your hormonal balance (↑ melatonin, ↑ leptin, ↑ growth hormone, ↑ serotonin, ↑ testosterone, ↓ cortisol, ↓ adrenaline, ↓ insulin).

Refresher #2: Your 6-Week Check-In

Go back to the "get prepped" instructions outlined for you in Chapter 6. Repeat your measurements and check your progress. Feel free to tell me about your results—just visit www.thehormonediet.com. I would absolutely love to hear from you.

From this point on, you should incorporate the following components of the Hormone Diet plan into your life as best you can. Hopefully they'll become regular habits you look forward to using.

- Maintain balance with an anti-inflammatory detox at least twice a year
- Recuperate and rejuvenate with hormone-balancing sleep
- Keep stress in check with meditation, visualization, massage, goal setting, and more
- Eat for hormonal balance and healthy weight maintenance
- Take your basic supplements for hormonal balance and good health
- Exercise and enjoy regular sex
- Look your best with all-natural skin care

Beyond these basic steps, you can continue progressing and modifying your wellness plan by tweaking your supplements to meet your changing needs, hormonal imbalances, or special health concerns. For instance, it's probably been a few weeks since you have looked at the Hormonal Health Profile results you recorded in your Treatment Pyramid. You might want to revisit them if you had more than one imbalance or if you are still experiencing symptoms. Go back to Chapter 13 and look into your next solution.

Most people will have lost 12 to 25 pounds and several inches by this point. Favorable changes will almost always occur in your body fat percentage, too. However, on the off chance that you are not happy with your progress, I encourage you to revisit the signs and symptoms of the fat-packing hormonal imbalances. If you have followed all three steps to a T and you still do not see the results you had hoped for, one of these hormone-hampering conditions or even a medication you are taking could be interfering with your results.

A recap of the fat-packing conditions (and their associated questions in the Hormonal Health Profile):

1. Insulin resistance discussed in Chapter 3 (Hormonal Imbalance 1)
2. Inflammation discussed in Chapter 1
3. Estrogen dominance explained in Chapter 3 (Hormonal Imbalance 7 and Hormonal Imbalance in men 11)
4. Stress discussed in Chapter 3 (Hormonal Imbalance 5)
5. Hypothyroidism covered in Chapter 4 (Hormonal Imbalance 13)
6. Menopause presented in Chapter 4 (Hormonal Imbalance 8, Hormonal Imbalance 9, and/or Hormonal Imbalance 11)
7. Andropause presented in Chapter 4 (Hormonal Imbalance 11)
8. Depression/anxiety discussed in Chapter 4 (Hormonal Imbalance 3)

If you suspect you are experiencing any one of these imbalances, visit your doctor to request the tests outlined in Appendix A. Specific supplements for these conditions (see Chapter 13) will also be helpful.

Refresher #3: Tips for a Metabolic Shake-Up

By now you have been following your Hormone Diet plan for a little over a month and a half. You've actually passed the daunting 21-day mark, the amount of time "they" say is required for your brain to turn a new task or approach into a habit. Now is a good time to take stock and assess your progress. How are you doing? Are you feeling good? Are you happy? Or are you feeling stuck?

Sometimes by week 5 or 6, weight loss may stall. If so, you've probably hit a weight-loss plateau. During such a plateau, weight reduction slows down or stops completely, reflecting the body's natural need to maintain constant equilibrium.

When we change our diet, cut our calories and begin a fitness plan, we typically alter our energy expenditure balance by taking in fewer calories than we burn. At the beginning, this imbalance is beneficial for fat loss, as the body taps into fat stores for fuel. But because our body prefers balance, it gradually adjusts by burning fewer calories in order to protect its reserves. This point is usually when our eating and exercise efforts stop producing the results we are looking for. If you follow my suggestion to wait until the fourth week of your new lifestyle to begin your exercise plan, however, a plateau will be unlikely because you'll enjoy a metabolic boost just at the right time.

Nonetheless, a weight-loss plateau may occur for these reasons:

1. Your body simply needs a "rest" period to adapt to calorie reduction.
2. Your current calorie intake may be in balance with your calorie expenditure.
3. You have reduced your calorie intake too much. Excess calorie cutting prompts your body to respond by slowing your metabolism to conserve calories. Note that you are also at risk of losing metabolically active muscle with excessive caloric restriction.
4. During weight loss, water is generated in the body as a normal part of fat metabolism. This process can lead to water-related weight gain.
5. A hormonal imbalance is interfering with your body's ability to burn fat.
6. For women, fluctuations of a few pounds may also be related to the menstrual cycle or water retention.

What Can You Do to Break Through?

In order to get past the plateau, the best approach is a multifaceted one. The two most important steps are altering your eating habits and changing your exercise program in ways that challenge your body and shake things up. You must also evaluate your lifestyle (honestly) and any negative symptoms you may be experiencing to determine whether one of your fat-burning foes is causing interference. Here are a few ideas to help you power past a plateau.

TAKE L-TYROSINE TO BOOST YOUR DOPAMINE. I spoke of the effects of dopamine on weight loss in Chapter 4. The trouble is, as you lose weight, this fat-loss friend tends to take a dip. It's just one of the ways your body works against you by attempting to maintain the status quo. But you can wake up your metabolism by supplementing with 1,000 mg of L-tyrosine each morning on an empty stomach. Since L-tyrosine increases the production of both dopamine and thyroid hormone, it could give you just the boost you need to push past your plateau.

MIX UP YOUR WORKOUT. Fire up your metabolism (and calorie expenditure) by increasing your activity level. This simple step can "reboot" your metabolism and restart your weight loss. For example, if you usually exercise for 20 minutes each day, try 25 to 30 minutes daily. If you're already exercising for a sufficient length of time, increase the intensity. Do 15 to 20 minutes of interval training instead of 30 minutes at a slower pace. Varying your workout routine can also help. Longer workouts are not always the answer, but 150 minutes per week does seem to be the magic number that sparks weight loss, according to studies.

TRY CARDIO FIRST THING IN THE MORNING ON AN EMPTY STOMACH. If you can manage it, try doing a 30-minute cardio workout (no longer!) first thing in the morning before breakfast. Why? In some cases, this technique may be just the trick your body needs to kick-start your metabolism.

PUMP SOME IRON. Remember, muscle is metabolically active tissue. Muscle mass determines our basal metabolic rate (i.e., the number of calories we burn daily while at rest). The more muscle we have, the more fat we can potentially burn, even while sitting around or sleeping. If your fat loss continues to stall, boost the intensity of your strength-training routine by increasing the amount of weight you lift. A personal trainer may be an excellent investment at this point, even for just a few sessions to get you back in gear and to make sure you are exercising at the right intensity.

DON'T BE AFRAID TO INTENSIFY YOUR WORKOUT (IF YOU ARE HEALTHY). Studies show that you need 150 to 200 minutes of exercise per week for weight loss. For an extra fat-burning boost, pump up the intensity of your cardio sessions with intervals, rather than making your workouts longer.

BE SURE TO REST AND RECUPERATE. Recovery is an essential part of your exercise program. Proper rest allows your muscle fibers to grow and prevents the elevation of cortisol and other stress hormones that can happen when we overtrain. Track your resting heart rate immediately after you wake up for a week or two. An increase from one week to the next could be a sign of overtraining. Remember, excess cortisol tears down the muscle tissue you've worked so hard to gain. Losing muscle will ultimately cause your metabolism to slow down.

MAKE SURE YOU ARE EATING THE RIGHT AMOUNTS AT THE RIGHT TIMES. Some of the biggest weight-loss mistakes are simply not eating enough calories, going too long without eating, or eating meals at irregular times. Skipping breakfast is the worst habit of all! Plenty of research shows that people who skip meals or slash too many calories are *more* obese and have an increased risk of type 2 diabetes and heart disease. If you're following the Hormone Diet eating plan, you should not be going too long without food. The program is designed to help you maintain stable blood sugar and create the perfect hormonal balance for fat loss. Eating the right foods every 4 to 5 hours reassures your body that food is plentiful. It also facilitates calorie burning and prevents metabolic decline.

KEEP A FOOD DIARY. If you feel your nutrition is off track but can't figure out where you're going wrong, try keeping a food journal. You may start to recognize dietary saboteurs, which can help you avoid them and get back on track. Have a professional nutritionist or naturopathic doctor assess your diet, if necessary.

IF YOU HAVE STUBBORN ABDOMINAL FAT, YOU MAY BE INSULIN RESISTANT. Your score from Hormonal Imbalance 1 in the Hormonal Health Profile and/or the results of your blood test from your Best Body Assessment will give you an indication of your insulin sensitivity. If you are insulin resistant, high insulin levels and excess weight will cause an accumulation of abdominal fat and will also impede further weight loss. A Glyci-Med diet is essential to remedy this condition, while supplements and strength training are important for improving insulin sensitivity. Supplement choices include CLA, chromium, alpha-lipoic acid, zinc, and magnesium, but you can review your complete list of options in Chapter 13. Note that this imbalance will take months to improve–trust the three steps and stick with the program!

JOIN A GROUP, GET A WORKOUT BUDDY, OR ASK FOR HELP. Studies show that people who have a support system tend to lose weight and keep it off, as they can share their diet ups and downs with others. Social support from a partner, friend, Web site, trainer, or workout partner can provide essential help and encouragement.

MAKE SURE THAT YOUR WEIGHT-LOSS EXPECTATIONS ARE REALISTIC. Safe weight loss is 1 to 2.2 pounds of fat per week. During the first few weeks of a weight-loss program, more weight may be lost, although most of it is water. After losing this initial weight, people tend to lose an average of 1 pound a week, which is still considered good progress (even a few pounds a month is good). Remember, 1 pound of body fat is equivalent to 3,500 calories, so losing 1 pound per week can mean cutting out 500 calories per day.

GET ORGANIZED. Make time for a good breakfast and travel with your own healthy snacks. Clear your cupboards of problem foods—you can't eat what's not there. Shop with the Hormone Diet eating plan in mind, and be sure you have plenty of healthy choices on hand to make meal and snack prep easy and convenient.

DRINK PLENTY OF WATER. As fat cells begin to shrink, they release toxins that need to be removed from your system by your liver, kidneys, and digestive tract. Studies show that if you don't take in enough water to support these processes, the toxins may interact with your hormones and cause increased fat storage or an inability to burn fat. Water can also help make you feel full and regulate your appetite, as many of us mistake thirst for hunger. To calculate how much water you need, multiply your body weight in pounds by 0.55. Divide the result by 8 to determine the number of cups you need to drink each day.

BE PATIENT AND STAY POSITIVE! A weight-loss plateau may take a few weeks to overcome, but you will get there. Stay focused on your goal and remember all the wonderful health benefits you are already enjoying thanks to the changes you have made to your lifestyle.

BEWARE OF COMMON DIET DEBACLES

- **Fat-free yogurt with added fruit.** Fat-free yogurt typically has 27 g carbs, 4 g protein, and no fat. Too many carbs! Plain yogurt is a much better bet, with 6 g protein, 6 g carbs, and a few grams of fat. Purchase plain yogurt and add your own fruit. If you really must have sweetened or flavored yogurt, mix it half and half with an unsweetened, plain one to decrease the amount of sugar per serving.

- **Packaged nuts (almonds, peanuts, etc.).** Most of these products contain hydrogenated oils or vegetable oils—no-no foods you need to avoid at all times. Instead, purchase raw nuts from a health food or bulk store.
- **So-called healthy breakfast cereals.** Take Smart Start cereal from Kellogg's, for example. It does offer more vitamins and minerals than other cereals, but it also contains a ton of sugar. The only breakfast cereal I recommend is Kashi GOLEAN or slow-cooked oatmeal. If you choose either of these options, you'll still need to add more protein to your breakfast (e.g., 2 or 3 egg whites) to remain in glycemic balance.
- **Too much fruit.** Fruits contain natural sugars and, just like anything else, too much is rarely a good thing. Aim for a maximum of three servings of fruit per day. At least one of these daily servings should be berries. Other choices include apples, pears, peaches, cherries, or grapefruit. Avoid raisins, dates, grapes, mangos, and melons (though watermelon is okay), and never eat your fruit on its own. Always have it with a food that contains fat and protein, such as a few nuts, some yogurt, or a piece of cheese.
- **Fizzy waters (Perrier, etc).** Although these contain few or no calories, they are very high in sodium, which can cause water retention and bloating. Choose sodium-free options or, better yet, drink pure water with lemon instead.
- **Coffee, lattes, teas, and more and more coffee.** Too much caffeine interferes with fat metabolism. It influences blood sugar and insulin balance and can contribute to an increase in abdominal fat. Although a little caffeine before a workout has been proven beneficial for weight loss, high amounts consumed throughout the day can do you more harm than

good. Instead, choose green tea, limit coffee to one a day, and always avoid sweet drinks such as caramel or vanilla lattes that are high in sugar and calories.

STEP UP YOUR STRESS-BUSTING STRATEGY, ESPECIALLY IF YOU HAVE STUBBORN AB FAT. Elevated cortisol inhibits thyroid function. As a result, cortisol is indirectly responsible for lagging metabolism, more water retention, and abdominal fat gain. Try meditation, visualization, or massage to help keep your cortisol in check. If you are under a lot of stress, consider Relora or one of the other supplements that lower stress, improve sleep, and reduce stress-related eating. Take another look at Chapter 13, Hormonal Imbalance 5, for a complete list of options.

GET A BLOOD TEST TO CHECK YOUR THYROID. Remember, your thyroid hormones govern your metabolism. If yours is sagging, TSH, free T3, and free T4 should be tested. Optimally, your TSH should be less than 2.0, not the previously accepted normal reading of 4.7. Note that thyroid problems occur more often in menopause and after pregnancy. You can revisit Chapter 13 for supplements to support a low thyroid hormone (Hormonal Imbalance 13) or talk to your doctor if further medical treatment is called for.

The key to your overall success is consistency. If you experience a setback, don't lose heart. Stay the course. Be kind to yourself, and remember, even if your weight has not budged recently, the healthy lifestyle changes you have made will benefit your body, mind, and soul for life.

If you are a doctor who would like to become certified in the Hormone Diet approach for your patients, or if you would like to become one of our patients, please visit www.thehormonediet.com.

UNDERSTANDING BLOOD TESTS

Visit your doctor at least once per year. *Always request a copy of your blood test results, and keep them in a folder.* Remember, significant changes can occur in your blood work from one year to the next without the appearance of obvious physical signs.

Tests for General Health, Immunity, and Wellness

- LIVER FUNCTION TESTS: AST, ALT, AND BILIRUBIN. These tests are used to identify liver disease and function. Your liver is vital for fat loss and wellness, as you've already discovered. Poor or "sluggish" liver function can interfere with fat loss, cause hormonal imbalances, and increase your risk of disease. The laboratory reference range covers normal values, but lower is better. Liver-cleansing herbs like those in Clear Detox—Hormonal Health, recommended as part of your detox, are essential if your liver enzymes are abnormally elevated. I recommend taking the liver-supportive herbs for at least 1 to 3 months and then retesting your enzymes to see if levels have improved.
- ZINC: Zinc is a cofactor involved in at least 70 different enzymatic reactions in the body. As an essential mineral involved in healthy immunity, blood sugar balance, thyroid function, collagen production, bone density, tissue healing and repair, antioxidant protection, prostate function, and growth hormone

and testosterone production, zinc is vital to good health. Zinc depletion is common with use of the birth control pill, corticosteroids, and diuretics. Its absorption is greatly compromised when your stomach acid (HCL) levels are low. Zinc deficiency causes decreased senses of taste and smell, poor wound healing, white spots in the fingernails, night blindness, low sperm count, hair loss, behavior or sleep problems, mental sluggishness, impaired immune function, and dermatitis. Optimally, your levels should be toward the high end of the laboratory reference range. You may add a supplement of zinc citrate if your zinc is low. Take it with food to avoid nausea.

- COPPER: Excess vitamin C and zinc interfere with copper availability. A deficiency of copper may result in anemia (indistinguishable from iron deficiency); impaired formation of collagen, elastin, and connective tissue proteins; osteoporosis; and arterial wall defects. It makes sense then if you have cardiovascular disease to monitor your copper levels closely. Although deficiencies are harmful, especially for cardiovascular health, it's more common to have excess copper due to medication use, supplements, or from copper leaching into drinking water from pipes. Symptoms of copper toxicity include depression, acne, and hair loss. If you find your copper is low, your multivitamin should provide all that you need. If your copper is too high, take zinc daily to encourage its depletion.

Tests for Glycemic Control, Fat Loss, Diabetes, and Heart Disease Risk

- FASTING GLUCOSE AND INSULIN. Glucose and insulin are implicated in many age-related diseases, such as type 2 diabetes, hypoglycemia, hypertension, heart disease, insulin resistance, and stroke. These tests require a fasting blood level, therefore a 10- to 12-hour fast is required before the collection of a blood sample. The optimal value for fasting blood glucose is less than 86 mg/dL. A value of less than 7 mU/mL is optimal for fasting insulin. Insulin resistance is associated with a glucose reading greater than 100 mg/dL and fasting insulin greater than 10 mU/mL. If your test is abnormal, use the recommendations in Chapter 13 for insulin imbalance in addition to the three steps.

- 2-HOUR POSTPRANDIAL GLUCOSE AND INSULIN. Simply have these two tests repeated 2 hours after you have eaten a very large breakfast (toast, orange juice, coffee, pancakes, syrup). The first sign of insulin resistance is elevated insulin *after* a meal *followed by high fasting insulin.* Insulin tends to be abnormal *long before* blood sugars start to rise typical of the diabetic state. Insulin resistance may be apparent with 2-hour glucose readings of more than 100 mg/dL and insulin levels of more than 60 mU/mL. If your test is abnormal, use the recommendations in Chapter 13 for insulin imbalance in addition to the three steps.

- FASTING GLUCOSE TO INSULIN RATIO. A value of fasting glucose divided by fasting insulin (using readings in US units) of less than 4.5 may indicate insulin resistance in nondiabetic individuals.

- FASTING TRIGLYCERIDES. Triglycerides are a particular type of fat present in your bloodstream that arises from fats or from carbohydrates taken in. Calories you ingest but that are not used immediately by tissues are converted to triglycerides and transported to your fat cells to be stored. Then, your hormones regulate the release of triglycerides from fat stores to help meet your body's needs for energy between meals. Levels greater than 100 mg/dL are associated with insulin resistance. If your test is abnormal, use the recommendations in Chapter 13 for insulin imbalance in addition to the three steps.

- FASTING CHOLESTEROL (TOTAL, HDL, AND LDL). An optimal HDL should be above 60 mg/dL. LDL should be between 80 and 100 mg/dL to be safe, and total cholesterol should be less than 180 to 200 mg/dL. If your cholesterol is too high, the three steps will help to lower your numbers. You might also want to look into supplementing with policosanols, PGX, or red yeast extract as natural alternatives to statins.
- URIC ACID. Normal levels are less than 0.35 mmol/L or 5.0 mg/dL. High levels of uric acid cause gout and are linked to increased heart disease risk; they're also a sign of insulin resistance. If your uric acid is imbalanced, you should consider the additional treatment options for inflammation and insulin imbalance in Chapter 13. Supplements of cherry juice and quercitin may also help to reduce uric acid.
- HbA1c LEVELS. This is an indicator of blood sugar control over the previous 120 days. Ideal levels are less than 4.6. If the number is higher, it indicates your blood sugar control over the previous months has been less than optimal. If your test is abnormal, use the recommendations in Chapter 13 for insulin imbalance.
- FASTING HOMOCYSTEINE (OPTIMAL VALUE: LESS THAN 6.3). Vitamin B_{12} (optimal value: more than 600) and folic acid (optimal value: more than 1,000) are useful tests to do along with this since they are involved in the process of metabolism necessary to reduce homocysteine levels, along with vitamin B_6 and a compound called trimethylglycine. Homocysteine is a protein that, if elevated in the blood, is a proven independent risk factor for heart disease, osteoporosis, Alzheimer's disease, and stroke. Homocysteine has been found to increase with insulin resistance and inflammation. Vitamin B_{12}, found only in animal-source foods, is necessary for the formation and regeneration of red blood cells. It also promotes growth, increases energy, improves sleep and cognition, and helps

maintain a healthy nervous system. Folic acid helps protect against chromosomal (genetic) damage and birth defects. It is needed for the utilization of sugar and amino acids, prevents some types of cancer, promotes healthier skin, and helps protect against intestinal parasites and food poisoning. Take a complex of vitamin B_6, vitamin B_{12}, and folic acid daily for at least 3 months before retesting your levels if your homocysteine is too high.

- HIGHLY SENSITIVE C-REACTIVE PROTEIN. Hs-CRP is a marker of inflammation and a risk factor for arterial disease. Levels tend to increase as body fat increases and with insulin resistance. An optimal value is less than 0.8 mg/L, although the Life Extension Foundation recommends less than 0.55 mg/L for men and less than 1.5 mg/L for women. This test is also important for breast cancer survivors and should be undertaken along with fasting and 2-hour postcarbohydrate challenge (PC) insulin level tests. High CRP or insulin is associated with increased risk of recurrence. If your hs-CRP test is abnormal, use the recommendations in Chapter 13 for inflammation.

- FERRITIN. Abnormally high levels of the storage form of iron (called ferritin) can increase the risk of heart disease in both men and women. It also appears to increase inflammation. Optimal levels should be close to 70 mcg/L in women and 100 mcg/L in men. Low levels of iron are associated with fatigue, hypothyroidism, decreased athletic performance, ADD/ADHD, restless leg syndrome, and hair loss. If your ferritin is too high, you should speak to your doctor about the possibility of donating blood; if too low, use a supplement of iron citrate with 1,000 mg of vitamin C. The citrate form of iron will not cause constipation and the vitamin C aids iron absorption.

- RBC MAGNESIUM. Magnesium is involved in over 300

enzymatic reactions in the body. Therefore, a deficiency of magnesium can result in the physical symptom of fatigue as bodily functions slow on a cellular level. Magnesium controls blood pressure and blood sugar balance. Optimal levels can assist in the prevention of muscle cramps or spasms, headaches and migraines, type 2 diabetes, and heart disease. Your multivitamin and your calcium-magnesium combination should replenish your magnesium levels if your stores are low.

Hormonal Assessments

Hormones are best tested in the morning. Menstruating women should go on day 3 of their cycle to look at estrogen and ovarian reserve and days 20 to 22 of their cycle to investigate progesterone (day 1 = first day of bleeding). Men and menopausal women can test on any day. Note that you can also assess your hormones via saliva or 24-hour urinary hormone analysis. This is argued to be the more accurate way to measure hormones because it looks at the free component of hormones rather than those bound to carrier proteins, as blood tests do. It is the free component of hormones that is biologically active. I use urine, saliva, and blood testing in clinical practice, however, especially when I want to assess the three types of estrogen or when someone is using BHRT, since only looking at blood values could result in overdosing.

- FOLLICLE-STIMULATING HORMONE (FSH) AND LUTEINIZING HORMONE (LH). These hormones are released from the pituitary gland and stimulate the ovaries and testes. High levels are found in menopause, infertility, amenorrhea, premature ovarian failure, or testicular failure. Low levels indicate pituitary dysfunction. If your FSH or LH is elevated you will need to replenish estrogen, progesterone, and/or testosterone. An excess of LH relative to FSH is common with polycystic ovarian syndrome (PCOS).

- DHEA-S. This is a precursor hormone to estrogen and testosterone. An adrenal hormone, it tends to naturally decrease as we age, is protective against the harmful effects of the stress hormone cortisol, is cardio-protective, and is crucial for a healthy body composition. Most antiaging programs recommend the use of DHEA; however, it should not be taken unless a true deficiency has been diagnosed with blood work, and follow-up testing should be completed to ensure an excess is not present. In some cases of PCOS it may be abnormally high, contributing to hair loss and male pattern baldness. Optimal levels should be 300 to 400 mcg/dL for men and 225 to 350 mcg/dL for women.
- CORTISOL. High levels (more than 15 mcg/dL) of cortisol are detrimental to almost every tissue and organ in the body. It causes destruction of muscle; increases calcium loss from bone; accelerates the process of aging; and is linked to memory loss, anxiety, depression, and low libido along with an increase in the deposition of fat around the abdomen. Low levels (less than 9 mcg/dL) indicate adrenal gland burnout. If your test is abnormal, use the recommendations in Chapter 13 for cortisol imbalance.
- CALCULATE THE DHEA/CORTISOL RATIO. The value of this ratio should optimally fall between 15 and 25 (i.e., the value of DHEA divided by cortisol). If your test is abnormal, use the recommendations in Chapter 13 for cortisol imbalance and DHEA.
- FREE AND TOTAL TESTOSTERONE. Many men with insulin resistance, obesity, or sleep apnea have low levels of testosterone, which is known to increase the risk of heart disease. This also influences erectile function, libido, sense of well-being, mood, and motivation. Maintaining testosterone levels is crucial if you want to build muscle and lose fat. Optimal free testosterone levels for men should be in the range of 7.2 to 24 mcg/dL; total testosterone should be 241 to 827 mcg/dL. In women, low

testosterone is damaging to bone density, a healthy libido, and aspects of memory (especially task-oriented memory). If testosterone is too high (often associated with PCOS or insulin resistance), hair loss, acne, increased risk of breast cancer, or infertility may occur. If your test is abnormal, use the recommendations in Chapter 13 for low or high testosterone.

- ESTRADIOL AND ESTRONE. Estrogen values will vary in women depending on their age and point in their menstrual cycle. The optimal value for estrogen is 180 to 200 pg/mL for premenopausal women and 60 to 120 pg/mL for women in their late 40s and older. Men's estradiol should be less than 40 pg/mL. In both sexes, high estrogen encourages fat storage. Elevated levels of estrogen in men are typically found in cases of increased abdominal obesity because the fat cells here encourage the conversion of testosterone to estrogen. High levels of estrogen and low levels of testosterone set the stage for sexual dysfunction and prostate conditions and promote weight gain in men. In women, excess estrogen is associated with PMS, weight gain around the hips, uterine fibroids and other gynecological conditions, and an increase in the risk of certain types of cancers. Before menopause, estrogen is naturally highest in the first half of the menstrual cycle; after menopause, levels are normally consistent and much lower. As estrogen levels decline, more abdominal weight gain can arise as estrogen does affect insulin sensitivity. Lower levels of estrogen are also associated with a decrease in serotonin. Recall from Chapter 3 that low estrogen can cause all of these symptoms: hot flashes, night sweats, urinary urgency and frequency, insomnia, depression, failing memory (especially when attempting to think of a word or name), hair texture and skin elasticity changes, a thickening waistline, vaginal dryness, and a missing "mojo." Low estrogen also increases the risk of heart disease, diabetes,

Alzheimer's disease, and osteoporosis. Evidently, estrogen is not all bad, but must be present in balance—not too high or too low. If your test is abnormal, use the recommendations in Chapter 13 for low or high estrogen.

- PROGESTERONE. Progesterone is naturally highest in the second half of the menstrual cycle and normal values can range widely. Progesterone is protective against anxiety, PMS, fibrocystic breast disease, and water retention. It encourages fat burning and is crucial for fertility. Progesterone is also protective of the prostate gland in men and may help to restore low DHEA levels. Decreased levels are associated with infertility, amenorrhea (lack of menstruation), fetal death, and toxemia in pregnancy. If your test is abnormal, use the recommendations in Chapter 13 for low or high progesterone.

- TSH, FREE T3, FREE T4, AND THYROID ANTIBODIES. These four tests are required to accurately assess the function of the thyroid gland, our master gland of metabolism. TSH should be less than 2.0 to be optimal, not the currently accepted 4.7 reported by most labs. T3 and T4 should be in the middle of your lab's reference range. Thyroid antithyroglobulin antibodies should be negative. Quite often I find elevated antibodies prior to abnormalities in TSH, T3, or T4, which indicates this may sometimes be the first step in the development of thyroid disease. Currently, it's estimated that 1 in 13 people have hypothyroidism, with the majority of cases being missed because of improper testing or interpretation of the test results. There is an increase in the risk of obesity, heart disease, and blood sugar abnormalities in hypothyroid cases. Hypothyroid patients also often have high levels of homocysteine and cholesterol. Also, if you are attempting to conceive, thyroid antibody abnormalities must be corrected to improve your chances of conception. If your test is abnormal, use the recommendations in Chapter 13 for low thyroid.

- REVERSE T3. This is a type of thyroid hormone the body will produce when under stress or when there is a deficiency of selenium. It is chemically similar to T3 (the active form of thyroid hormone) but is inactive and therefore does not have the metabolic benefits of T3. If your test is abnormal, use the recommendations in Chapter 13 for cortisol imbalance and low thyroid hormone activity and take a 200 mcg supplement of selenium daily.

- 25-HYDROXYVITAMIN D_3. Vitamin D has proven immune-enhancing, cancer-protective, bone-building, and insulin-regulating benefits. It is also important during pregnancy. Your levels should be over 125. If your vitamin D is low, add a 1,000 IU supplement of vitamin D_3 per day to your regime, in addition to your multivitamin and calcium-magnesium supplement. You will receive more than this amount of vitamin D_3 from the Clear Essentials—Morning and Evening packs.

- PROLACTIN. Elevated prolactin is associated with abnormal lactation, infertility, and amenorrhea. Prolactin can also be elevated in hypothyroidism when TSH is high. In men, the normal range is 2.17 to 17.7 ng/mL, and in women it is 2.8 to 29.2 ng/mL. If your prolactin is abnormally elevated, you may use the herb chasteberry (*Vitex agnus cactus*) to lower it.

- SHBG. Sex hormone-binding globulin binds with testosterone and makes it less bioavailable. SHBG increases with aging, liver disease, insulin resistance, and low-protein diets. Decreased levels will be found in hirsutism, obese postmenopausal women, and women with diffuse hair loss. If your test is abnormal, use the recommendations in Chapter 13 for insulin imbalance.

- IGF-1. This is a marker of human growth hormone (HGH) status. Because it remains constant in the blood longer than HGH (which tends to fluctuate in response to various stimuli), it is a more accurate indicator of HGH deficiency, and is also more precise for monitoring HGH therapy than is testing HGH directly. An optimal IGF-1 value will range between 200 and 300 ng/mL. Growth hormone is essential for maintaining healthy bones, skin, and hair, as well as strong, lean muscle mass. It tends to naturally decrease as we age; however, conditions such as sleep deprivation, diabetes, hypothyroidism, some cases of osteoporosis, anorexia, and insulin resistance can cause levels to decline more rapidly. If your test is abnormal, use the recommendations in Chapter 13 for low growth hormone.

Optional Advanced Functional Medicine Testing

The following tests are very useful if you can afford them. You may visit www.thehormonediet.com to request kits for the tests and complete many of them at home. Otherwise, I recommend visiting a naturopathic or integrated medical practitioner in your area.

From Metametrix Clinical Laboratory (www.metametrix.com)

URINARY ESTROGEN METABOLITE TESTING

To assess your risk of developing estrogen-sensitive cancers or recurrence of these types of cancer, I highly recommend the Estronex 2/16 test from Metametrix Clinical Laboratory. It measures the ratio of two critical estrogen metabolites from a single urine specimen. One metabolite, 2-hydroxyestrone (2-OHE1), tends to inhibit cancer growth. Another, 16-alpha-hydroxyestrone (16-A-OHE1), actually encourages tumor development. Estronex 2/16 ratios less than 2.0 indicate an increased long-term risk of breast, cervical, and other estrogen-sensitive cancers. It is your biochemical individuality and lifestyle habits that determine which of these metabolites predominates. Luckily, abnormal test results are modifiable with the three-step approach. If your test is abnormal, use the recommendations in Chapter 13 for high estrogen.

IGG ANTIBODY FOOD ALLERGY TESTING

We know that about 60 percent of the population suffers from unsuspected food reactions that can cause or complicate health problems.

Less common but widely recognized immediate food sensitivities, such as the reaction to peanuts or shellfish, are IgE-mediated responses. IgG antibodies are the most common type of immune-related food allergy. They are associated with "delayed" food reactions that can also worsen or contribute to many different health problems. Reactions are more difficult to notice since they can occur hours or even days after consumption of an offending food. Food antibody profiles clearly identify those foods that may be causing health problems. It can help to achieve positive outcomes sooner, especially when combined with the detox diet.

ORGANIC ACIDS TEST

From a single urine specimen, this test can assess the following:
- Fatty acid metabolism
- Neurotransmitter metabolism
- Carbohydrate metabolism
- Oxidative damage
- Energy production
- Detoxification status
- B-complex sufficiency
- Intestinal dysbiosis due to bacteria and yeast
- Methylation cofactors
- Inflammatory reactions

From Doctor's Data, Inc. (www.doctorsdata.com)

COMPREHENSIVE STOOL ANALYSIS

Comprehensive Digestive Stool Analysis uses advanced methods to evaluate digestion, absorption, pancreatic function, and inflammation, in addition to bacterial balance, yeast, and parasitic infection. This profile features exclusive new markers for assessing irritable bowel syndrome, inflammation, colorectal cancer risk, pancreatic insufficiency, and infection. If your results are abnormal, use the recommendations outlined in Chapter 8 on the anti-inflammatory detox, which can improve your symptoms by addressing the five keys to healthy digestion.

URINARY OR FECAL HEAVY METAL ANALYSIS

This test from Doctor's Data looks for the presence of abnormal amounts of metals in the urine or stool, including mercury, lead, cadmium, arsenic, and others. If you have had mercury fillings; flu shots; worked with metals, plastics or ceramics; smoked; or possibly been exposed to contaminated drinking water, invest in this test. Heavy metals influence the function of every cell in the body and greatly increase risks for hormonal imbalance, aging, heart disease, inflammation, and cognitive problems. Search out a qualified integrated medical practitioner to help you with the process of heavy metal detoxification if your results are abnormal. I recommend investigating EDTA suppositories from www.detoxamin.com.

From SpectraCell Laboratories (www.spectracell.com)

VITAMIN AND MINERAL LEVELS IN THE BLOOD CELLS

The FIA (Functional Intracellular Analysis) provides unique insights into the metabolic functions of a variety of vitamins, minerals, antioxidants, and other essential micronutrients, and identifies deficiencies that reflect each person's unique biochemical requirements. SpectraCell's FIA provides you with the next generation of micronutrient analyses based on requirements within your actual cells, rather than just in your bloodstream, for adequate nutritional support for optimal cell function. For example, a more accurate and clinically meaningful determination of folic acid status is gained from measuring its levels within the blood cells, rather than in the serum, which fluctuates daily depending on your intake of foods and nutrients.

The SpectraCell Laboratories report will itemize the supplements you will need to take for at least 6 months to replenish your deficiencies. At that point you should repeat the test.

The Fat-Packing Hormonal Imbalances:
A Review of Diagnostic Tests

Should you wish to request further investigation by your doctor for one or more of the fat-packing hormonal imbalances and their complications, I have summarized the tests and the most common expected results to confirm a diagnosis.

EXCESS INSULIN/INSULIN RESISTANCE

Test	Result Indicating Presence of Insulin Resistance
Fasting glucose and insulin	Abnormally elevated glucose and/or insulin
2-hour PC glucose and insulin	Abnormally elevated fasting glucose and/or insulin
Fasting cholesterol panel (total, HDL, LDL)	Elevated total and LDL; low HDL
Triglycerides (TGs)	Often elevated
Uric acid	Often elevated
Homocysteine	Often elevated (> 7)
Hs-CRP	High (> 0.8)
Free and total testosterone (blood or saliva)	Elevated in women; low in men
SHBG	Often elevated
DHEA-S (blood or saliva)	Elevated in women; low in men
Estradiol (blood, saliva, or urine)	Elevated in men
Ferritin	Often elevated
Vitamin B_{12}	Low (< 600)
RBC magnesium	Often low
Folic acid	Often low (< 1,000)
Liver function tests: AST, ALT, GGT	One or more liver enzymes may be abnormally elevated
Zinc and copper	Copper tends to be high and zinc low in insulin-resistant patients.
25-hydroxyvitamin D_3	Often low
Fasting glucose and insulin	Normal or abnormally elevated fasting glucose and/or insulin (abnormal results are more likely in men with this condition)
HbA1c	Often elevated

EXCESS ESTROGEN/ESTROGEN DOMINANCE
(LOW TESTOSTERONE OR ANDROPAUSE IN MEN)

Test	Result Indicating Presence of Estrogen Dominance/Low Testosterone (Men)
2-hour PC glucose and insulin	Normal or abnormally elevated glucose and/or insulin (abnormal results are more likely in men with this condition)
Hs-CRP	High (> 0.8)
SHBG	Elevated
Estradiol (blood, saliva, or urine)	Elevated
Estrone (blood, saliva, or urine)	Elevated
Estriol (blood, saliva, or urine)	Possibly low
Progesterone (blood, saliva, or urine)	Possibly low
DHEA-S (blood or saliva)	Normal or low
Cortisol (blood or saliva)	Normal or elevated
Testosterone (blood, saliva, or urine)	Women: normal, low with stress, elevated with insulin resistance; Men: low
Specialized testing: urinary estrogen metabolite excretions From Metametrix Labs (the Estronex test)	Elevated levels of harmful estrogen metabolites in the urine
Zinc, copper, magnesium	Zinc low, copper high, magnesium low

EXCESS CORTISOL (STRESS)

Test	Result Indicating Presence of Excess Cortisol (Stress)
Fasting glucose and insulin	Normal or abnormally elevated glucose and/or insulin
2-hour PC glucose and insulin	Normal or abnormally elevated glucose and/or insulin
Estradiol (blood, saliva, or urine)	Normal or elevated
Estrone (blood, saliva, or urine)	Normal or elevated
Estriol (blood, saliva, or urine)	Normal or possibly low
Progesterone (blood, saliva, or urine)	Normal or likely low
DHEA-S (blood or saliva)	Normal or likely low
Cortisol (blood or saliva)	Normal or elevated—or suppressed in very late stages of burnout

Test	Result Indicating Presence of Excess Cortisol (Stress)
Testosterone (blood, saliva, or urine)	Women: normal, low with stress, elevated with insulin resistance; Men: low
Hs-CRP	High (> 0.8)
Specialized testing: salivary cortisol profile—4-point collection of cortisol and DHEA throughout the day	Imbalanced pattern or release; elevated cortisol and suppressed DHEA; low DHEA and cortisol in late stages of burnout

HYPOTHYROIDISM

Test	Result Indicating Presence of Hypothyroidism
Fasting glucose and insulin	Normal or abnormally elevated glucose and/or insulin
2-hour PC glucose and insulin	Normal or abnormally elevated glucose and/or insulin
Thyroid panel (TSH, free T3, free T4)	Elevated TSH (> 2) and low free T3 and free T4. One, two, or all of these abnormalities are common.
Reverse T3	Normal or abnormally elevated (when selenium deficiency or stress is a factor)
Thyroid antibodies	Elevated or normal
Homocysteine	Often elevated (> 7)
Cholesterol panel (total, HDL, LDL)	Total and LDL cholesterol are often elevated. HDL may be normal or low.
Ferritin	Often low (< 70)
Vitamin B_{12}	Often low (< 600)
Folic acid	Often low (< 1,000)
Progesterone (blood, saliva, or urine)	Often low
Estradiol and estrone (blood, saliva, or urine)	May be elevated or normal in women; normal or elevated in men
Cortisol (blood or saliva)	Often high
DHEA-S (blood or saliva)	Often low
Prolactin	Often high
Zinc	Often low
Specialized testing: urinary heavy metal analysis (to rule out mercury toxicity as a cause of thyroid suppression)	Often mercury is elevated

LOW SEROTONIN

Test	Result Indicating Low Serotonin
Fasting glucose and insulin	Normal or abnormally elevated glucose and/or insulin
2-hour PC glucose and insulin	Normal or abnormally elevated glucose and/or insulin
Hs-CRP	Often high (> 0.8)
Cortisol (saliva or blood)	Often high (or low in the late stages of burnout)
DHEA (saliva or blood)	Often low
Free testosterone (blood, saliva, or urine)	Often low
Progesterone (blood, saliva, or urine)	Often low
Estradiol (blood, saliva, or urine)	Normal or low
Specialized testing: urinary neurotransmitter analysis from Neuroscience Laboratories	Deficient serotonin; dopamine and noradrenaline may also be imbalanced.

MENOPAUSE

Test	Result Indicating Menopause
Fasting glucose and insulin	Normal or abnormally elevated glucose and/or insulin
2-hour PC glucose and insulin	Normal or abnormally elevated glucose and/or insulin
Hs-CRP	High (> 0.8), especially if overweight
FSH and LH	Elevated
Estradiol (blood, saliva, or urine)	Low
Estrone (blood, saliva, or urine)	Normal, low, or elevated (if estrogen dominant from excess body weight, alcohol intake, or exposure to environmental xenoestrogens)
Estriol (blood, saliva, or urine)	Low
Progesterone (blood, saliva, or urine)	Low
DHEA-S (blood or saliva)	Often low
Cortisol (blood or saliva)	Normal or elevated—or suppressed in very late stages of burnout
Testosterone (blood or saliva)	Often low or may be elevated if insulin resistant

MENOPAUSE (continued)

Test	Result Indicating Menopause
Fasting cholesterol panel (total, HDL, LDL)	Possible elevated total and LDL; low or normal HDL
Specialized testing: urinary neurotransmitter analysis from Neuroscience Laboratories	Often serotonin is low; dopamine and noradrenaline may also be imbalanced

INFLAMMATION

Test	Result Indicating the Presence of Inflammation
Fasting glucose and insulin	Abnormally elevated glucose and/or insulin
2-hour PC glucose and insulin	Abnormally elevated glucose and/or insulin
Highly sensitive C-RP	High (> 0.8)
Homocysteine	High (> 7)
Vitamin B_{12} and folic acid	Both often low
Cholesterol panel (total, HDL, LDL)	Possibly elevated total and LDL; low or normal HDL
Uric acid	Often elevated
Immunoglobulin panel (blood) for IgE, IgG, and IgM	Normal or abnormal
Ferritin	Can be high (> 110 in women; > 170 in men)
25-hydroxyvitamin D_3	Often low
Red and white blood count: CBC	Normal; WBC may be suppressed if there is an underlying autoimmune component
Liver function tests: AST, ALT, GGT	Normal or elevated
IgG food allergy testing	Elevated results possible for several different foods
Antigliadin antibodies to rule out celiac disease	Normal or positive
ANA, rheumatoid factor (Rh factor), and thyroid antibodies to assess risk of an autoimmune disease	Normal or positive
Estrogen, testosterone, and progesterone	Imbalanced (maybe high or low)
Cortisol and DHEAs	DHEA low, cortisol may be high or low

TACKLING TOXINS IN YOUR SPACE

When we think about pollution, we usually think about smog, acid rain, CFCs, or other forms of outdoor air pollution. But chemical substances in the air inside our homes also affect our health. Considering that we spend 80 to 90 percent of our lives indoors, household air quality and circulation have huge implications for our well-being. Many studies from both the United States and Canada have shown that exposure to pollution is greater in the home than outdoors. Somewhat unexpectedly, though, researchers found exposure was primarily linked to personal-care products and household cleaners rather than to pesticides or weed killers frequently stored in garages.

Toxin exposure from our environment is a major concern. In fact, the Canadian Environmental Protection Act (CEPA) was developed in 1988 to form strategies to limit our exposure to harmful substances. According to CEPA, we have the potential to be exposed to over 23,000 known chemical compounds through consumer products and industrial processes. Although some are considered safe, others present in many common household products can cause harmful side effects, such as breathing difficulties, fatigue, rashes, headaches, hormonal disruption, compromised immunity (irritated mucus membranes in the respiratory tract, which then increase the risk of viral and bacterial infections), and even increased risk of certain types of cancers. One 15-year study found that women who worked at home had a 54 percent higher death rate from cancer than those who worked outside the home. Given that the National Institute of

Occupational Health and Safety found 884 chemicals out of 2,893 analyzed to be toxic, a high incidence of cancer occurrence should not be surprising.

Your Toxin Solution: Detoxify Your Space

Prevention is your best defense. This involves making environmentally conscious choices and assessing your current living space for possible offenders. To start, purchase a HEPA air filter to clean the debris out of the air in your home. Special filters can also be fitted to your furnace to remove allergens from the air. Next, take a detoxifying tour of your home to create simple solutions to diminish your exposure to dangerous chemicals.

1. Bathroom and Kitchen (Cleaning Products and Kitchenware)

You should choose household and laundry cleaning alternatives that are less toxic than standard products. Examples include Kosher Soap, Citra-Solv, borax, That Orange Stuff, and Nature Clean. For your laundry, consider the nontoxic household products by Seventh Generation (www.seventhgeneration.com). (Note: This site also provides a very useful download, "Guide to a Toxin-Free Home." Click on Living Green to gain access to the document.) Also, purchase personal-care products (shampoos, makeup, lotions, etc.) in glass containers as often as possible—they will be less likely to contain phthalates that leach from plastics.

For cooking, avoid aluminum pots and pans because using these materials has been associated with an increased risk of Alzheimer's disease (and the same goes for antiperspirants that contain aluminum). Limiting or eliminating your exposure to Teflon-coated pans may not be such a bad idea either, as the chemical used to make the nonstick substance is currently being studied for potential health risks.

You can purchase reverse osmosis water systems to attach to your tap in the kitchen for drinking water (see the Resource section). It is much cheaper than a unit for the whole house. I also recommend getting a showerhead from the health food store to reduce your exposure to chlorinated hydrocarbons.

2. Living Room, Den, or Family Room (Furniture, Carpeting, and TV)

Unfortunately, much furniture and many TVs emit chemicals of great concern, such as flame retardants (PBDEs) or perfluorinated chemicals (PFOAs). PBDEs build up in breast milk and can increase the risk of neurological problems in children, whereas PFOAs have been found to be carcinogenic in animal studies. Chemically conscious furniture companies include IKEA, Herman Miller, and Steelcase. They make an effort to manufacture products low in chemical emissions and toxins. When purchasing a TV, Samsung Electronics or Sony models may be your best choices.

Depending on the source, carpets can possess a sea of harmful chemical pollutants including PBDEs, PFOAs, polyvinyl chloride (PVC) plastic (phthalates), or pesticides. PVC is toxic to the reproductive system and is linked to asthma, as are many of the chemicals previously mentioned. Again, IKEA has made excellent changes in their manufacturing processes to reduce the risk of chemical exposure. The manufacturers Shaw and Interface have also taken some steps to reduce harmful chemicals in their products.

3. The Office (Computers and Other Electronic Equipment)

Many computers and other electronic equipment release harmful chemicals similar to those present in carpets and furniture. Apparently, electronic cables contain the highest amount of harmful PVC (phthalates). If you are concerned, chose Dell. They report a policy to phase out all restricted chemicals. Hewlett Packard, Apple, and IBM also have public policies to phase out "some" or "most" harmful chemicals.

4. Bedroom (Mattress)

In an effort to reduce the number of deaths or injuries caused by mattress fires ignited by cigarettes, a standard was enacted in 1973 calling for preventative measures. This resulted in flame-retardant chemicals such as boric acid/antimony, decabromodiphenyl oxide, zinc borate, melamine, PBDEs, PVC, and formaldehyde being added to mattresses. Unfortunately, these same flame-retardant chemicals are linked to cancer, SIDS, prenatal mortality, reduced fertility, neuro-logical disorders, and other negative effects. You may wish to look for a chemical-free, wool mattress.

Sealy and Serta apparently are in the process of making changes to their mattresses, though they don't yet completely meet safety stan-dards. If you have already invested in a quality mattress but are unsure of the chemical content, an activated carbon blanket can reduce your exposure to toxic mattress fumes (visit www.nontoxic.com).

Other Steps to Reduce Your Exposure to Toxic Chemicals

- Air out your dry cleaning or, better yet, choose a dry cleaner that uses nontoxic products.
- Sleep on white or organic bedding that is free of dyes that can be absorbed through your skin.
- Golf courses are extremely high in pesticides. Take your shoes off at the door after you've played a round to avoid tracking in pesticides. Keep your golf equipment in the garage, away from your kids and pets.
- Don't smoke, and minimize your exposure to secondhand smoke.
- Reduce or stop using pesticides and herbicides for home, lawn, garden, and pet care wherever possible. Try nontoxic alternatives.
- Avoid polycarbonate plastic baby and sports/water bottles

and other products made of polycarbonate that might come in contact with food. These can leach bisphenol A.

- Make sure that PVC plastic "cling" wraps you put in contact with food do not contain phthalates (ask the manufacturer).
- Never microwave foods in plastic containers that may leach harmful compounds. Store foods in glass containers.
- Keep your home well ventilated when vacuuming, cleaning, painting, or doing arts and crafts to clear out indoor air pollutants that get stirred up during these activities, and air out vapors from glues, paints, resins, and lacquers used in craft and home projects.
- If pregnant, avoid pumping fuel, remodeling your home, painting, and hobbies that involve solvents and glues. Be careful to use nontoxic nail and hair products.
- Avoid the use of synthetic chemical air fresheners, fabric softeners, and fragrances.

You may wish to visit these additional Web sites for more information and sources of ecofriendly products.

- www.naturallifemagazine.com: A source of articles on sustainable living.
- http://cleanproduction.org/Home.php: Click on Safer Products Project for a room-to-room tour of the home to learn about specific products and also how products from various manufacturers rank according to whether or not they are adhering to measures to avoid high-risk, hazardous chemicals in their products.
- www.gaiam.com/category/eco-home-outdoor.do: An array of ecoconscious home and outdoor products for those who wish to enjoy a backyard, kitchen, and furniture without the use of harsh chemicals or unsustainable production methods.

APPENDIX C

THE HORMONE DIET RECIPES

- All the recipes serve one person unless otherwise mentioned. Simply double the recipes should you wish to serve two people.
- Choose organic ingredients whenever possible.
- Even though 100 percent whey protein isolate powder is derived from dairy, it's permitted during the detox step (when dairy is not otherwise allowed). If you suspect you are sensitive to dairy, choose an alternate protein powder such as bean, rice, or soy for your recipes during your detox step. After your detox, try reintroducing whey as a "test" food and note how your body responds.
- ✿☺ When you see these symbols next to a recipe, the recipe is compatible with both Step 1 (the anti-inflammatory detox) and Step 2 (the Glyci-Med approach).
- ✿ When you see this symbol next to a recipe, the recipe is suitable only for the Glyci-Med approach because it contains ingredients that are to be avoided during your detox step.
- You are free to add a mixed green salad to any of the meals.
- Please note that the nutrition information for each meal will vary depending on the brands you choose. Visit www.calorieking.com to check the nutrition content of almost any food.
- A note about chia: Should you choose to use this gluten-free, high-fiber, high-omega-3 grain in your smoothies rather than flaxseeds, it will result in a less "grainy" texture because it mixes more completely than flaxseeds do.

BREAKFAST OPTIONS

☼☺ Pure Energy Smoothie

¼	cup raspberries
¼	cup sliced strawberries
¼	cup blueberries
2	tablespoons chia or ground flaxseeds
¾	cup low-fat plain soy milk
4	ice cubes
1	serving whey protein powder (vanilla)

Place all the ingredients except the protein powder in a blender and blend at high speed until smooth. Then add the protein powder and lightly blend it in to stir it into your drink.

Nutrition Information:

Calories 313 | Carbohydrates 30.5 g | Protein 26.8 g | Fat 9.3 g | Fiber 9 g

☼ ☺ Açaí-Avocado Smoothie

¼	cup peeled and sliced avocado, frozen
1	Sambazon Açaí Smoothie Pack, frozen
1	tablespoon chia or ground flaxseeds
	Water to desired consistency
1	serving whey protein powder (vanilla)

Place all the ingredients except the protein powder in a blender, add the desired amount of water, and blend at high speed until smooth. Then add the protein powder and lightly blend it in to stir it into your drink.

Nutrition Information:

Calories 395 | Carbohydrates 40.5 g | Protein 30 g | Fat 12.5 g | Fiber 6.5 g

TIPS FOR MAKING SUPER SMOOTHIES

- Freeze your fruit—including your bananas and avocados (peel and cut them into pieces prior to freezing) or add ice to your smoothies to make them refreshing.

- Blend the ingredients before adding your protein. Do not overblend the protein. Just lightly blend it to stir it into your drink; otherwise you damage the protein molecules.

- I prefer the use of ground flaxseeds over flaxseed oil. However, the seeds do change the consistency of your smoothie. If you don't like the flaxseeds, you may use 1 tablespoon of flaxseed oil instead. Keep your ground flaxseeds or flaxseed oil in a tightly sealed container in the freezer. If your shake tastes "fishy," it is very likely your flaxseeds or flaxseed oil has gone rancid and will need to be tossed out.

- You may add water or ice to any smoothie to thin it out. Do not add more juice or soy milk since this will increase the calorie content of your drink.

- Add 2 tablespoons of lecithin to any smoothie to boost your memory and muscle-enhancing acetylcholine.

- To increase the fiber content of your smoothies, add 1 to 2 tablespoons of wheat or oat bran.

- Add 4 grams of ı-glutamine powder to any smoothie to enhance growth hormone, tissue healing, and repair.

✿ ☺ Blueberry-Avocado Smoothie

¾   cup blueberries, frozen
¼   cup peeled and sliced avocado, frozen
1   tablespoon chia or ground flaxseeds
    Water to desired consistency
1   serving whey protein powder (vanilla)

Place all the ingredients except the protein powder in a blender, add the desired amount of water, and blend at high speed until smooth. Then add the protein powder and lightly blend it in to stir it into your drink.

Nutrition Information:

Calories 313 | Carbohydrates 25.5 g | Protein 29 g | Fat 10.5 g | Fiber 9.2 g

✿ ☺ Antiaging Smoothie

½   cup raspberries
½   cup blueberries
½   cup sliced strawberries
¼   cup blackberries
1   cup water
2   teaspoons flaxseed oil
1   serving whey protein powder (vanilla)

Place all the ingredients except the protein powder in a blender and blend at high speed until smooth. Then add the protein powder and lightly blend it in to stir it into your drink.

Note: You may also use 1½ cups of a frozen four-berry mixture instead of adding the four berries separately.

Nutrition Information:

Calories 340 | Carbohydrates 30.4 g | Protein 26.9 g | Fat 11.8 g | Fiber 9.3 g

✿ Dopamine Delight Smoothie

½   small banana, peeled and frozen

1   tablespoon chia or 2 teaspoons flaxseed oil

½   teaspoon ground cinnamon

¾   cup soy milk (vanilla or plain)

1   double shot (approx. ¼ cup) espresso (preferably organic)

1   serving whey protein powder (vanilla)

Place all the ingredients except the protein powder in a blender and blend at high speed until smooth. Then add the protein powder and lightly blend it in to stir it into your drink.

Nutrition Information:

Calories 337 | Carbohydrates 26.9 g | Protein 32.7 g | Fat 10.9 g | Fiber 7.9 g

✿ ☺ Super Satisfying Shake

½   small banana, sliced, or ½ cup diced pineapple

¼   cup sliced strawberries

¼   cup sliced mango

1   tablespoon chia or ground flaxseeds

1   cup water

1   teaspoon flaxseed oil

1   serving whey protein powder (vanilla)

Place all the ingredients except the protein powder in a blender and blend at high speed until smooth. Then add the protein powder and lightly blend it in to stir it into your drink.

Nutrition Information:

Calories 355 | Carbohydrates 31.3 g | Protein 27.6 g | Fat 13.2 g | Fiber 6.6 g

☼ ☺ **Serotonin-Surge Smoothie**

¾ small banana, sliced

1 tablespoon almond butter

2 teaspoons chia or flaxseed oil

1 teaspoon cocoa powder

¾ cup low-fat plain soy milk

1 serving whey protein powder (vanilla)

Place all the ingredients except the protein powder in a blender and blend at high speed until smooth. Then add the protein powder and lightly blend it in to stir it into your drink.

Nutrition Information:

Calories 389 | Carbohydrates 34.5 g | Protein 33.8 g | Fat 12.5 g | Fiber 8.0 g

☼ ☺ **Testosterone-Surge Smoothie**

1 cup blueberries

½ banana, peeled and frozen

2 tablespoons ground flaxseeds

1 cup plain low-fat soy milk

1 serving whey protein powder (vanilla)

Place all the ingredients except the protein powder in a blender and blend at high speed until smooth. Then add the protein powder and lightly blend it in to stir it into your drink.

Nutrition Information:

Calories 334 | Carbohydrates 33.0 g | Protein 27.0 g | Fat 10.4 g | Fiber 9.5 g

✿ ☺ Anti-Inflammatory Smoothie

½   cup blueberries
½   cup raspberries
½   small banana, peeled and frozen
¼   cup diced pineapple
2   tablespoons chia or ground flaxseeds
3   ice cubes
½   cup pomegranate juice
1   serving whey protein powder (vanilla)

Place all the ingredients except the protein powder in a blender and blend at high speed until smooth. Then add the protein powder and lightly blend it in to stir it into your drink.

Nutrition Information:
Calories 343 | Carbohydrates 35.7 g | Protein 29.5 g | Fat 9.2 g | Fiber 10.5 g

✿ Awesome Omelette
(Make it a ✿ ☺ meal without the rye toast)
1   tablespoon extra-virgin olive oil
¼   cup diced green bell pepper
¼   cup diced red bell pepper
    A few slices of red onion, chopped
½   cup sliced mushrooms
1   large omega-3 egg
3   large egg whites
2   teaspoons crumbled goat cheese
1   slice rye toast (optional)

1. Heat the olive oil in a small skillet over medium heat. Add the green and red peppers, onion, and mushrooms, and sauté until the vegetables soften.

2. Meanwhile, beat the egg and the egg whites with a wire whisk in a small bowl until blended.
3. When the vegetables are soft, transfer them to another bowl and set aside.
4. Pour the egg mixture into the skillet and cook for several minutes over medium heat until the eggs are set.
5. Spread the vegetables evenly on one side of the cooked egg, top with the goat cheese, and use a spatula to fold the omelette in half over the vegetables. Enjoy with a piece of rye toast—after your detox stage.

Nutrition Information:
Calories 337 | Carbohydrates 31.0 g | Protein 24.0 g | Fat 13.0 g | Fiber 4.6 g

✿ Lovely Leptin Lastin' Satisfaction
½	cup raspberries
¼	cup unsweetened applesauce
½	cup low-fat plain yogurt
½	cup cottage cheese (1% fat)
2	tablespoons chia or ground flaxseeds
3	coarsely chopped walnuts (or 2 cashews)

1. Place the raspberries and applesauce in a blender and blend for a few seconds until smooth.
2. Combine the raspberry and applesauce mixture, yogurt, cottage cheese, and chia or ground flaxseeds in a serving bowl. Top with the chopped nuts and enjoy.

Nutrition Information:
Calories 328 | Carbohydrates 30.9 g | Protein 21.8 g | Fat 13.0 g | Fiber 11.0 g

☼ **Eggscetylcholine Pocket**

½   cup canned black beans, drained and rinsed
¼   cup salsa
1   large omega-3 egg
2   large egg whites
      Salt and pepper to taste
1   teaspoon extra-virgin olive oil
1   ounce shredded Cheddar cheese
½   whole wheat, high-fiber pita

1. Combine the beans and salsa in a bowl.
2. In another bowl, beat the egg, egg whites, salt, and pepper with a wire whisk until blended.
3. Heat the oil in a small skillet over medium heat. Add the egg mixture and cook for a few minutes, until the egg is almost set.
4. Sprinkle the shredded cheese over the top and stir in the bean mixture. Cook for another minute, until the cheese is melted.
5. Place the mixture in the pita pocket. Enjoy!

Nutrition Information:
Calories 387 | Carbohydrates 39.0 g | Protein 29.1 g | Fat 12.7 g | Fiber 10.0 g

✿ ☺ Balsamic Vinegar and Olive Oil Dressing

Serves 4

1–2	tablespoons balsamic vinegar (or apple cider vinegar)
¼	cup extra-virgin olive oil
½–1	teaspoon mustard powder
	Maple syrup or honey to taste
	Sea salt and pepper to taste

Combine the vinegar, olive oil, and mustard powder in a glass jar. Add the maple syrup or honey to your desired sweetness—keep in mind that less is more! Add sea salt and pepper to taste. Cover the jar and shake well to mix. This homemade dressing is good to have on hand and will keep in the fridge.

✿ ☺ Greek Salad Topped with Grilled Chicken Breast

3	cups mixed greens
½	green bell pepper, diced
½	red bell pepper, diced
½	cup halved or quartered cherry tomatoes
¼	cup sliced red onion
1	teaspoon fresh chopped dill
½	teaspoon fresh or ⅛ teaspoon dried basil
3	pitted black olives
1	cup peeled and sliced cucumber
4	ounces grilled boneless, skinless chicken breast, thinly sliced on the diagonal
1	ounce feta cheese, crumbled
2	teaspoons Balsamic Vinegar and Olive Oil Dressing (see above)

(continued)

Mix the greens, green pepper, red pepper, tomatoes, onion, dill, basil, olives, and cucumbers in a large bowl. Top with the grilled chicken slices, feta cheese, and salad dressing.

Nutrition Information:
Calories 420 | Carbohydrates 43.7 g | Protein 30.0 g | Fat 14.0 g | Fiber 7.0 g

✿ ☺ Curried Tuna-Chia Salad

1	can (4 ounces) light tuna in water (about ½ cup drained)
1	tablespoon low-fat mayonnaise (canola oil –based)
¼	teaspoon curry powder
½	tomato, chopped
½	cup peeled and chopped cucumber
½	cup diced green bell pepper
½	cup diced red bell pepper
¼	cup chopped onion
1	dill pickle, chopped
1–2	tablespoons Balsamic Vinegar and Olive Oil Dressing (see page 415)
1	tablespoon chia

1. Place the tuna in a small bowl and flake it with a fork. Add the mayonnaise and curry powder to the tuna, combine them well, and then set aside.
2. In a medium-size bowl, combine the tomato, cucumber, green and red peppers, onion, and pickle. Toss with the dressing.
3. Serve on a plate with a scoop of the tuna mixture on top, sprinkle with the chia, and enjoy!

Nutrition Information:
Calories 336 | Carbohydrates 29.0 g | Protein 29.0 g | Fat 11.5 g | Fiber 8.0 g

✿ ☺ Antioxidant Chicken Salad

- 3 cups baby spinach
- 4 ounces grilled boneless, skinless chicken breast, thinly sliced on the diagonal
- 2 or 3 thin slices red onion
- ½ cup raspberries or blueberries
- 1 cup strawberry halves
- 1 tablespoon Balsamic Vinegar and Olive Oil Dressing (see page 415)
- ⅛ avocado, peeled and sliced

Combine the spinach, chicken, onion, raspberries or blueberries, and strawberries in a salad bowl. Top with the dressing and avocado.

Nutrition Information:

Calories 335 | Carbohydrates 20.0 g | Protein 32.0 g | Fat 14.0 g | Fiber 8.0 g

✿ ☺ Goat Cheese, Green Pea, and Spinach Frittata

- 1 large omega-3 egg
- 3 large egg whites
- 1 ounce goat cheese
- 1 tablespoon chopped onion
  Sea salt and pepper to taste
- ½ cup frozen green peas
- 1¼ cups frozen spinach
- 1–2 teaspoons extra-virgin olive oil
- 1 slice whole grain toast (optional in the Glyci-Med stage)

1. Preheat the oven to 350°F.
2. Beat the egg and egg whites in a medium-size bowl with a wire whisk until blended. Mix in the cheese, onion, salt, pepper, peas, and spinach.

(continued)

3. Spread the olive oil in a small ovenproof skillet and add the egg mixture.
4. Bake for 15 to 20 minutes, or until the frittata is fully set. Enjoy with a slice of whole grain toast—if you are not on your detox.

Nutrition Information:
Calories 403 | Carbohydrates 39.0 g | Protein 29.0 g | Fat 14.5 g | Fiber 9.0 g

✿ ☺ California Avocado and Chicken Salad
Serves 4

	Sea salt and pepper to taste
2	large boneless, skinless chicken breasts
1	tablespoon peeled and crushed fresh ginger
2	teaspoons extra-virgin olive oil
4	tablespoons freshly squeezed lime juice
3	tablespoons fresh chopped cilantro
5	cups fresh greens (any kind except iceberg lettuce)
1	avocado, peeled and sliced
2	peaches, peeled and sliced
2	tablespoons chopped red onion

1. Preheat the oven to 350°F.
2. Sprinkle salt and pepper on the chicken and bake until cooked through but still moist (30 to 40 minutes). Remove from the oven and, when cool enough to handle, cut into bite-size chunks, and set aside. (The chicken can be cooked a day in advance.)
3. Combine the ginger, olive oil, lime juice, cilantro, and salt and pepper to taste in a salad bowl and mix well. Add the greens and toss with the dressing.
4. Divide the greens among four plates and arrange the avocado, peaches, and chicken on each plate. Sprinkle with the onion and serve.

Nutrition Information (per serving):
Calories 410 | Carbohydrates 42.0 g | Protein 31.0 g | Fat 13.1 g | Fiber 6.0 g

✿ Sweet Potato, Squash, and Ginger Soup

(Remove the cheese to make it a ✿ ☺ meal)

Serves 4 or 5

1	large sweet potato, peeled and cubed
1	small butternut squash, peeled and cubed
2	carrots, peeled and thinly sliced
	1-inch piece fresh ginger, peeled and sliced
1–2	teaspoons curry powder (optional)
6	cups vegetable stock
1	pear, cored, peeled, and sliced
1	apple, cored, peeled, and sliced
2	large onions, chopped
2	tablespoons extra-virgin olive oil
3	tablespoons apple juice or white wine
1	teaspoon sea salt
	Black pepper to taste
1¼–2½	cups organic pressed cottage cheese

1. Place the sweet potato, squash, carrots, ginger, and, if desired, curry powder in a large saucepan. Add the vegetable stock. Cover, bring to a gentle boil, and then reduce the heat and simmer for about 30 minutes or until all the vegetables are soft.
2. Place the pear, apple, onions, olive oil, and apple juice or wine in a separate saucepan and cook over medium heat until soft (5 to 10 minutes).
3. Add the cooked pear and apple mixture and the salt and pepper to the saucepan with the vegetables, and mix well. Once all the ingredients are thoroughly cooked, purée in a food processor or with a hand blender.
4. Serve topped with ¼ cup (for women) or ½ cup (for men) of the cottage cheese.

Nutrition Information (per serving):

Calories 360 | Carbohydrates 49.0 g | *Protein 24.0 g (*if the cheese is added) | Fat 8.0 g | Fiber 6.0 g

✿ ☺ **Lovely Lentil Soup**

Serves 4

2	tablespoons extra-virgin olive oil
1	sweet potato, peeled and diced
1	large onion, chopped
4	cloves garlic, minced
	1-inch piece fresh ginger, peeled and minced
1	tablespoon curry powder
1	teaspoon cinnamon
1	teaspoon sea salt
1	cup dry red lentils
4	cups vegetable stock
2	tablespoons tomato paste

1. Heat the olive oil in a large saucepan over medium heat. Add the sweet potato, onion, garlic, and ginger, and cook until the vegetables are softened.
2. Stir in the curry powder, cinnamon, and sea salt, and cook for a few more minutes.
3. Add the lentils, vegetable stock, and tomato paste, and mix well. Bring to a gentle boil, reduce the heat, and then simmer covered for 30 minutes or until the lentils are cooked. Remove from the heat and serve.

Nutrition Information (per serving):
Calories 325 | Carbohydrates 44.5 g | Protein 16.0 g | Fat 9.0 g | Fiber 7.5 g

✿ Zippy Three-Bean Salad

(Skip the cheese to make it a ✿ ☺ meal)

⅓ cup canned kidney beans, drained and rinsed

⅓ cup canned black beans, drained and rinsed

¼ cup canned chickpeas, drained and rinsed

1 small red bell pepper, chopped

2 ounces low-fat Cheddar or Colby cheese

   A few slices red onion, chopped

2 cloves garlic, minced

½ teaspoon dried coriander

   Pinch of cayenne pepper, or to taste

   Pinch of ground cumin

2 tablespoons freshly squeezed lemon juice

1 tablespoon extra-virgin olive oil

1 teaspoon apple cider vinegar

   Salt and pepper to taste

Combine all the ingredients in a bowl and enjoy.

Variation: For a bean dip, purée all the ingredients and enjoy with raw vegetables such as sliced bell peppers and carrot and celery sticks.

Nutrition Information:

Calories 395 | Carbohydrates 45.2 g | Protein 26.0 g | Fat 12.0 g | Fiber 9.5 g

✿ Warm Black Bean and Turkey Salad

(Remove the cheese to make it a ✿ ☺ meal)

1	teaspoon extra-virgin olive oil
½	cup diced green bell pepper
½	cup diced red bell pepper
¼	cup chopped onion
1–2	cloves garlic, minced
½–1	teaspoon dried basil
½–1	teaspoon dried dillweed
¼–½	teaspoon dried oregano
	Pinch cayenne pepper, or to taste
3	ounces lean ground turkey
¼	cup salsa
¼	cup canned black beans, drained and rinsed
	Sea salt and pepper to taste
1	teaspoon hot pepper sauce such as Tabasco (optional)
3	cups mixed greens
1	ounce Cheddar cheese, grated

1. Heat the olive oil over medium-high heat in a skillet and add all the veggies, herbs, and spices. Sauté until the peppers and onions are soft.
2. Add the ground turkey and cook until it browns. Drain thoroughly.
3. Add the salsa and black beans and continue cooking until they are warmed through.
4. Add salt and pepper and, if desired, the hot sauce, and mix well.
5. Serve over the mixed greens and top with the cheese.

Nutrition Information:

Calories 383 | Carbohydrates 37.7 g | Protein 29.6 g | Fat 12.6 g | Fiber 8.0 g

✿ India-Style Chicken Pita Pocket with Side Salad

Pita Pocket:

4	ounces grilled boneless, skinless chicken breast, cubed
1	medium stalk celery, chopped
2	cashews, chopped
1	tablespoon low-fat plain yogurt
1	teaspoon Dijon mustard
¼–½	teaspoon curry powder
1	high-fiber whole wheat pita

Side Salad:

2	cups mixed greens
½	cup sliced, peeled cucumber
3 or 4	halved or quartered cherry tomatoes
1	tablespoon Balsamic Vinegar and Olive Oil Dressing (see page 415)

1. Combine the chicken, celery, cashews, yogurt, mustard, and curry powder in a bowl.
2. Cut the pita in half, and spoon the mixture into the pita pocket.
3. Toss the salad ingredients together and serve with the chicken pita pocket. (You may enjoy any type of green salad with this dish).

Nutrition Information:

Calories 409 | Carbohydrates 38.0 g | Protein 29.0 g | Fat 14.0 g | Fiber 9.0 g

✿ Zesty Chicken Salad

(Skip the cheese to make it a ✿ ☺ meal)

1½	teaspoons freshly squeezed lime juice
1½	teaspoons apple juice
1½	teaspoons sesame oil
1½	teaspoons tamari soy sauce
2	cups raw spinach
4	ounces grilled boneless, skinless chicken breast, thinly sliced on the diagonal
1	ounce low-fat Swiss cheese, grated
1	medium apple, cored, peeled, and sliced
1	tablespoon finely chopped green onion

1. To make the dressing, combine the lime juice, apple juice, sesame oil, and soy sauce in a small bowl and whisk until well blended.
2. Place the spinach leaves on a plate and add the chicken, cheese, and apple. Sprinkle the green onion on top, toss with the dressing, and serve.

Nutrition Information:

Calories 380 | Carbohydrates 38.6 g | Protein 29.7 g | Fat 12.8 g | Fiber 6.0 g

✿ **Easy Caesar Salad**

2   cups torn romaine lettuce

4   ounces grilled boneless, skinless chicken breast

1   slice whole grain toast cut into even cubes (for croutons)

2   tablespoons prepared Caesar salad dressing (canola- or
     olive oil–based)

1   tablespoon grated Parmesan cheese

Assemble the lettuce, chicken, and croutons on a plate. Toss with the
dressing, top with the cheese, and enjoy.

Nutrition Information:

Calories 392 | Carbohydrates 34.0 g | Protein 29.0 g | Fat 15.6 g | Fiber 7.0 g

DINNER OPTIONS

✿ ☺ **Mediterranean Tilapia**

4½   ounce tilapia fillet

1½   teaspoons extra-virgin olive oil

½   tomato, sliced

4   pitted black olives, sliced

1. Preheat the oven to 375°F.
2. Place the tilapia fillet in a small, shallow baking dish and brush with
   the olive oil.
3. Top the fillet with the sliced tomato and olives and bake in the oven
   until the fish flakes easily with a fork and is opaque, 10 to 20 minutes.
4. Serve with a side salad tossed with Balsamic Vinegar and Olive Oil
   Dressing (see page 415) and a baked sweet potato or steamed brown
   basmati rice.

Nutrition Information:

Calories 400 | Carbohydrates 45.8 g | Protein 29.9 g | Fat 13.5 g | Fiber 6.0 g

✿ ☺ Veggie Chili

Serves 4

2	teaspoons extra-virgin olive oil
1	large onion, chopped
1	green bell pepper, chopped
4	ounces mushrooms, sliced
½	package (or 6 to 8 ounces) extra-firm tofu, cubed
1	can (28 ounces) crushed tomatoes, pureed
1	can (15 ounces) red kidney beans, drained and rinsed
3 or 4	cloves of fresh garlic, chopped
2	tablespoons chili powder
1	teaspoon dried basil
1	teaspoon dried oregano
1	teaspoon nutmeg
½	teaspoon crushed chiles, or to taste
1	tablespoon blackstrap molasses
1	tablespoon apple cider vinegar

1. Heat the olive oil over medium heat in a large, heavy saucepan, and sauté the onion, green pepper, mushrooms, and tofu until the vegetables are soft.
2. Add all the remaining ingredients and cook until heated through (10 to 20 minutes) and serve.

Variation: For a nonveggie version, substitute cooked cubed turkey breast for the tofu.

This makes a lot of chili! You can freeze it in individual portions or it will keep in the fridge for up to 5 days.

Nutrition Information (per serving):
Calories 401 | Carbohydrates 43.0 g | Protein 28.0 g | Fat 13.0 g | Fiber 9.0 g

✿ ☺ Anti-Inflammatory Curry

1–3	cloves of garlic, minced
½	cup chopped broccoli
½	cup snow peas
1	green onion, sliced
	Sea salt and pepper to taste
1	red bell pepper, sliced
1½	teaspoons curry powder
2	tablespoons chopped cashews
½	teaspoon peeled and minced fresh ginger
1	small jalapeño pepper, minced
1	teaspoon extra-virgin olive oil
4	ounces boneless, skinless chicken breast, cut into bite-size pieces
¼–½	cup vegetable stock, if necessary for moisture
½	cup cooked brown basmati rice

1. Combine the garlic, broccoli, snow peas, green onion, salt and pepper, bell pepper, curry powder, cashews, ginger, and jalapeño in a bowl. Mix well and let marinate for 10 to 30 minutes.
2. Heat the olive oil in a small skillet over medium heat. Add the chicken and sauté until lightly browned.
3. Combine the vegetables and chicken in a large, heavy saucepan. Simmer covered for 10 minutes or until the chicken is fully cooked, adding the vegetable stock if necessary. Serve over the rice.

Variation: As an alternative to rice, you may have this with one small peeled and cubed sweet potato cooked with the curry.

Nutrition Information:
Calories 465 | Carbohydrates 56.0 g | Protein 29.0 g | Fat 14.0 g | Fiber 5.5 g

☼ ☺ Sweet Garlic Chicken Stir-Fry

2	teaspoons extra-virgin olive oil
1	small zucchini, sliced
1	cup diced red bell pepper
½	cup diced yellow bell pepper
½	cup fresh pineapple, diced
2	cloves garlic, minced
¼	cup vegetable stock, if necessary for moisture
4	ounces boneless, skinless chicken breast, sliced
2	cups spinach
¼	cup cooked brown basmati rice

1. Heat the olive oil over medium heat in a large skillet or wok. Add the zucchini, red and yellow bell peppers, pineapple, and garlic. Cook until the vegetables are tender, adding the vegetable stock if necessary.
2. Stir in the chicken and cook for a few minutes.
3. Add the spinach and cook until it is wilted and the chicken is cooked through. Serve over the rice.

Nutrition Information:

Calories 402 | Carbohydrates 43.0 g | Protein 29.0 g | Fat 12.7 g | Fiber 8.0 g

☼ ☺ Grilled Halibut with Rice and Broccoli

Sauce for the Rice and Broccoli:

- ¼   cup sliced cherry tomatoes
- 1   tablespoon chopped fresh basil
- ½   green onion, thinly sliced
- 1½   teaspoons extra-virgin olive oil
       Salt and pepper to taste

Fish:

- 1   teaspoon fennel seeds
- ½   tablespoon freshly squeezed lemon juice
- 1½   teaspoons extra-virgin olive oil
       Sea salt and pepper to taste
- 4   ounce halibut fillet
- ½   cup cooked brown basmati rice
- 1   cup broccoli, steamed

Note: Be sure to prepare your brown rice and steamed broccoli so that they are done when the fish is ready.

1. To make the sauce, heat the tomatoes, basil, green onion, and olive oil in a saucepan over medium-high heat until the vegetables are soft. Set aside.
2. To make the fish, prepare the grill and place a rack 4 inches above the coals.
3. Toast the fennel seeds in a small skillet over medium heat until fragrant.
4. Combine the lemon juice, toasted fennel seeds, olive oil, salt, and pepper in small bowl.
5. Put the fish in a glass dish and brush the mixture over both sides to coat it evenly. Let it marinate for 15 minutes at room temperature.
6. Place the fish on the hot grill and cook until done through (10 to 15 minutes).

(continued)

7. Meanwhile, reheat the sauce. Serve the fish with the sauce spooned over the rice and broccoli.

Nutrition Information:
Calories 393 | Carbohydrates 38.8 g | Protein 30.7 g | Fat 12.8 g | Fiber 5.0 g

☼ ☺ **Super Salmon Salad**

4–6	spears of asparagus, steamed and sliced
1	can (4 ounces) wild salmon
¼	cup chopped or sliced tomato
2	tablespoons chopped green onion
1 or 2	cloves garlic, minced
1	tablespoon tamari soy sauce
1	teaspoon extra-virgin olive oil
3	cups mixed greens

Mix the asparagus and salmon together. Add the tomato, green onion, garlic, soy sauce, and olive oil to the salmon mixture. Chill and serve over the mixed greens.

Nutrition Information:
Calories 319 | Carbohydrates 26.0 g | Protein 29.0 g | Fat 11.0 g | Fiber 13.0 g

☼ ☺ Baby Spinach with Grilled Ginger Scallops

Serves 2

1	tablespoon minced sweet onion
2	tablespoons freshly squeezed lime juice
½	cup fresh grapefruit juice
1	tablespoon peeled and grated fresh ginger
3	tablespoons tamari soy sauce
1	tablespoon honey
½	teaspoon Dijon mustard
	Sea salt to taste
1	tablespoon extra-virgin olive oil, divided
8	large sea scallops
1	pound organic baby spinach leaves

1. Put the onion, lime juice, and grapefruit juice in a small skillet, bring to a boil over medium heat, and cook for 1 to 2 minutes.
2. Combine the ginger, soy sauce, honey, and mustard in a small bowl, add to the skillet, and warm through. Remove from the heat and mix in the sea salt and 1½ teaspoons of the olive oil.
3. Heat the remaining 1½ teaspoons of the olive oil in a large skillet. When it's hot, place the scallops in the skillet and sear them by cooking for 30 seconds to 1 minute on each side. Add the sauce and simmer over low heat for 1 to 2 minutes.
4. Meanwhile, pile the spinach leaves on 2 plates. Immediately serve the scallops on top of the spinach, divided between the plates.

Nutrition Information (per serving):

Calories 337 | Carbohydrates 30.0 g | Protein 25.3 g | Fat 10.4 g | Fiber 4.0 g

✿ Carb Craving Shepherd's Pie

Serves 2 (Leave out the spelt flour to make it a ✿ ☺ meal)

2	medium sweet potatoes
1	teaspoon butter
1	tablespoon extra-virgin olive oil
10	ounces lean ground turkey
3	cloves garlic
1	onion, chopped
1	teaspoon sea salt
	Black pepper to taste
¼	teaspoon thyme
1	tablespoon spelt flour (optional)
1	cup vegetable stock
1	teaspoon Worcestershire sauce
1	cup frozen peas and carrots

1. Bake the sweet potatoes, remove the skins, and mash the flesh with the butter (you should have about ½ cup of mashed potato). Set aside.
2. Preheat the oven to 400°F.
3. Heat the olive oil in a skillet. Add the turkey, garlic, and onion and cook until the turkey is lightly browned.
4. Add the salt, pepper, thyme, and, if using, the flour, and mix well.
5. Stir in the vegetable stock and cook until thickened.
6. Stir in the Worcestershire sauce and the peas and carrots, and cover and simmer for 20 minutes.
7. Transfer the turkey mixture to a baking dish and spread the reserved mashed sweet potatoes on top.
8. Put the shepherd's pie in the oven, bake for 15 minutes, and serve.

Nutrition Information (per serving):
Calories 413 | Carbohydrates 43.0 g | Protein 31.0 g | Fat 13.0 g | Fiber 6.0 g

✿ Beef Fajita with Side Salad

Side Salad:

2	cups torn romaine lettuce leaves or mixed greens
½	peach, peeled and sliced
2–3	thin slivers red onion
1	tablespoon Balsamic Vinegar and Olive Oil Dressing (see page 415)

Fajitas:

1½	teaspoons freshly squeezed lemon juice
1–2	teaspoons chili powder
1–2	cloves garlic, minced
¼	teaspoon dried red pepper flakes
¼	teaspoon ground cumin
¼	teaspoon paprika
	Sea salt and pepper to taste
1	teaspoon extra-virgin olive oil
4	ounces lean eye of round beef, cut into thin strips
½	cup sliced green bell pepper
½	cup sliced red bell pepper
¼	medium onion, chopped
½	tomato, chopped
¼	cup salsa
1	medium whole wheat tortilla wrap

1. Prepare the side salad by combining the greens, peach, and onion. Toss with the dressing just before serving.
2. Combine the lemon juice, chili powder, garlic, red pepper flakes, cumin, paprika, salt, and pepper in a bowl and set aside.
3. Coat a skillet with the olive oil and place over medium-high heat. Add the beef and stir-fry until browned.
4. Add the green and red peppers and the onion, and stir-fry until the vegetables are cooked to the desired tenderness and beef is cooked through.

(continued)

5. Mix in the tomato and salsa and stir until heated through.
6. Spoon the mixture onto the tortilla and roll it up. Serve with the side salad.

Variation: Substitute the beef with chicken for a chicken fajita.

Nutrition Information:

Calories 383 | Carbohydrates 39.5 g | Protein 29.7 g | Fat 11.8 g | Fiber 6.0 g

✿ Quick-and-Easy Pasta with Tomato Sauce

Serves 2

	Whole wheat or kamut pasta
1	tablespoon extra-virgin olive oil
½	pound ground turkey
1	onion, chopped
1	bottle (25 ounces) organic sugar-free tomato pasta sauce made with olive oil
2	cups broccoli, steamed and pureed
1	clove garlic, minced
1	teaspoon dried oregano
1	teaspoon dried parsley

1. Prepare the pasta according to the package instructions, making each serving the size of your fist (approximately ½ cup). Cook until it is soft but still firm. (Overcooking pasta raises its glycemic index.)
2. Heat the olive oil in a saucepan and sauté the turkey and onion until the turkey is cooked.
3. Add the tomato sauce, broccoli, garlic, oregano, and parsley and simmer until heated through.
4. Serve the pasta topped with the sauce.

Variation: For a vegetarian option, substitute 1½ cups of pressed cottage cheese for the turkey. Place the cottage cheese on top of the cooked pasta, pour the hot tomato sauce over the cheese, and stir it up. The cheese will melt and you'll have a tasty high-protein, high-fiber meal. Note: Do not use this as your protein source during your detox Day 14 when you will be testing wheat.

Nutrition Information (per serving):
Calories 400 | Carbohydrates 44.0 g | Protein 29.0 g | Fat 13.0 g | Fiber 8.0 g

SNACK OPTIONS

✿ The Simply Bar
A gluten-free, dairy-free, wheat-free, easily digested, high-protein bar that's perfect as a midday snack. It is available in some health food stores or you can visit www.wellnessfoods.ca or www.thehormonediet. com. Choose peanut butter, ginger-flax, or cocoa-coffee flavors—they're the lowest on the glycemic index according to Cathy Richards, creator of the bar.

✿ ☺ Elevate Me! Bar
All-natural, gluten- and wheat-free protein and whole-fruit energy bar. It contains 16 grams of protein and 35 grams of carbs, making it a good choice for a postworkout snack. For women, half a bar would be a snack; men can eat the whole bar. Choose from the flavors that are lowest in carbs: Cocoa Coconut Cluster, All Fruit Original, Banana Nut Bread, or Matcha Green Tea with Cranberries. Visit www.prosnack.com.

✿ ☺ **Black Bean Dip or Burrito Filling**

Serves 4 or 5

1	can (15 ounces) of black beans, drained and rinsed
1	medium onion, chopped
2	cloves garlic, minced
2	teaspoons cumin
1	teaspoon coriander (optional)
½	teaspoon cayenne pepper
½	teaspoon sea salt
2	tablespoons extra-virgin olive oil

Blend all the ingredients in a food processor. Eat as a dip or as a filling for a burrito. You may top the burrito with salsa, 1 tablespoon of guacamole, or 1 ounce of grated low-fat cheese. Store dip in the fridge in a sealed container.

Nutrition Information (per serving):
Calories 208 | Carbohydrates 25.0 g | Protein 15.7 g | Fat 5.0 g | Fiber 4.1 g

✿ ☺ **Curried Chickpea Dip**

Serves 4 or 5

1	can (15 ounces) organic chickpeas, drained and rinsed
¼	cup extra-virgin olive oil
2	tablespoons freshly squeezed lemon juice
½	teaspoon curry powder
½	teaspoon garam masala spice
2 or 3	cloves garlic, peeled
½	teaspoon sea salt
	Black pepper to taste
1	teaspoon cayenne (optional)
½	cup freshly chopped cilantro

1. Purée the chickpeas, olive oil, lemon juice, curry powder, garam masala, garlic, salt, pepper, and, if using, cayenne in a food processor until smooth.
2. Add the cilantro and pulse a few times to combine.
3. Transfer the dip to a bowl. Eat ½ cup as a veggie dip or spread. Store dip in the fridge in a sealed container.

Nutrition Information (per serving):
Calories 245 | Carbohydrates 25.2 g | Protein 24.0 g | Fat 5.4 g | Fiber 4.1 g

✿ ☺ Quick Trail Mix
Quick Trail Mix

  3   tablespoons dry-roasted soy nuts
  1   tablespoon dried unsulfured cranberries or cherries

Mix the ingredients together and enjoy!

Nutrition Information:
Calories 203 | Carbohydrates 22.3 g | Protein 13.0 g | Fat 6.9 g | Fiber 3.1 g

✿ ☺ Hummus and Veggies
Serves 4

Hummus and Veggies

      Unlimited sliced red, yellow, and green bell peppers; celery sticks; broccoli; carrot sticks; etc.
  1   can (15 ounces) organic chickpeas, drained and rinsed
  2   tablespoons chia
  1   tablespoon plus 1½ teaspoons extra-virgin olive oil
1–3   teaspoons tahini
      Sea salt and pepper to taste

(continued)

1. Slice and cut the vegetables for dipping.
2. Place the chickpeas, chia, and olive oil in a food processor and blend until smooth.
3. Add the tahini and enough water to achieve the desired thickness.
4. Add the salt and pepper to taste and pulse to blend thoroughly.

Variations: Hummus is a very versatile dish; you can add curry, spinach, garlic, roasted red bell peppers, and many other ingredients for different variations on this fantastic snack choice.

Nutrition Information (per serving):
Calories 205 | Carbohydrates 24.0 g | Protein 16.0 g | Fat 6.0 g | Fiber 8.6 g

✿ Almond Butter Protein Bars

Makes 5 bars

2	cups oatmeal
½	cup sliced almonds
¼	cup ground flaxseeds
2	tablespoons lecithin
5	scoops whey protein powder (vanilla)
¼	cup almond butter
¼–½	cup water

1. Combine the oatmeal, almonds, flaxseeds, lecithin, and protein powder in a large bowl.
2. In a separate bowl, mix together the almond butter and water until blended.
3. Combine the almond butter mixture with the dry ingredients and mix well.
4. Place plastic wrap in the bottom of an 8-inch square pan, making sure there is enough to wrap over the top.
5. Place the mixture in the pan and press flat with the overhanging plastic wrap.

6. Put the pan in the freezer for 1 hour and then store in the refrigerator before slicing into 5 bars.

Nutrition Information (per serving):
Calories 225 | Carbohydrates 13.3 g | Protein 17.0 g | Fat 6.0 g | Fiber 5.0 g

✿ Berry-Apple Ricotta Cheese

½	cup low-fat ricotta cheese
½	cup strawberry halves
½	apple, sliced
1	tablespoon ground flaxseeds or chia

Mix together the ricotta cheese, strawberries, apple and ground flaxseeds or chia in a bowl. Eat and enjoy!

Nutrition Information:
Calories 219 | Carbohydrates 22.0 g | Protein 18.0 g | Fat 6.5 g | Fiber 5.2 g

✿ Simple Apple Snack
(Remove the cheese and use more nuts to make it a ✿ ☺ snack)

1	apple (organic)
1	ounce (or 1 slice) low-fat Swiss cheese
10	raw almonds

Enjoy!
You can change this snack by choosing 5 walnuts, 7 cashews, 8 pecans, or 1 tablespoon of sunflower seeds. You can also increase the amount of nuts you eat and eliminate the cheese (i.e., 12 almonds, 9 cashews, 11 pecans, 8 walnuts).

Nutrition Information:
Calories 165 | Carbohydrates 11.9 g | Protein 9.0 g | Fat 9.0 g | Fiber 4.5 g

✿ Berry-Pecan Mix

½	cup cottage cheese or ricotta cheese (1% fat)
½	cup sliced strawberries
¼	cup blueberries
2	ounces low-fat plain yogurt
1	tablespoon chia (or wheat bran—a fat-free option)
1	tablespoon chopped pecans

Place the ricotta, strawberries, blueberries, yogurt, and chia in a blender and blend until smooth. Top with the chopped nuts.

Nutrition Information:
Calories 252 | Carbohydrates 23.4 g | Protein 17.1 g | Fat 10.0 g | Fiber 4.8 g

✿ Healthy Nacho Snack

12	blue corn tortilla chips
½	cup shredded low-fat Cheddar or Colby cheese
¼	cup canned black beans, drained and rinsed
¼	cup salsa
½	tablespoon guacamole

Place the tortilla chips on a plate. Top with the shredded cheese and the beans. Bake or broil for a few minutes, until the cheese is melted. Use the salsa and guacamole as dips.

Nutrition Information:
Calories 202 | Carbohydrates 22.6 g | Protein 12.6 g | Fat 6.8 g | Fiber 4.1 g

A Healthy Tasty Treat

☼ Erin's Healthy Muffins
Makes 24 medium-size muffins

Dry ingredients:

1½	cups organic slow-cooking oats
1½	cups fresh or frozen blueberries
1	cup freshly ground flaxseeds
1	cup whole grain spelt flour
1	cup grated carrots
½	cup crushed walnuts (or almonds or pumpkin seeds)
3	tablespoons dried cranberries or chopped dried organic apricots
4	teaspoons aluminum-free baking powder
1	teaspoon ground cinnamon

Wet ingredients:

1	cup organic soy milk
½	cup unsweetened crushed pineapple
2	omega-3 eggs
3	large egg whites
4	tablespoons blackstrap molasses
3	tablespoons extra-virgin olive oil
1	teaspoon vanilla extract

1. Preheat the oven to 350°F.
2. Butter two muffin pans (for 24 muffins).
3. Combine the dry ingredients in a large bowl.
4. Combine the wet ingredients in a small bowl by hand or with an electric mixer.

(continued)

5. Combine the wet and dry ingredients and mix well.
6. Spoon the batter into the greased muffin pans, filling each cup about two-thirds full.
7. Place in the oven and bake for about 25 minutes.

Nutrition Information:
Don't worry about it. Enjoy your treat—you've earned it!

Your Detox Shopping List

Type of Food	Suggestions
Grain products	Brown rice, basmati rice, rice pasta, rice crackers
	Millet, quinoa, buckwheat or other gluten-free options
Condiments	Tamari (wheat-free soy sauce)
	Almond butter
	Honey (for your salad dressing only)
	Maple syrup (for your salad dressing only)
	Extra-virgin olive oil
	Apple cider vinegar
	Balsamic vinegar
	Hummus—any flavor (just watch for unhealthy oils!) or make your own
	Salsa (ensure no sugar added)
	Cocoa powder (preferably organic)
	Vegetable stock (preferably organic)
	Low-fat mayonnaise
	Tomato paste
	Blackstrap molasses
	Black olives
	Dijon mustard
	Worcestershire sauce
	Organic canola oil
	Sesame oil

Type of Food	Suggestions
Spices	Cinnamon
	Ginger (whole root)
	Ground mustard powder
	Chili powder
	Cumin
	Fresh garlic
	Sea salt
	Fresh ground pepper
	Curry powder
	Basil
	Oregano
	Nutmeg
	Crushed chiles
	Thyme
	Ground turmeric
	Ground coriander
	Anise
	Cayenne pepper
	Dill
Drinks, Milks, and Special Cheeses	Organic unsweetened soy milk (Soy Nice)
	Herbal teas, green tea
	Carbonated water/sodium-free soda water
	Purified water/reverse osmosis water
	Pure fruit juices (not from concentrate, nothing added)
	Goat cheese
	Sheep or goat feta cheese

Type of Food	Suggestions
Vegetables (The detox recipes call for these vegetables— though you can certainly include any vegetable except corn)	Frozen peas and spinach
	Canned tomatoes (large size, preferably organic)
	Sweet potatoes
	Broccoli
	Cauliflower
	Zucchini
	Tomatoes
	Asparagus
	Cucumber
	Baby spinach
	Baby carrots
	Cherry tomatoes
	Mushrooms
	Red and green bell peppers
	Mixed greens
	Red onion
Fruits (All fruits are okay *except for* grapes, melons [water-melon is allowed], raisins, and dates)	Frozen blueberries, strawberries, mango, raspberries, and pineapple
	Bananas
	Lemons
	Dried apricots
	Dried cranberries
	Avocado
	Mango
	Apples
	Peaches
	Bananas
Nuts/Seeds	Raw almonds (unsalted)
	Raw cashews (unsalted)
	Raw walnuts
	Raw pecan pieces
	Soy nuts (roasted)
	Chia and/or flaxseeds
	Sliced or slivered almonds
	Almond butter

Type of Food	Suggestions
Protein	Choose fresh options according to the recipes you wish to try (chicken breasts, ground turkey, scallops, shrimp, tilapia, etc.)
	Liquid egg whites
	Eggs
	Tempeh (usually found in the freezer at your health food store)
	Canned light tuna in water
	Canned wild salmon in water
Beans	Black beans
	Kidney beans
	Chickpeas
	Lentils (red or green—dried)
	Bean dips (or make your own!)
Options for On the Go	The Simply Bar (high-protein bar)
	Elevate Me! Bar (protein/energy bar)

Foods to Add to Your Kitchen—After Your Detox

Type of Food	Suggestions
Grain products	Stonemill bread (glycemically tested)
	Whole wheat pasta
	Rye crackers (Wasa or Ryvita)
	Kamut pasta (Sayoba)
	Whole grain or sprouted-grain tortillas
	100% rye bread (Dimpflmeier bread)
	Kashi GOLEAN Cereal
	Ezekiel bread (Foods For Life)
	High-fiber, whole wheat pita
	Spelt whole grain flour
Dairy products (preferably organic)	Pressed cottage cheese (Organic Meadows)
	Low-fat Cheddar or Colby cheese
	Low-fat cottage cheese
	Plain yogurt

ACKNOWLEDGMENTS

I cannot thank my family and friends enough for putting up with the rigors of my work schedule. Tim, Mom, Simon, Maria, Bruce, Betty, Mari, and the Martin family, I love you. Thank you for your support. Cynthy, Lise, Lorri, Tim Thorney, and PG, you have helped me more than you will ever know.

I wish to thank my patients for enriching my learning and my life in so many ways. I am honored to have the opportunity to care for each and every one of you. A special note to Silvia Presenza, Jeffrey Long, Natalie Shay, and author Caroline Van Hasselt—your support is an incredible source of inspiration for me.

Next, a *huge* thank you to Andrea Ritter for your editing skills, input, and ideas. Thank you for working so hard on such a short timeline. Your contributions have been an immense help in making this book better.

Sandro Sagrati, the value of our friendship and your faith in me is something I cannot begin to measure. You have been instrumental in not only making this book better, but also in continuing to make *me* a better person. Dr. Jan Dorrell, you are a wonderful friend and doctor. I am honored to have had your expertise and contribution on this project.

Thank you to Chantal Richard for your friendship, editing, and encouragement. In front of me is the copy of *On Writing Well* that you gave me years ago along with the note, "I hope this book inspires you as much as it inspires me. You *will* be published someday." All

I can say is thank you. Your belief in me has made a difference.

I wish to thank personal trainer and sports and conditioning coach Reggie Reyes for his input with the exercise component of this program—and for helping with the setup of the training studio at Clear Medicine.

Thank you to my agent, Rick Broadhead. Without you none of this would have been possible. Thank you to Rodale for seeing the potential in this project. A special message of gratitude to Denise McGann for her editorial input and to my publicist, for being instrumental in getting this approach "out there."

A sincere message of thanks to Jonathon Wright, MD, for taking the time out of his incredibly busy schedule to read this book, share his knowledge, and offer his suggestions.

Thank you to Jason Gee, certified strength and conditioning specialist, and personal trainer Vanessa Bell for posing as fitness models and for helping me with the exercise terminology when I was on such a tight deadline. And, to a multitalented osteopath, Sam Gibbs, thank you for your photography skills and for keeping me healthy—I am very grateful.

To Lucia—thank you for your help with this project and my clinic, Clear Medicine.

Lastly, thank you, the reader, for picking up this book. By doing so, you have helped me to fulfill my life's purpose—to inspire others to achieve better health.

RESOURCES

(Please look for the resources for specialized medical testing in Appendix A)

Heavy Metal Detox
    Detoxamin: EDTA suppositories: www.detoxamin.com

Infrared Sauna
    Infrared Saunas: www.saunaray.com

Natural Lubricants
    Hathor: www.hathorbody.com
    O'My: www.omyonline.com

Body Fat/Composition Analyzer
    Tanita: Home body-fat analyzer: www.tanita.com

Natural Skin Care and Makeup
    Naturopathica: Environmental Defense Facial Mask:
        www.naturopathica.com
    Be.Products Company: Skin care made from natural food: www.befine.com
    Caudalie: Toxin free skin care: www.caudalie-usa.com
    Juice Beauty: Toxin free skin care: www.juicebeauty.com
    John Masters: Toxin free skin and hair care: www.johnmasters.com
    Burt's Bees: Natural skin care: www.burtsbees.com
    Alba Organics: Sugar Cane Body Polish, Kukui Nut Organic Body Oil:
        www.albaorganics.com (Unlike the two products listed here, all Alba
        products may not be free of harmful methylparabens and propyl
        parabens.)
    Dr. Hauschka Skin Care: www.drhauschka.com
    Jane Iredale: Mineral makeup: www.janeiredale.com

Supplements

Zenbev: Natural source of tryptophan to boost serotonin, reduce anxiety, sleep disruption, and depression: www.zenbev.com

Wobenzym N: One of the top selling natural anti-inflammatory enzyme formulas in the world www.wobenzym-usa.com; www.thehormonediet.com or www.clearmedicinestore.com

Clear Detox—Homonal Health, Clear Detox—Digestive Health, Clear Essentials—Morning and Evening: www.clearmedicinestore.com or www.thehormonediet.com

Carlson Fish Oils: www.carlsonlabs.com

Nordic Natural Fish Oils : www.nordicnaturals.com, www.clearmedicinestore.com

Jarrow: www.jarrow.com

Genuine Health: (Proteins+, all natural whey protein isolate supplement and Greens+, green food supplements): www.genuinehealth.com

New Chapter: www.newchapter.com

AOR: www.aor.ca; www.thehormonediet.com or www.clearmedicinestore.com

Doctor's Choice: Dream Protein (all natural whey protein supplement): www.thehormonediet.com or www.clearmedicinestore.com

Pure Encapsulations: (G.I. Fortify and Liver-G.I. Detox): www.purecaps.com

Seditol Natural sleep aid containing Magnolia Bark Extract: www.thehormonediet.com or www.clearmedicinestore.com

Glyci-Med Forte: Olive and avocado oil supplement to aid weight loss: www.thehormonediet.com or www.clearmedicinestore.com

Metagenics: www.metagenics.com, www.thehormonediet.com, or www.clearmedicinestore.com

Life Extension Foundation: www.lef.org

Specialty Foods

Green and Blacks: Organic chocolate: www.greenandblacks.com

NewTree: Fine Belgian dark chocolate: www.newtree.com

Cocoa Camino: Organic fair-trade chocolate: www.cocoacamino.com

The Simply Bar: Gluten-free protein bar: www.wellnessfoods.ca; www.thehormonediet.com or www.clearmedicinestore.com

Acai Canada Inc.: Açaí berry products: www.acaicanada.com

Sambazon: Açaí concentrate: www.sambazon.com

Navitas Naturals: Goji Power: www.navitasnaturals.com

Pom Wonderful: Pomegranate juice: www.pomwonderful.com

La Tortilla Factory: Pitas, wraps, and gluten-free products: www.latortillafactory.com

Muzi Teas: Green tea: www.muzitea.com

Mr Pita: Low-carb, high-protein pita: www.mrpita.ca

Organic Meadow: Organic pressed cottage cheese:
www.organicmeadow.com

Liberté: Organic yogurt: (this brand has the right balance of protein and
carbs): www.liberte.qc.ca/en/home.ch2

Kashi Company: GOLEAN high-protein, high-fiber cereal: www.kashi.com

Dimpflmeier Bakery: 100% rye bread: www.dimpflmeierbakery.com

Food For Life Baking Co.: Ezekiel breads: www.foodforlife.com

Bob's Red Mill Natural Foods: Gluten-free and other grain products
www.bobsredmill.com

So Nice: Unsweetened organic soy milk: www.sonice.ca

PROsnack Natural Foods: Elevate Me! (organic whole-food and protein
bar): www.prosnack.com

Relaxation Aids

Somerset Entertainment: Sonic Aid (meditation and sleep CD series by Dr.
Lee Bartel): www.somersetent.com

Toxin-Free Household Cleaning Products

Nature Clean: www.naturecleanliving.com

Attitude: www.thegoodattitude.com

Seventh Generation: www.seventhgeneration.com

Organic Cotton Bedding and Mattresses

The Guide to Less Toxic Products (provides numerous sources):
www.lesstoxicguide.ca

Health Information Resources

Life Extension Foundation: www.lef.org

Mary Shomon's thyroid health Web site: www.thyroid.about.com

SeaChoice: Healthy seafood choices: www.seachoice.org

Harvard School of Public Health: The Nutrition Source
www.hsph.harvard.edu/nutritionsource/index.html

Whole Foods Market: Tasty soup recipes!: www.wholefoodsmarket.com/
recipes

Slice—Health Inspired Food: www.sliceofhealth.com

Environmental Working Group: Information about cosmetics, seafood
safety, etc.: www.ewg.org

Calorie King: Nutrition information database: www.calorieking.com

Glycemic Index and GI Database (University of Sydney):
    www.glycemicindex.com
American Journal of Clinical Nutrition Glycemic Load Chart:
    www.ajcn.org/cgi/content/full/76/1/5#SEC2
International Hormone Society: www.intlhormonesociety.org
Clear Medicine: www.clearmedicinestore.com

INDEX

Underscored page references indicate sidebars. **Boldface** references indicate photographs and illustrations.

Hormone Diet Three-Step Fix
  expected results from, 133
  preparing for, 134–45
  renew and revitalize, 35
    Anti-Inflammatory Detox, 170–201
    sleep improvement, 149–69
    stress relief, 202–21
  replenishment and hormone balance,
      35–36
    advanced supplement plan, 280–305
    basic supplement plan, 270–79
    Glyci-Med Dietary Approach,
      240–69
    understanding nutrition mistakes,
      224–39
  restore strength, vigor, and radiance,
      36–37
    better sex, 308–9, 308–17
    exercise, 308–9, 317–27
    Hormone Diet exercise
      prescription, 328–54
    natural skin care, 355–68
    refreshers, 369–81
  for reversing muscle loss, 124–25
  tips for, 132–33
Hormones. *See also specific hormones*
  effect on weight loss, 14
  in endocrine system, 16–17
  functions of, 14–15, 18
  interactions among, 54–55
Hot bath or shower, for improving sleep,
      161
Hot flashes, 168, 296, 297
Hot Hormone Foods, 243–44
Hummus
  Hummus and Veggies, 437–38
Hunger
  from calorie-restricting diets, 30
  from excess insulin, 58
  from high cortisol, 152
  with insulin resistance, 3
Hydrolyzed milk protein, for treating
  excess cortisol, 292–93
  excess progesterone, 298
Hyperthyroidism, 82
Hypothalamus, 16, 16, 17, 29, 78, 81, 83,
      107, 150, 314
Hypothyroidism
  author's vs. standard treatment of, 3–4
  causes of, 82–84
  diagnosis of, 85

incidence of, 18, 82
oversleeping and, 158
progesterone deficiency from, 88
review of diagnostic tests for, 398
symptoms of, 1–2, 82, 84
untreated, consequences of, 85

I
Immune system
  food sensitivities and, 174
  inflammation and, 24, 25, 26
  progesterone and, 27, 87, 89
Indole-3-carbinol, for treating
  excess estrogen, 295
  low testosterone, 298
Indoor pollution, 401–2
Inflammation
  abdominal fat and, 112
  adipokines and, 122
  AGEs causing, 239
  chronic
    causes of, 26–28
    reducing, for total wellness and fat
      loss, 35
  conditions associated with, 24, 26, 28
  fats and, 266
  foods causing, 224–27
  food sensitivities and, 174–75
  function of, 24–25
  future treatments for, 23, 24
  high-fat proteins causing, 261
  Hormonal Health Profile for
      assessing, 39–40
  muscle loss from, 124
  obesity and, 25
  PPARs and, 23
  reducing, with
    exercise, 319, 328
    fish oils, 275
    Glyci-Med Dietary Approach, 241
    probiotics, 178
    repair of digestive-tract wall, 178–79
  review of diagnostic tests for, 400
  supplements for treating, 188, 283–85
  testing for, 28
Infrared sauna, for detox and sleep
      improvement, 161, 162
Inositol, for low serotonin, 289
Insomnia. *See* Sleep deprivation
Insulin
  artificial sweeteners and, 233
  balanced, benefits of, 57

Vitamin or mineral deficiency. *See also* Nutrient deficiencies
    oversleeping and, 158
Vitex, for treating
    low dopamine, 288
    low progesterone, 297
Vivanno, Starbucks, 259

W

Waist circumference, for measuring body fat, 116, 120
Waist-to-hip ratio
    indicating insulin sensitivity, 142
    for measuring body fat, 116, 120, 121
Walking, benefits of, 194
Warning scores, in Hormonal Health Profile, 52
Water drinking, 244, 250, 379
Weight gain
    from artificial sweeteners, 232–33
    from deficient thyroid hormone, 21
    after dieting, 31, 32, 125
    hormonal changes with, 112
    with hypothyroidism, 1
    from low serotonin, 99, 101
    with polycystic ovarian syndrome, 3
    potential causes of, 131
    from sleep deprivation, 150–51, 152
    from stress, 65
Weight loss. *See also* Fat loss
    from Anti-Inflammatory Detox, 190
    dieting alone as ineffective for, 31–33
    dopamine for, 105–6
    effect of hormones on, 14, 15, 18
    fats for, 264
    ghrelin interfering with, 78
    hormonal balance for, 5
    from Hormone Diet, 35, 37, 373
    insulin resistance preventing, 60
    obstacles to, 13–14
    safe weekly amount of, 378–79
    sleep aiding, 152

Weight-loss plateau, tips for overcoming, 374–81
Weight maintenance, keys to, 33–35
Weight on scale, muscle affecting, 135
Weight training. *See* Strength training
Whey protein
    in basic supplement plan, 272, 276, 279
    in detox, 406
    in smoothies, 408
White-noise machine, for sleep improvement, 156
White tea extracts, in skin-care creams, 364
Wobenzym, for reducing inflammation, 284
Workouts. *See also* Hormone Diet exercise plan
    eating before and after, 245–46, 261, 323–24, 330–31
    in hormonally balanced day, 370, 371
    lengthening, for boosting metabolism, 376
    mistakes with, preventing fat loss, 319–27
Wrinkles, 358, 359, 364

X

Xenoestrogens, estrogen dominance from, 73

Y

Yeast infections, probiotics preventing, 178
Yoga
    benefits of, 326–27
    in Hormone Diet exercise plan, 330

Z

Zenbev, for low serotonin, 288–89
Zinc
    for excess insulin, 286
    for low testosterone, 299

Dr. Natasha Turner is one of Canada's leading naturopathic doctors and natural health consultants. She is clinic director and founder of Clear Medicine—a wellness boutique in Toronto. As an expert in nutrition and natural health, she is regularly featured in print and on television. Her experience has contributed to the design and development of two commercial weight-loss programs, which have helped to transform an abundance of lives. She also frequently lectures to both the public and health care providers on topics related to healthy hormonal balance. She lives in Toronto.

Visit her Web site: www.thehormonediet.com.